# BIOETHICAL DECISION MAKING IN NURSING

**GLADYS L. HUSTED, PhD, MSNEd, RN,** is professor emeritus of nursing at Duquesne University, Pittsburgh, Pennsylvania. She received a master's in nursing education from the University of Pittsburgh, where she also completed her PhD in curriculum and supervision. She was awarded the title of School of Nursing Distinguished Professor in 1998. She has retired from full-time employment at Duquesne University but continues to teach part time in the MSN and PhD programs. Her main area of expertise is in bioethics. She continues to write and consult. Her other areas of expertise are in curriculum design, instructional strategies, and theory development. Dr. Husted's website can be accessed at www.duq.edu /nursing/faculty/husted

**JAMES H. HUSTED** is an independent scholar. He is a member of the American Philosophical Association and the North American Spinoza Society. He has been a member of the high IQ societies, Mensa and Intertel. He was the philosophy expert for Dial-An-M for Mensa, as well as the philosophy editor of *Integra*, the journal of Intertel.

**CARRIE J. SCOTTO, PhD, RN,** is an associate professor at the University of Akron School of Nursing, where she teaches pathophysiology and pharmacology. She earned her BSN and MSN from the University of Akron and her PhD from Duquesne University. As an educator and clinician, she has a vested interest in bioethics. She has served more than 20 years at the bedside as a critical care nurse. Her research related to adherence to prescribed treatment for cardiac patients and therapeutic clinical interventions for critically ill patients has been presented nationally and is published in professional journals. She is a member of Sigma Theta Tau International, American Association of Critical-Care Nurses, American Association of Cardiovascular and Pulmonary Rehabilitation, and Preventive Cardiovascular Nurses Association.

**KIMBERLY M. WOLF, PhD, PMHCNS-BC,** is a psychiatric-mental health clinical nurse specialist at Hennepin County Medical Center, Minneapolis, Minnesota, and the psychiatric-mental health nurse practitioner track director at the University of North Dakota, Grand Forks, North Dakota. She also teaches part time as an adjunct faculty in the nursing department at Duquesne University, Pittsburgh, Pennsylvania. She received a master's degree in science in advanced practice psychiatric-mental health nursing from the University of North Dakota. She received a PhD from Duquesne University in 2013. She enjoys her work as a full-time provider in the busy urban county hospital but also values actively teaching in master's and doctoral programs. Her interest areas are bioethics, cultural competency, and psychiatric-mental health advanced practice nursing.

*Contributor*
**SUZANNE EDGETT COLLINS, JD, PhD, MPH, RN,** is a nurse-attorney with experience in the areas of medical and nursing malpractice, legal and bioethics education of allied health care practitioners, and consultation practice in licensure defense, health law/policy, and health care risk management. She is a professor in the Department of Nursing at the University of Tampa. Her particular areas of expertise focus on the intersections of law, ethics, health policy/economics, and nursing. Her research interests include issues of nursing law and ethics, patient safety and nursing error, and social and behavioral issues among nurses, including topics such as rule bending, practice act violations, and facilitators/barriers to new nurse retention. She has published on the topics of nursing law and ethics and has been a presenter at educational conferences.

# BIOETHICAL DECISION MAKING IN NURSING

## FIFTH EDITION

Gladys L. Husted, PhD, MSNEd, RN

James H. Husted

Carrie J. Scotto, PhD, RN

Kimberly M. Wolf, PhD, PMHCNS-BC

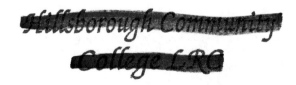
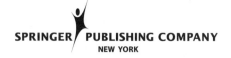
SPRINGER PUBLISHING COMPANY
NEW YORK

Copyright © 2015 Springer Publishing Company, LLC

Springer Publishing Company, LLC
11 West 42nd Street
New York, NY 10036
www.springerpub.com

Acquisitions Editor: Joseph Morita
Composition: Graphic World Inc.

ISBN: 978-0-8261-7143-6
e-book ISBN: 978-0-8261-7144-3
Instructors Manual: 978-0-8261-3014-3

Instructors Materials: Qualified instructors may request supplements by e-mailing textbook@springerpub.com:

14 15 16 17 / 5 4 3 2 1

The author and the publisher of this Work have made every effort to use sources believed to be reliable to provide information that is accurate and compatible with the standards generally accepted at the time of publication. Because medical science is continually advancing, our knowledge base continues to expand. Therefore, as new information becomes available, changes in procedures become necessary. We recommend that the reader always consult current research and specific institutional policies before performing any clinical procedure. The author and publisher shall not be liable for any special, consequential, or exemplary damages resulting, in whole or in part, from the readers' use of, or reliance on, the information contained in this book. The publisher has no responsibility for the persistence or accuracy of URLs for external or third-party Internet websites referred to in this publication and does not guarantee that any content on such websites is, or will remain, accurate or appropriate.

**Library of Congress Cataloging-in-Publication Data**

Husted, Gladys L., author.
  Bioethical decision making in nursing / Gladys L. Husted, James H. Husted, Carrie J. Scotto, Kimberly M. Wolf. -- Fifth edition.
      p. ; cm.
  Preceded by Ethical decision making in nursing and health care / by James H. Husted, Gladys L. Husted. 4th ed. c2008.
  Includes bibliographical references and index.
  ISBN 978-0-8261-7143-6 -- ISBN 978-0-8261-7144-3 (e-book)
  I. Scotto, Carrie J., author. II. Wolf, Kimberly M., author. III. Husted, James H. Ethical decision making in nursing and health care. Preceded by (work): IV. Title.
  [DNLM: 1. Ethics, Nursing--Case Reports. 2. Decision Making--ethics--Case Reports. 3. Models, Theoretical--Case Reports. WY 85]
  RT85
  174'.2--dc23
                                        2014036197

Printed in the United States of America by McNaughton & Gunn.

# CONTENTS

## SECTION I: THE BASICS OF BIOETHICAL DECISION MAKING

## SECTION II: BEYOND THE BASICS—AN EXTENDED PERSPECTIVE

## SECTION III: CASE STUDY ANALYSES

# LIST OF CASE STUDY DILEMMAS*

*See Section III: Analysis of Dilemmas.

# LIST OF FIGURES AND TABLES

# PREFACE

## FOCUS OF A FIELD OF STUDY

Every science and every art arises from imagination and reason. Each is inspired by need and curiosity to serve a purpose. Human beings desired to navigate the seas, and someone created celestial navigation. Curious about living things, someone created biology. Someone created mathematics for the purpose of computation. Someone created medicine from a need to alleviate suffering and to bring about healing.

## EVERYDAY ETHICS

We make so many decisions in any given day—how we perform at work, how we engage with others, and so on—and virtually never stop to think about whether these decisions are ethical. Many such decisions are not dilemmas, meaning that the choice is clear-cut because you know what you should do, but they are ethical decisions nevertheless. The ethical decisions of everyday life are not the subject of this book, but it is important that everyone becomes more aware of the pervasiveness of ethics in one's daily life. The purpose of this book is to help nurses and all health care professionals recognize the importance of ethics to their professions and know how to resolve ethical dilemmas when the choice is not clear.

## THE ORIGIN OF ETHICS AND THE UNDERPINNINGS OF SYMPHONOLOGY

Ethics originally was meant to be a search for, or a science of, the good life or the successful life. The first major ethicist of the Western world, Socrates (464–399 BC), described ethics as an examination of life, as a way of making life worth living.

Socrates's ethical work was twofold: (a) to establish and define ethical terms to provide a common language in which ethics could be discussed and (b) to understand ethics as contextualized, meaning we should recognize that actions that are right in one circumstance may be wrong in another. For example, violence against another for no purpose is wrong, whereas self-defense against an attack is justifiable. Thus, a blanket condemnation of violence is a mistake. The context determines its ethical quality.

After Socrates, Plato (427–347 BC) shifted the theme of ethics away from identifying the good life—a life worth living—to identifying the "good," that is, the true nature of goodness itself. Ultimately, this shift displaced concern for the good life, nearly driving it out of ethics. This issue persists today as many health care decisions focus on what should be done as opposed to what should be done *for this patient in these circumstances.* Concern for life is central to the health care setting—the realm of bioethics. Concern for the good life is central to human existence—the realm of ethics—and to achievement of life goals and flourishing.

Fortunately, Aristotle (483–322 BC) brought the concerns of human life back as the central subject matter of ethics. His focus on the golden mean and virtue contributed greatly to the theory of symphonology.

Aristotle's theory of ethics as a science of successful living and Socrates's emphasis on context provided a strong foundation for a practice-based ethic. It is unfortunate that the interest of Socrates and Aristotle in defining, understanding, and living by the meaning of ethical terms has largely been forgotten in modern ethical systems while Plato's quixotic theory of ethics as a search for an unknown and unknowable "good" has become the almost exclusive concern of ethics.

Benedict Spinoza (1632–1697) contributed the virtue of desire as the essence of the human person. He asserted that if desires are directed by an objective awareness, this will establish the intelligible sequences that characterize a life lived according to the nature of a living rational being.

## BIOETHICS

Bioethics is the branch of ethics that investigates problems arising from medical and biological research and clinical practice. It includes issues of individual care and broader concerns such as access to health care, confidentiality, genetic testing, and resource allocation (Johnson, 2011). This book presents a system to guide health care professionals in providing ethically sound care.

*Symphonia* is a Greek word meaning "agreement." *Symphonology* is the study of agreements and the elements necessary to form agreements. Within the health care arena, symphonology is the study of agreements between health care professionals and patients and the ethical implications of those agreements.

Symphonology is a practice-based ethical system appropriate for practicing health care professionals. It is a normative approach to ethics that looks at how people should act within a given context and contributes to the value of character. Symphonology is in opposition to a descriptive approach, which is more scientific, and studies what people think is right. Symphonology delineates standards of professional behavior based on the preconditions necessary for professional agreement and interaction. These standards are then applied within a contextual understanding. The goal is to bring about optimal interactions in the health care setting that result in optimal patient care outcomes.

Achieving optimal care for patients is central to the purpose of all health care professionals and institutions and is, therefore, indispensable to professional bioethics. Within the realm of symphonology, excellent patient care is only one aspect of the outcome. It is the nature of an agreement that both parties will benefit. Symphonology, which is based on agreements, promotes the welfare of both the patient and the health care professional. A high degree of personal and professional development is fostered through the use of sound bioethics in practice. As the patient receives optimal care, the professional matures in knowledge, skill, and professional satisfaction. This dual benefit is achieved through a symphonological ethic.

Although ethical problems faced by nurses are the primary focus here, symphonology can be applied to any heath care professional. The only adjustment required is consideration of the education, experience, and role of each professional involved. The theory is also applicable to any patient population, regardless of age, disease, competency, and cultural background.

## THE RETURN TO LIFE AND FLOURISHING

In this book, we turn away from seeking an unobtainable good and return to a concern for life. Like the ethicists of the past, we are concerned not only with life but with a flourishing life and the achievement of happiness. We approach life as it is experienced, as a journey accompanied by tears and smiles, by conflict and harmony. We begin amid life in all its complexity, discussing what we bring to life's journey: human virtues, their relation to the health care setting, their development, and what they make possible. We discuss individual rights, the necessary foundation for an ethic of human life. Human virtues and individual rights are the foundations for ethical actions.

As individuals, a majority of our achievements come to us through cooperation with others. This cooperation occurs through agreement (thus, the name *symphonology*). The professional agreement between a nurse and patient perfectly illustrates the achievement that results from cooperation. For each, nurse and patient, great value is achieved from cooperation as each brings his or her virtues and considers the rights of the other.

From this vantage point, we analyze the decline of ethics from an individual pursuit into an exclusively social context, where societal standards dictate whether something is right or wrong. We then examine the absurd, but commonly held, idea that the emotions of an individual can provide guidance for the resolution of complex ethical dilemmas. We will see that the emotional response of one or a few is often the basis for ethical decisions even at the expense of virtue and human rights. Here, ethics has reached a dead end.

Because of "the increasingly complex nature of care and provider demands in health care settings, the potential for ethical conflicts for nurses and nursing students continues to rise" (Hutchinson, Shedlin,

Gallo, Krainovich-Miller, & Fulmer, 2014, p. 58). Add this to the current state of bioethics and clinical practice and it becomes essential for all health care professionals to understand their own ethical beliefs. If you do not understand why you consider one action right and another action wrong, your disadvantage is obvious. You will not be able to interact on an equal footing with your colleagues, whose rationalizations can seem plausible. You will not be able to objectively and effectively defend the actions you take. You will have no objective means of moral self-defense.

We have included numerous dilemmas in this book as a way of providing practice in ethical decision making. We offer resolutions to most of these dilemmas, realizing that being in an actual situation may change the information sought and therefore alter the resolution found. However, in the Study Guide that appears at the end of Chapters 3 through 12, there will be one case for which the analysis appears only in the instructor's manual. In this book, we examine a variety of bioethical dilemmas from patients' conflicts about their own care to withdrawing all life supports. We demonstrate the relevance of bioethical standards to these, and by extension to all, bioethical dilemmas. We examine how to define and understand bioethical standards in different contexts in order to use them effectively in ethical decision making. In this way, even the novice health care professionals will have the tools to examine and manage ethical issues with their patients.

Because all the key concepts listed in the chapters are terms that require precise definitions, we have provided a glossary for your use.

## NOTES

1. The pronoun *she* is used to designate the health care professional. This convention is for the reader's ease of understanding and to keep understanding in context. The singular is preferred to the plural because professionals are individuals, and a practice-based ethic is, and ought to be, an individualistic ethic. On the other hand, we almost invariably use the pronoun *he* to designate the patient, again for the same reason.
2. There are certain subjects we will return to numerous times. This is especially true of virtue, individual rights, and bioethical standards. The reason for this is that these facts serve different functions in different aspects of the nurse–patient interaction—and because this will make discussions in later chapters easier to understand.
3. Case studies will be used throughout the book to show how to apply concepts and also to illuminate pertinent concepts that recur in health care. (For those who have used the book before, you will notice that self-assertion is no longer discussed. We have incorporated self-assertion into freedom, including short-term, single events; the here and now control of one's actions; and extended sequences of events, including those sequences that extend over a lifetime.)

4. Four humorous vignettes are included throughout the book. It is important that the reader recognize the seriousness of humor and the lessons that can be learned from these vignettes. In the case of these vignettes, the learning takes place effortlessly if the mind is open to the lesson behind the humor. All of them will have a certain designation so that they are easily recognized. The humor reveals the obvious from the obscure.

5. Although the aspects of context are very important and need to be considered in each analysis of what one is to do in the situation, we have not isolated these aspects in the resolutions except for one case in Chapter 5 to show how it could be done. The reason for not doing each analysis with the aspects of the context illuminated is that, with the analysis of the standards, the context is revealed through the standards. For educators, you may want to propose that students isolate these aspects in their discussion of the standards.

## DIGITAL SUPPLEMENT

There will be a continuation of a digital supplement for educators who adopt this book for classroom use. It has been expanded and increased in ways to teach the concepts and relate them to the health care setting. This online instructor's manual, which can be obtained from Springer Publishing Company, LLC, by e-mailing textbook@springerpub.com, provides a wealth of information for instructors to plan their teaching activities and to enhance active learning for students. It will assist faculty in preparing for class and decrease preparation time.

The online instructor's manual includes:

- **Chapter Summaries:** To assist faculty in quickly identifying chapter themes and purposes.
- **Major Focus Areas:** To help in identifying key elements in each chapter and to pinpoint content essential to classroom instruction.
- **Classroom Activities:** To enhance active engagement of the learner through classroom activities (two to four activities are included per chapter that can be used in a traditional or online class format). Directions are included for conducting these activities.
- **Unresolved Cases:** At the end of Chapters 3 through 12, there will be one case whose resolution will appear only in the instructor's manual, which is new to this edition.
- **Test Bank:** To enhance the evaluative process by providing test questions for each chapter. The test bank questions at the end of each chapter use the two types of questions that now appear on the NCLEX exam: single answer and select all that apply.

How faculty use this information, especially the activities, depends on classroom variables: level of students, time available, and what fits best with class discussions.

## REFERENCES

Hutchinson, K., Shedlin, M. G., Gallo, B., Krainovich-Miller, B., & Fulmer, T. (2014). Ethics in-the-round: A Guided peer approach for addressing ethical issues confronting nursing students. *Nursing Education Perspectives, 35*(1), 58–60.

Johnson, L. (2011). *A life-centered approach to bioethics: Biocentric ethics.* New York, NY: Cambridge University Press.

Spinoza, B. (1949). *Ethics.* (J. Gutmann, Ed.). New York, NY: Hafner Publishing. (Original work published 1675.)

# ACKNOWLEDGMENTS

I, **Gladys,** wish to acknowledge my gratitude to the following people:

My daughter, her husband, and my two granddaughters, who bring me an abundance of joy and constant support.

My many friends who have supported me through this process, **but especially Carroll Miller, my long-time colleague and friend.**

My former students, now my friends and coauthors, for taking the theory to the next level and for being such great partners with whom to write.

---

I, **Carrie,** wish to acknowledge my gratitude to the following people:

My husband, Mark; my daughter, Kelly; and my son, Kevin, who always believe the best about me.

---

I, **Kim,** wish to acknowledge my gratitude to the following people:

My four children, my daughter-in-law, and my grandson, who are the true loves of my life.

My boyfriend and his two daughters, my parents, my friends, and my coworkers, who have supported me through this process.

---

We wish to thank:

The students who, over the years, have served as crucibles for refining the dominant ideas in this book.

Joe Morita for his editorial assistance.

And most of all to my (Gladys's) husband, James Husted, with whom we conceived, brought to life, and nurtured the theory of symphonology so that it has become an essential guideline for human life and interaction. Jim has gifted us with his astounding intelligence and his boundless wit. His good humor has created a place where one may fearlessly consider the more and the better in life. He has lived well and inspires us to do the same.

And finally to Charlie-Charlie, to whom this book is dedicated.

# ONE

# ETHICAL FOUNDATIONS

## OBJECTIVES

- Describe the purpose of ethics and bioethics.
- Define ethics and bioethics.
- Discuss the process of understanding the human nature of yourself and others.
- Examine the essential nature of human behavior.
- Examine bioethics as the foundation of health care practice.
- Define symphonology.

## THE PURPOSE OF ETHICS

Ethics, like every science, arose from the necessity of analyzing and coming to understand some part of our world. Ethics is that part of our world that is concerned with making decisions and taking actions in the face of adversity or opportunity. Ethics deals with alternatives, and the central alternative is between that which is beneficial and that which is harmful. In an ethical context, that which makes life more perfect is beneficial. That which makes life less perfect is harmful. Ethics is a study of how decisions and actions can move a human life from a state of lesser perfection to a state of greater perfection (well-being and flourishing), or how decisions can cause a human life to move from a state of greater perfection to a state of lesser perfection (loss and stagnation). In the context of an individual's life, discounting the influences of unpredictable chance, a failed life is one that a person looks back on with regret for the way one has lived it. A successful life is a life that one experienced as having been lived well. A rational ethical system is a science of living well.

1

## BIOETHICS

Bioethics places particular emphasis on situations in which one person is extremely vulnerable, the goals to be pursued are crucial, and the dilemmas to be resolved are extraordinarily complex (Husted & Husted, 2008).

Bioethics is ethics as it relates to the health care professions. Bioethics places particular emphasis on situations in which one person is extremely vulnerable, the goals to be pursued are crucial, and the dilemmas to be resolved are extraordinarily complex (Husted & Husted, 2008).

Bioethics came into existence as an independent discipline around 1970 as a result of pharmacological and technical advances in health care. As it became possible to save and prolong lives that were previously beyond hope, questions arose as to whether it was actually beneficial to do so. "Bioethics should not tell [patients] what to do, but it should provide them with tools and skills in reasoning and ways to improve their own decisions" (Perring, 2005, p. 63).

The fundamental elements of a sound bioethics include the nature and needs of human beings, the purpose and function of a health care system, and an awareness of the dignity of individuals. The values that the biomedical sciences offer those who can profit from them are complex and vitally important. At the same time, the threat to a patient's values is very real. The relationship between the health care professional and patient is extraordinarily intimate. This calls for a decision-making method that is patient centered and practice based.

## UNDERSTANDING SELF AND OTHERS

Because ethical decision making involves choosing actions to promote and enhance human life, it is important to understand yourself and others in the human context. To understand how this is accomplished, we first consider a curious paradox. A paradox is a statement that is seemingly contradictory or incongruent with itself or with what is known.

Benedict Spinoza (1632–1677) was a pioneering ethicist who used two facts that seemingly contradict each other to show how we develop self-understanding. Consider these true statements:

- To make a hammer, it is necessary for a person to be able to work iron.
- For a person to be able to work iron, he or she needs a hammer.

From this it would seem that no one can work iron and that there can be no such thing as a hammer. A person must have a hammer to make a hammer. Therefore, it seems that it is impossible either to make or to have a hammer. Yet, hammers do exist, and people do work iron.

Hammering was first accomplished by people using whatever tools were already at hand; most likely, stones were used. Over time, tools were improved upon until they had a primitive type of hammer with which iron could be worked. The better they became at working iron, the better hammer they were able to produce. The better hammer they could produce, the better they became at working iron.

The process of achieving an understanding of self and others is very similar to the process of making a hammer. In her earliest years, a person learns what a person is by observing others. By examining the nature of mature, independent people, she discovers her own nature; she comes to know what she is: a person. As with Spinoza's hammer, learning about herself and others is a seesaw process—back and forth—comparing other people to herself, comparing herself to other people. In learning what other people are, she comes to understand what she is in ways that she could not without her knowledge of other people. In learning what she is, she comes to understand other people in ways that she could not without self-understanding.

She knows others as persons before she knows herself. All persons are unique and complex and therefore difficult to understand. To understand them, she can compare their similarities and differences to herself, using her own characteristics as a standard by which she can evaluate the various characteristics of others. Then she can evaluate her own characteristics by using what she has learned of the nature of others as a standard for herself.

After a period of personal development, by observing others, a person gains a better understanding of herself by noting her similarities to, and differences from, other persons. Then she looks into herself and gains a better understanding of others by observing how they are similar to, and different from, her. This process continues and expands until the observer has gained a multifaceted understanding of human nature.

## THE BASIS OF HUMAN BEHAVIOR

Through observing others, one can discover what characteristics people have in common and the variations of these characteristics. Through interaction and reflection, one discovers the meaning that concepts, experiences, and circumstances have for others and how they came to have such meanings. This understanding goes far to explain how personal meaning is expressed in human behavior.

The process of developing human character, as described earlier, is initially unconscious and unintentional. A child does not consider the behavior of others and compare it to her own on a conscious level. As a person matures, she begins to actively choose behaviors that resonate with what she knows about herself and others. These choices are based on her understanding of herself, her desires and purposes, and her ability to reason and to act. To develop ethical integrity and a strong character, she chooses behaviors that will bring benefit to her life and the lives of others and avoids those behaviors that lead to harm. Human behavior develops in the context of an individual life through interaction with others and the environment and subsequent reflection on those interactions. Human behavior is the expression of ethical choices. Human behavior expresses the essential nature of the person.

Achieving ethical integrity is certainly the desire of most people. However, the human condition is unpredictable. Observations, experiences, and circumstances can lead an individual to choose and develop habits of thinking and behavior that promote good. In the same way, people can be led to develop habits of thinking and behavior that lead to deterioration, loss, and harm.

## ETHICS AS THE FOUNDATION OF HUMAN CHARACTER

To understand the importance of personal ethics, we consider this question: Would one need to be concerned with ethics if one were marooned alone on an island? Survival is the fundamental ethical concern. If one does not survive, there are no choices of behavior to be made. Ethics has to do with benefit and harm. One who is alone, marooned on an island where survival is a constant concern, will have to be excessively concerned with benefit and harm.

Being marooned would be a test of character. Strength of character develops over time as one establishes habits of thought and action directed toward benefit. A person with strong character is said to be virtuous.

### Virtue

Virtue is the means by which ethical choices are made.

In reality, virtue is a dynamic mechanism that requires great objectivity, clear thinking, and commitment to achieving benefits.

A nurse who is nurturing is a virtuous nurse. It takes knowledge about the patient, knowledge about the situation, and rational thought to discern the most beneficial course of action—the virtuous action, the ethical action.

As every nurse knows, ethical action does not result from simple dichotomous choices. Virtue is the means by which ethical choices are made. Virtue is often thought of as a static condition. A virtuous person is considered somewhat withdrawn from worldly affairs, pursuing introspection. A virtuous person may be one who is concerned with careful rule following. In reality, virtue is a dynamic mechanism that requires great objectivity, clear thinking, and commitment to achieving benefits. Aristotle demonstrated the complexity of arriving at an ethically justifiable decision with his doctrine of the *golden mean*. Aristotle proposed that a virtue is a middle ground between two extremes. The extremes are vices. The *golden mean* is the midpoint among three possible attitudes. One attitude leads to a deficit of action, less than what is called for in the situation. For example, a nurse may show indifference to her patient when he needs her attention. The second attitude leads to an excess of action. For example, a nurse may be overbearing and controlling in relation to her patient, denying him the ability to control his situation. The virtue that is a mean between these two vices is nurturing. A nurse should not be indifferent, but attentive. A nurse should be attentive but not domineering. A nurse who is attentive is nurturing. A nurse who is nurturing is a virtuous nurse. It takes knowledge about the patient, knowledge about the situation, and rational thought to discern the most beneficial course of action—the virtuous action, the ethical action.

Virtues are those aspects of character that are based on rational thought and rational desires. Virtuous actions require an objective understanding of reality and clear thinking. Survival on a deserted island would almost certainly depend on the development of certain virtues such as fortitude, objectivity, diligence, prudence, and commitment. Repeated decisions and choices would be required to pursue benefit and avoid harm. Clearly, one alone on an island has to be concerned with ethics.

It follows, then, that all people everywhere must be concerned with survival and flourishing (living a successful and rewarding life) and therefore must rely on ethics. It is not necessary to have two or more people involved to understand the importance of ethics. In fact, if an individual marooned on an island did not need ethical awareness, no one ever, under any circumstances, would have any need for ethics. What is needed by a person in a downtown crowd is needed more so by a person marooned and alone. The ethical nature of a person is expressed in the decisions that person makes. We must all make decisions and choices to make life better. We strive to prevent life from deteriorating. We plan on ways to survive and to attempt, always, to achieve happiness.

## THE ETHICAL FOUNDATIONS OF HEALTH CARE PRACTICE

Human action is behavior that expresses the nature of the human being. Human actions are behaviors directed by reason. A person's ability to act is known as *agency*. The human possessing agency is known as an *agent*. In nursing, a person who has lost agency is known as a *patient*. A patient enters the health care setting because he has lost his power of agency—his power to take actions. A nurse is there to supply his agency—to do for him the things that need to be done that he cannot do for himself because of his disability or lack of knowledge.

> Ethics is a system of standards to motivate, determine, and justify actions taken in the pursuit of vital and fundamental goals.

Ethics is a system of standards to motivate, determine, and justify actions taken in the pursuit of vital and fundamental goals. Vital goals are those that are concerned with the preservation and enhancement of life. Vital goals are similar for most people: We desire to eat; we have the need to breathe and to grow. Fundamental goals are those that promote the essence of what it is to be human and what it is to be a specific individual. Our fundamental goals are those devoted to using our resources to achieve our optimal individual potential as human beings. These goals vary to a greater extent. For example, one person may have the desire to regain his ability to walk, whereas another may prefer to use his time and strength in another way. A patient is one who has lost his ability to pursue his vital and fundamental goals on his own.

> When an ethical system is fully developed, it provides a framework for what is appropriate to human motivations and value-oriented action and how these relate to the human condition.

When an ethical system is fully developed, it provides a framework for what is appropriate to human motivations and value-oriented action and how these relate to the human condition. It examines the processes of decision making and the ways in which agents reach, or fail to reach, their goals. A well-developed ethical system is concerned with the nature of the goals that agents pursue. It indicates the ways these goals might best be pursued. Ethics examines the right and wrong of the decisions and choices agents make regarding their actions and interactions. Therefore, ethics has a practical purpose. This purpose is to guide actions toward the good. The purpose is to increase or recapture the patient's ability to flourish and, in some cases, to survive.

## PRACTICE-BASED ETHICS VERSUS RULE-BASED ETHICS

*That which is the goal of practice ought to be the goal of ethics.*

Every health care professional should ask herself whether a professional ethic exists to serve her patient's life, health, and well-being or whether bioethics is a machine to create assembly line products. That which is the goal of practice ought to be the goal of ethics. Ethics, as well as practice, can help heal disabilities and nurture the resources needed for successful living.

Like the interaction between players on a professional sports team, the ideal interaction between a nurse and a patient is an uninterrupted series of comprehensible, causal, sequential events. The events are comprehensible in that both the patient and the nurse understand what is happening. They are casual, meaning the events are planned and controlled because of an intended outcome. They are sequential in that their consecutive timing is purposeful in order to achieve a desired outcome.

A strong bioethical system will lead the ethical agent to action that benefits her patient. It serves as a defense against being mandated to do what is wrong. It can be a positive means to increase success in the health care arena. Clearly this last perspective is the most rewarding, productive, and mature view of bioethics. This is the perspective taken by a practice-based ethic. Bioethical decision making is a skill. Like every skill, practice improves performance. When performance is improved, the well-being of patients is improved.

A practice-based ethical decision maker is very much like a skilled pool player. An unskilled pool player merely attempts to put a ball into a pocket. An unskilled decision maker decides on what seems best at the time and acts on it. A skilled pool player sets up shots and tries to put a ball into a pocket while leaving the cue ball in a strategic position for the next shot. Principles and theories guide the skilled pool player to take the specific actions that will bring about the long-term win. There is no list of rules that he follows to bring about the same outcome in each game.

*A skilled decision maker works to master the process of bioethical decision making.*

A skilled decision maker makes decisions purposefully. A skilled nurse makes decisions based on the needs and purposes of her patient and on what is necessary to accomplish them. Like the pool player, she applies principles and theories to achieve the specific outcome for her specific patient. Certainly, a skilled nurse does not provide the same set of actions for every patient. A skilled decision maker works to master the process of bioethical decision making. She will not assume that intuitive "knowledge" and the conditioned behavior that she has learned in childhood is adequate for successful interaction with patients in the health care setting. She knows there is no list of specified actions that will meet the needs of every patient. How then do health care professionals make decisions?

## TRADITIONAL ETHICAL MODELS

Ethical models currently used in health care systems are based on the work of early philosophers and used by many as ways to make health care decisions for patients. These models will be discussed in detail in Chapter 6, but here we can consider the basic ideas that drive current ethical decision-making models. This brief overview of the contemporary systems is offered to help motivate readers to entertain the idea that something different, more relevant, and beneficial is possible to guide nursing practice.

The four most prominent ethical systems today are:

- Deontology: a duty ethic. This method is driven by human "moral sense" that is supposed to be an analog with our five senses. Human moral sense proposes that human beings innately know what is right and what is wrong. Instinctively knowing the right course of action, each person then has the duty to carry out that action. An ethical action is determined by whether it is in response to a duty, without regard to the consequences of action. Although many people believe they have a sense of moral right and wrong, it is not a concrete sense. Even if we instinctively know that violence is wrong, still we would defend ourselves against an attacker.
- Utilitarianism: an ethics of utility, *utility* being defined as "the greatest good for the greatest number." The standard by which an ethical action is measured is whether, in the circumstances, it brought about the greatest good for the largest possible number of beneficiaries. This precludes concern for one's individual patient. A nurse would not leave a bleeding patient because it was time to give medications to her other patients.
- Social/cultural relativism: the current opinions of society or the culture regarding what is right or wrong, beneficial or harmful for all individuals. What is commonplace in a particular social group may develop according to convenience or the whims of a leader. In some societies slavery or female circumcision is accepted and encouraged. These things change over time and have no meaning in supporting an individual person's desires, motivations, and purposes.
- Emotivism: ethical nonnaturalism—the theory that ethics has nothing to do with the world we live in. In other words, emotivists believe we cannot find right and wrong in reality. They also embrace ethical noncognitivism, meaning that ethical terms cannot be defined or understood. Ethical decision making is a matter of taste or convenience.

Therefore, the only possible source of ethical guidance is from our emotions. That which feels right to us is right. However, what feels right to a nurse may not feel right to a patient.

Clearly, in the health care system, a much more practical and reliable system is necessary. Instead of these methods that ignore the individual and rely on whims and emotions, what is called for is a way to ensure action and interaction on behalf of a patient. The nurse is meant to provide this but cannot do so through these traditional ways. How then can she proceed?

## SYMPHONOLOGY: A PRACTICE-BASED, PATIENT-CENTERED ETHIC

Optimal nursing practice is founded on ethical analysis and interaction. Symphonology, which is a system of ethics based on the terms and presuppositions of agreement, is concerned with ethical decisions and agreements. The standards of symphonology are not chosen conveniently, emotionally, or arbitrarily. They are based on internal and external realities that are essential to human development, fulfillment, and flourishing.

Symphonological practice begins with the nurse's awareness of the nature of her patient. By the time someone becomes a nurse, she has a great deal of experience in understanding human nature. She has spent years serving others and herself and has made her way through countless situations requiring virtue. For a nurse to practice her profession with skill, she needs some knowledge of her patient, but she must begin with her knowledge of herself.

A nurse sharpens her understanding of her patient's characteristics by knowing herself. By the time she begins practicing, she:

- Is aware of who she is and has a desire to maintain and develop herself.
- Realizes her power to act for herself to bring about her own purposes and to lead a successful life.
- Accepts the need for a true and objective understanding of her world.
- Has recognized her desire to attain good and to avoid harm.
- Has committed herself to attaining and maintaining what she values.

Now she observes her patient and discovers:

- The pleasure he takes in being who and what he is.
- His desire for freedom and the pleasure he takes in actions that bring about his desires and purposes.
- His motivation to gain a true and objective understanding of his world.
- The actions he takes to achieve benefit and to avoid harm.
- His commitment to acting in ways that bring about and maintain what he values.

Through this process, she gains a better understanding of her patient. She recognizes that he, his motivations and desires, may be different from her own. However, as she gains knowledge of his desires, motivations, and commitments, she is able to act confidently *on his behalf* and to justify her actions. The actions she takes will be those that help him achieve his desires, support his motivations, promote his commitments, and improve his agency. "The purpose of Symphonology is to return the patient to a state of agency where he can be his own agent to the extent possible in the context" (Husted, Husted, & Scotto, 2013, p. 523).

With each patient she cares for, the nurse's process of knowing herself and learning about her patient continues and expands until she reaches her fullest ethical understanding, the widest understanding she is able to gain of herself and of others. The more knowledge she gains of herself, the greater her understanding of others. The more knowledge she gains of others, the greater her understanding of herself. In this way she prepares herself for strong ethical practice. Without knowledge of self and others, ethical (good) actions cannot be determined.

Within the symphonological system, the considerations of self and others are the standards by which ethical action is planned and evaluated. The standards listed here are familiar to most health care professionals; however, in this book we adjust the traditional definitions to clarify the application of the term as it relates to an individual person. In symphonology, the bioethical standards are not concrete concepts but are considered characteristics possessed by all persons. This is discussed further in Chapter 4.

- Autonomy: the uniqueness of the individual, including the understanding that a person has a desire to maintain and develop himself.
- Freedom: the individual's right to take action for himself in order to bring about his own purposes.
- Objectivity: the individual's capacity for true and objective understanding of his world.
- Beneficence: the individual's desire to attain good and to avoid harm.
- Fidelity: the individual's commitment to attaining and maintaining what he values.

Symphonology offers a practice model based on ethical action, guided by standards that represent human characteristics. Decisions are made and actions are taken on behalf of the patient to promote his individual life and purposes.

## MUSINGS

A degree of misdirection exists in contemporary nursing ethics. The focus is almost exclusively on what nurses ought to do, with little emphasis on how the nurses, themselves, should be. Consequently, practitioners may believe that character is not an issue and that doing the right thing (according to rules predetermined by others) is what matters (Tunna & Connor, 1993, p. 26).

For symphonology, character matters, and what follows is the intention to benefit those with whom one has agreement. (This is primarily one's patients, but it extends to those with whom one works and/or teaches.) Patients entrust nurses with their health, well-being, and life. Nurses, practicing nursing, make an implicit promise that the patient is justified in believing that the nurse will be worthy of this trust. Character can, and following the tenets of the contemporary ethical systems cannot, justify a patient's confidence.

> For symphonology, character matters, and what follows is the intention to benefit those with whom one has agreement.

## STUDY GUIDE

1. Discuss the paradox of the hammer as it relates to personal human development.
2. Explain how understanding yourself and others is interdependent.
3. Describe how virtue is a dynamic process rather than a static condition.
4. Think about what the desert island scenario has to do with your own practice and your life.
5. What is the importance of practice-based bioethics?
6. From your own experience, what is the value of agreements?

## REFERENCES

Husted, G. L., & Husted, J. H. (2008). The ethical experience of caring for vulnerable populations: The symphonological approach. In M. de Chesnay (Ed.), *Caring for the vulnerable: Perspectives in nursing theory, practice, and research* (2nd ed., pp. 103–113). Boston, MA: Jones and Bartlett.

Husted, G. L., Husted, J. H., & Scotto, C. (2013). Ethics and the advanced practice nurse. In A. Joel (Ed.), *Advanced practice nursing* (3rd ed., pp. 522–543). Philadelphia, PA: FA Davis.

Perring, C. (2005). Expanding the repertoire of bioethics: What next? *The American Journal of Bioethics, 5,* 63–65.

Tunna, K., & Conner, M. (1993). You are your ethics. *The Canadian Nurse, 89,* 25–26.

# TWO

# THE ETHICAL JOURNEY TAKEN BY THE PATIENT AND NURSE

## OBJECTIVES

- Discuss the importance of the ethical journey that the nurse and patient take together.
- Define ethical justification.
- Recognize the relationship between desire, reason, and purpose.
- Interpret the meaning of the definition of nurse and the definition of patient.
- Explain the importance of the rights agreement as a singular term.
- Relate the caveman scenario to human rights.

## MAKING PREPARATIONS FOR THE JOURNEY OF PATIENT AND NURSE

Every day a nurse interacts with her patients and takes action. In the nature of action and interaction, it is possible for intentions to be right but consequences and outcomes to go wrong. Unknown conditions and unforeseeable events occur at times and affect the consequences of action and interaction, thereby influencing the outcomes. It is even possible, although extremely unusual, for intentions to be wrong and for consequences and outcomes to be favorable. In general, evasion, deception, and coercion, by their mischievous natures, do not tend to serve human action and life.

*For all of these reasons, ethics has traditionally been called the practical science. The ability to engage in processes of ethical analysis is known as practical reason. "[Because] ethics is fundamentally a practical discipline [it is] concerned with what we should do and how we should live." (Churchill, 1989, p. 28)*

## FINDING THE RIGHT DIRECTION TO GUIDE DECISION MAKING

It is important to recognize an ideal ethical decision. An unflawed ethical decision is one that:

- One is going to act upon (it is more than just thinking about it or theorizing about it).
- Will guide one's actions to a justifiable end.
- Actually affects one's life and one's character over a span of time.
- Will give one a reason to believe that one's actions will make life better (the patient's life and one's own life).
- Will allow and enable one to change one's direction as appropriate and necessary while one is acting on it.

Each of these points is essential to producing a flawless decision, including the last point. There is a difference between being able to change the direction of actions when the direction proves to be mistaken and being tied into a course of action without having the awareness or the power to change it. This difference matters in whatever one does in one's life: being aware of the necessity to change and being able to make the decision to change is imperative in ethical decision making.

To be able to change one's direction is, of course, indispensable to clinical practice. It is also indispensable to a symphonological ethical system. One whose professional practice is such that once the direction of action is set, it is unchangeable, is a person who, to that extent, is incompetent. The same is true of one's ethical practice. A professional has a responsibility to interact with patients and to take action to assist them in avoiding possible failures and in bringing about potential positive outcomes, thereby ensuring patients' sustained success in the health care system.

These criteria point to an indispensable criterion for a professional ethic: A nurse has a responsibility to interact with a patient as a person, to interact as a thinking, desiring, feeling human being with another. A professional does credit to herself and her profession only when she remembers that she is a human being and that her patient is a human being and when her actions are those of one human being interacting with another.

A professional does credit to herself and her profession only when she remembers that she is a human being and that her patient is a human being and when her actions are those of one human being interacting with another.

Human beings make mistakes. A human being can make a decision and come to realize that she has made the wrong decision. When this happens, she can do one of three things:

1. She can make herself unconscious and refuse to let herself know that her decision is a bad one.

2. She can subtly change the definition of one or more terms describing what she is doing so that she can falsify it to herself or others.
3. She can admit her mistake and change her direction.

This third action is the desirable action, the ethical action. However, under contemporary ethical systems, that is, non-practice-based ethics, this latter alternative happens only by accident; therefore, it seldom happens.

## SELF-DETERMINATION

*Art does not tolerate "anyhow," "in general," "approximately." "More or less" is the enemy of art.*

—Stanislavski, 1963, p. 108

This quote describes how a nurse may see her patient. A nurse knows, or comes to know, a great deal about patients, but she knows about each specific patient only in terms of "more or less." Not, "Don is . . .," but, "This type of patient is . . ." The patient knows far more about his own life and values than his nurse does. This is why the patient is the final authority and why a nurse must strive to learn as much as possible about each of her patients.

> The patient knows far more about his own life and values than his nurse does. This is why the patient is the final authority and why a nurse must strive to learn as much as possible about each of her patients.

A nurse has a blueprint of generalized knowledge of persons, conditions, and generalities. Although invaluable, the blueprint is not complete. It consists of knowledge, not of each specific patient, but of wide-ranging abstractions. A virtuous nurse knows that "more or less" is not a complete blueprint of any individual.

Picture a person's arrival at several forks in a road (Figure 2.1). It was a nurse's generic knowledge that allowed her to get this far, but to get to her intended destination, she now needs more knowledge. A nurse at a patient's crossroads is bewildered—and possibly even unaware that she is bewildered. However, the patient has the necessary, narrower, and more specific knowledge that is essential in choosing the right fork. The patient is a person who knows or who can come to know which of the forks to take.

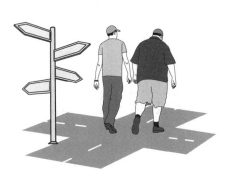

**FIGURE 2.1** The journey.

When a nurse's professional action is effective, it is intelligible and logical. It is obvious that she knows what she is doing. What she is doing is under her direction and control and therefore under her patient's direction and control. She is efficient and purposeful. Her actions are connected in a chain of sequences that are linked together by her concern for her patient's well-being and her sustained awareness of each patient's uniqueness. She is not comforted by acting on the basis of possibly irrelevant, generalized abstractions. When a system does not require sustained awareness of an individual's uniqueness, the system does not encourage comprehensive concern and produces episodic interactions based on something outside of the nurse–patient relationship.

## IMPORTANCE OF JUSTIFICATION

An ethical decision by which the nurse's patient loses the advantages of interacting within meaningful causal sequences is a flawed decision. The loss of understanding causal sequences inspires the feeling of having lost control and of being at the mercy of chance.

Human action and human life are enormously enhanced through objective and rational ethical interactions. This type of interaction will produce a series of sequential interactions that make understanding and continuing progress toward goals possible. A nonobjective and irrational ethical system of interacting, taking action, and making decisions will produce quite the opposite. Efficacy will be hampered by unease and resentment as interactions arise spontaneously and then dwindle away into distrust. Ethical agents will not devote their causal abilities to bring things about on a productive and continuing basis.

An appropriate ethical decision is one that:

- Preserves the understandability that is found in the circumstance.
- Enables the nurse (and therefore the patient) to retain control of the events involved in a purposive process.
- Supports the continuation of causal chains that enable the patient to realize his purpose.

An appropriate ethical decision is a decision that, when carried out into action, sustains intelligible causal sequences. It is a decision that is successful. The action it produces sustains progress and moves forward toward positive outcomes.

A justifiable ethical decision is a decision that a nurse or patient can explain in terms of, or as related to, an agreed-upon purpose. It is one that enables each of them to explain the reasons for his or her decision and subsequent actions.

Within a practice-based bioethic, if a health care professional can develop the ability to justify objectively (i.e., to explain) ethical decisions, she has, by that very fact, developed the ability to make appropriate decisions (i.e., logical, useful decisions). It is not possible to make consistently appropriate decisions without the ability to justify objectively those decisions. It is imperative to be able to justify and to explain her decisions in a logical and intelligible manner to herself, her patient, and other health care professionals to be confident and to continue to make such decisions.

To develop the ability to make justifiable practice-based bioethical decisions, a nurse must have a sound ethical orientation toward her role—her obligations that go with her role. This must be derived from the nature and purpose of her profession. Such an ethical orientation and the relation between her ethical system and her professional role make hers a practice-based ethical system. If she has this orientation, she can begin any ethical journey with calm assurance and confidence.

A justification is a description of how an action achieves a purpose that is formulated in a decision or an agreement. To perform an operation, it is justifiable to use a scalpel. It would not be justifiable to use a retractor or forceps without a scalpel, because these alone would not achieve the operation's purpose. To fight a staphylococcal infection, it is justifiable to use an antibiotic. It would not be justifiable to simply beat a drum, to vigorously excise the affected part, or to apply a tourniquet. These examples refer to technical justification and are not the current topic of concern. The topic at hand is that of ethical justification. An ethical justification is a description of how an action assists in the development or happiness of a human by preserving and/or enhancing his life or how an action serves to respect his rights.

> To develop the ability to make justifiable practice-based bioethical decisions, a nurse must have a sound ethical orientation toward her role—her obligations that go with her role. This must be derived from the nature and purpose of her profession.

> An ethical justification is a description of how an action assists in the development or happiness of a human by preserving and/or enhancing his life or how an action serves to respect his rights.

## PURPOSE AND JUSTIFICATION

> It is necessary to justify ethical actions in terms of ethical purposes. It is also necessary to justify ethical purposes.

It is necessary to justify ethical actions in terms of ethical purposes. It is also necessary to justify ethical purposes. If the actions necessary to accomplish a purpose are inappropriate given the context, then, of course, the purpose is not justifiable. If the actions, for instance, would violate someone's rights, they are, to say the least, inappropriate. An ethical purpose is not justified if the time and resources necessary to achieve it could be devoted to more vital and fundamental purposes with greater values. A justifiable action, then, is an action that will accomplish a justifiable purpose.

Following is a perceptual and concrete-level example of the justifiable: All things being equal, to catch a ride to a restaurant 10 miles from home, knowing you will have to walk 10 miles back, may not be easy to justify rationally. In comparison, walking 1 mile to a restaurant and 1 mile back is easy to justify. The first action will bring one from a condition of greater perfection (hungry but energetic) to a condition of lesser perfection (well fed but exhausted). The second action will bring one from a condition of lesser perfection (hungry but energetic) to a condition of greater perfection (well fed, relaxed, and still energetic).

To act in a way that will strengthen the agency and enhance the patient's life is justifiable.

To act in a way that will undermine or weaken one's own life or the life of one's patient is not justifiable. To act in a way that will undermine the conditions that make agency possible is not justifiable. To act in a way that will strengthen the agency and enhance the patient's life is justifiable.

It is justifiable to act only when one knows what one is doing and that what one is doing makes sense and has purpose.

If that which one's patient desires increases the ability to achieve that which is desirable, then this desire is justified. If it decreases this ability, then it is not. To act against one's knowledge and awareness when this action will negatively affect the life of one's patient or one's own life cannot be justified. It is justifiable to act only when one knows what one is doing and that what one is doing makes sense and has purpose.

## DESIRE, REASON, AND PURPOSE

Without a motivating desire, nothing is important. Desire keeps one knowledgeable about oneself. In a very strong sense, one's desires sum up the evidence of who the person is. One relates to things in the world through various forms of desire (or aversion—the desire to avoid). Without a relation to things in the world, one would be aware of nothing. Desire, however, does not tell one about the conditions under which one desires something, whether one can achieve one's desire, or the best way to attain the desire. Therefore, desire must always be subject to reason. Reason is an instrument that nature has provided to determine what is truly desirable and the best means of achieving it.

A purpose must always be achieved through the exercise of reason. It cannot be achieved through desire alone.

Reason, or unreason, writes one's biography. Reason gives human life all of its meaning. The betrayal of reason brings life's tragedy. A decision must always be justified through the exercise of reason. It cannot be justified through desire alone. Desire alone will not produce intelligible decisions or actions. Desire responds to outside stimuli. It does not express the character of an agent. An agent is one whose actions are motivated and guided by reason. In itself, desire is not a virtue. Reason—and only reason—has the resources necessary to define desire, to defend itself, and to defend an agent's capacity to desire and to act. A purpose must always be achieved through the exercise of reason. It cannot be achieved through desire alone.

## ROLE OF PATIENT AND NURSE

A patient is one who has lost or suffered a decrease in his agency and who is therefore unable to take the actions on his own accord that his survival or flourishing requires.

A patient is one who has lost or suffered a decrease in his agency and who is therefore unable to take the actions on his own accord that his survival or flourishing requires. The fact that patients are persons who have suffered a decrease in their agency and are vulnerable is established by the fact that they are patients. As patients, they remain vulnerable, more vulnerable than they were before they became patients.

Health care professionals possess an undesirable degree of power over patients. They may be tempted to take actions that can be justified only through rationalization. They are also sometimes motivated to take irrelevant, ritualistic actions. They unfortunately often have little concern for the ethical meaning of their actions. They may see little need for ethical doubt, analysis, or decision. Their ethical concerns may be obscure or misguided. All of this increases the potential vulnerability of patients. The nurse (or any health care professional) is the agent of a patient, doing for the patient (given her education and experience) what he would do for himself if he were able. As the agent of a patient, a nurse must decrease in every way open to her the vulnerability of the patient.

Two theories of nursing espouse the concept of agency: Orem's self-care deficit nursing theory (SCDNT) and Husted and Husted's symphonological bioethical theory. Dr. Gladys Husted explained to me their rationale for the use of the terms *agent* and *agency:*

> We decided on agent since we did not go along with the idea
> of the nurse or any health care professional (HCP) being a
> surrogate—one who acts for another. We believe that the patient
> is his or her own agent and acts for self when possible—and
> the entire role of the HCP is to return the person to his/her
> own agency—where the person can once again be his or her
> own agent [to the extent possible] and make decisions for self.
> (G. Husted, personal communication, August 25, 2011, as cited
> in Berbiglia, 2012, pp. 3–4)

Consider this case: Mr. Dietrich is hospitalized in the final stages of cancer and probably will not live out the week. All his desires and intentions have been interrupted. As with every human being, the processes of thought, choice, decision, and action are natural to Mr. Dietrich, but now he cannot translate these into action. Mr. Dietrich's power of agency is nullified, and all his purposeful and goal-directed actions are disorganized and frustrated. To seek values and to arrange these values into a more perfect life is natural to all humans, but Mr. Dietrich can seek only to rid himself of disvalues in his current condition.

Mr. Dietrich expects beneficence from his nurse. He cannot know, and he probably would not believe, that his nurse would make an ethical decision involving him without objectively knowing why that decision was made. To do so would be a failure of beneficence. Mr. Dietrich, like every patient, assumes beneficence on the part of his nurse. His physician has ordered physical therapy for him, but he does not want to go. His nurse assumes that the physician has some reason for the therapy and decides that she will not question the order. She decides Mr. Dietrich should go to therapy. When she makes this decision, she is not acting as the agent for Mr. Dietrich.

Health care professionals possess an undesirable degree of power over patients.

The nurse (or any health care professional) is the agent of a patient, doing for the patient (given her education and experience) what he would do for himself if he were able.

Can the nurse justify her decision to insist that Mr. Dietrich undergo the ordered therapy? She must remain unaware because the order is, in fact, inappropriate. In fact, it seems obvious, that it is an inappropriate order—irrelevant, at best, to Mr. Dietrich's circumstances. Mr. Dietrich would have no reason to imagine that his nurse has no clear awareness of the relationship between the decision to make him endure the pain of therapy and the purposes that are appropriate to his context. There is no ethical justification for Mr. Dietrich's nurse to remain unaware. Yet, all too often, ethical decisions suffer this sort of defect. A nurse has an ethical responsibility to be aware of her patient's uniqueness and his specific context.

Generally, a nurse will learn from experience what is to be done, but no one can function well without an open and clear awareness of what she is doing and why she is doing it. In addition, the nurse's role as the agent of her patient is difficult. Her environment is filled with distractions. However, even under conditions that make appropriate ethical decisions seem impossible, a nurse can make ethical decisions that are justifiable. These are decisions made even in crisis conditions on the basis of what the circumstances, her preexisting knowledge, and her present awareness allow. These are the best decisions that can be made, although they cannot be made with perfect assurance, serenity, or consistency. All that can ever be asked of a nurse is that she makes decisions justified by her effective analysis of the circumstances, her preexisting knowledge, and her present awareness of the patient.

> Generally, a nurse will learn from experience what is to be done, but no one can function well without an open and clear awareness of what she is doing and why she is doing it.

Justifiable ethical decision making is quite possible—and in most situations, it is not even difficult. However, it is impossible to achieve if based on hunches, intuitions, traditions, or even laws. These "imply a psychology of moral motivation in which anxiety and dependence are the primary [ethical] motivators" (van Hooft, 1990, p. 210). Anxiety and dependency do not justify ethical decisions.

> Anxiety and dependency do not justify ethical decisions.

## ETHICAL INDIVIDUALISM AND THE LAW

> Every patient who enters the health care system, concerned for his survival and well-being, enters as an ethical individualist.

Every patient who enters the health care system, concerned for his survival and well-being, enters as an ethical individualist. Many lawsuits have originated over the failure of the health care system to recognize this. Virtually every law that relates to these issues sanctions the patient's ethical individualism. The law recognizes, among other things:

- A patient's legal right to give an informed consent. No one has a legal right to treat a patient without his consent. No one has a legal right to obtain a patient's consent without the patient's knowing to what he is giving his consent.
- A patient's legal right to refuse treatment.
- A patient's legal right, postmortem, to be protected against the "harvesting" of organs.

- The legal right of children to receive medical attention, regardless of the wishes of their parents.
- A patient's legal right to confidentiality.
- An individual's legal right to refuse to donate organs (e.g., bone marrow) to a relative.
- A patient's legal right not to participate in research against his wishes.
- A patient's legal right to be protected against malpractice or wrongful death.

Ethical individualism is desirable and proper, but this is not because it is sanctioned by the law. Individual rights are not produced by law. Rather, laws are purposeless and unintelligible if they are not derived from individual rights (Guido, 2013). Laws gain purpose and become logical when they develop from individual rights. Contemporary medical law is desirable and proper because it is sanctioned by ethical individualism. Each of the previously stated rights had to be recognized as an ethical right before it was enacted as a legal right. However, be advised that the legal system is not always consistent in the use of individual rights and ethical individualism in the development of legal rights and law.

*Laws gain purpose and become logical when they develop from individual rights.*

## HUMAN RIGHTS

### THE FIRST HUMOROUS VIGNETTE: THE CAVEMAN

One day, many thousands of years ago, two cavemen passed each other on a forest pathway. One caveman struck the other with a club and knocked him down. There was nothing unusual about this; it had happened many times before and happened many times since. But this day, something world-historic happened. The victim, holding his bloodied head, looked up and asked the fateful question, "Why did you do that?" This was history's first demand for an ethical justification. The aggressor, a thoughtful chap as cavemen go, replied to his victim's query with the remark: "I harm you so that you will have no power to harm me. It is terribly unfortunate that you and I cannot leave each other alone, each of us free to do what he wants to do. Someday, we ought to give some thought to this." As time passed, the human race began to form the idea of individual rights, including the right to be left alone. It is an idea with a very rocky history and one that is far from completely formed. But it is a reality. It does motivate and control a considerable amount of human interaction and can be observed in operation constantly and everywhere today, especially in the health care arena. It is the irreplaceable reality serving as the foundation of humanity's ethical existence.

## THE IMPORTANCE OF RIGHTS AS A SINGULAR

Rights is the product of an implicit agreement among rational beings, made and held by virtue of their rationality, not to obtain actions nor the products or conditions of action from one another, except through voluntary consent objectively gained.

Rights* is the product of an implicit agreement among rational beings, made and held by virtue of their rationality, not to obtain actions nor the products or conditions of action from one another, except through voluntary consent objectively gained. In other words, rights is an agreement that a person will not force another to take action, unjustly deprive another of any value his effort has produced, or place another in any circumstance without the voluntary consent of that other and that the consent is gained with full awareness. This agreement establishes the practice of acting together only on the basis of the informed and voluntary consent of everyone involved, without force or deception.

Rights pertains to an individual's freedom of action. An individual has a right to make free choices among alternatives and to act on these choices based on his or her own desires, purposes, and values as long as these choices and actions do not interfere with the rightful choices and actions or violate the rights of another. The first great creation of ethics that made all the rest possible is the creation of individual rights. The scope of ethics then expanded from this. It began by making trust between rational beings a natural, expected, and essential reality. Individual rights and explicit agreements make productive interaction between ethical agents possible.

## AGENCY, RIGHTS, AND THE ETHICAL INTERACTION

Strictly speaking, rights exist only in situations in which more than one person is involved. A right is a right against another person—a right not to be aggressed against.

Let's say Debbie is stranded alone on a desert island. There is no possibility of a division of labor, and there are no tools of civilization available to her; therefore, survival is a pressing problem for Debbie. Under these circumstances, does Debbie have a right to do whatever she wants to do? In these highly unusual circumstances, Debbie has the right to do whatever she has the power to do, and her right to take action is unlimited. Strictly speaking, rights exist only in situations in which more than one person is involved. A right is a right against another person—a right not to be aggressed against. So when speaking of "one's rights on a desert island," the term *rights* is used in an extended sense to refer to what would be equivalent to rights among a number of people.

Debbie has the right to pursue any value that she has reason to believe will bring her benefit and the right to avoid anything that would lead to her detriment. She has as much the right to take action to pursue her values as she has the right to exist and survive. The fact that Debbie, a thinking,

---

*As the reader proceeds through the text, the necessity of regarding "rights" as a singular concept, denoting a single, noncomplex agreement, will become more obvious.

valuing person actually exists, is exhaustive evidence that it is right that she should exist. The fact that she is, by nature, a being to whom the pursuit of values is appropriate is conclusive evidence that it is right that she pursue that which she values.

Debbie has the right to be the person she is. Any alternative to this principle is not logical or rational, so Debbie has a right to do whatever she has the power to do. Nothing she does can violate the rights of another. There is no other on the island.

If the scenario changes and one day someone else (Michelle) happens to wash ashore, this principle remains intact. However, two significant changes have occurred:

1. As rational beings, Michelle and Debbie have an obligation not to violate each other's rights. Regardless of whether or not they violate each other's rights, the obligation remains. The obligation is there, not by virtue of any arbitrary decision either might make, but by virtue of their defining characteristics, by virtue of the rational nature of Debbie and Michelle. As a consequence of this, each has an obligation to honor the agreements that she makes with the other.
2. Debbie's and Michelle's experience of existence has been greatly enhanced because they now have each other.

If the inhabitants of the island number two or number in the millions, nothing essentially changes. Whether one is Debbie, Michelle, or one of a million, the ethical principles governing the situation remain the same. One does not lack any rights that others possess, and one has no right that others lack. If any ethical circumstance that might apply to a particular individual is, all things being equal, right or wrong, it can only be because it is right or wrong universally, for every ethical agent.

## SOLITUDE AND SOCIETY

In a state of solitude, a person has a right to do whatever he desires. An individual has this right because no one else is relevantly involved, so there is no possibility of violating the rights of others. However, when ethical agents live and interact together, the benefit of the rights agreement is so great and so obvious, and the detriment of not having this agreement is so manifestly ruinous, that the agreement literally "goes without saying." It is, in various ways, the basis of all benevolence, justice, and cooperation among people.

As cavemen became more and more rational, people began to give some thought to rights and the idea caught on. People began to form this agreement among themselves. Eventually, it formed, naturally and spontaneously, without words, simply as a matter of course. It is an agreement to forgo aggression in favor of communication, agreement, cooperation, and interaction. As reason began to enlighten their lives,

**TABLE 2.1** ENHANCEMENT OF HUMAN LIFE

Cooperation is possible, and human action is predictable.

There is a natural benevolence among humans, and trust in the goodwill of others is reasonable.

Integrity, reason, and respect for the rights of a reasoning being support interaction.

Foresight, purposeful interaction, and cooperation based on an exchange of values are possible.

People can foresee the probable consequences of their actions.

cavemen realized that aggression was dysfunctional and that cooperation produced human progress and well-being. The practice of recognizing individual rights spread, and it continues to do so because it makes sense and serves human purpose and flourishing. When this agreement is put aside, there is nothing whatsoever to protect people against each other's brutal irrationality or to ensure good faith and justice in interactions and actions. Individual rights is necessary and purposeful and a reality that one experiences every day.

The recognition of rights is an essential element of the ethical interaction between agents. It is an original and implicit agreement that shapes every future agreement. It is an agreement that agreements will be kept. The violation of rights produces aggression and coercion. The recognition of rights produces justice and trust. It is easy to see that without the recognition of rights, trust is a fatal illusion. Justified trust, in its turn, produces ethical interaction. As ethical agents become aware of the benefits of trading values that they possess or can produce for values they do not possess or cannot produce, the existence of a justified trust makes trade and interaction their most significant asset. Human life is enhanced through cooperation, agreements, trust, and trading values.

*Human life is enhanced through cooperation, agreements, trust, and trading values.*

## TRUST AND OBLIGATION

The word *profession* comes from a Latin term meaning "to make a public declaration." The difference between a nurse and a restaurant worker, or a prima donna at the opera, or an interior decorator, or a sales clerk is that the nurse is a professional and the others are not. The nurse has professed that she will be a nurse, and because of this, she has taken on the responsibilities and obligations of taking action as a professional. She has, in essence, made an agreement to take on the responsibilities and obligations of being a professional nurse. A nurse understands that completing one's established "duties" as a professional nurse is an obligation, but she likely does not understand what establishes whether something is an obligation or not. One's emotions do not establish what is or is not an obligation. The sentiments of society do not establish what is or is not an obligation. A professional's obligation is not to her subconscious, her emotions, or society, nor is it blindly following her "duty" without reference to the context and consequences of her actions. Then what are her obligations? Her obligations are to be true to the agreement she has made with her patient, which basically means to benefit and not harm and to allow the patient (to the extent possible) to be in charge of his own destiny.

A nurse understands that trust is essential when taking action as a professional. "[I]n addition to the inherent vulnerability of patients, trust itself involves vulnerability and dependency" (Dinc & Gastmans, 2013, p. 509). If a nurse exclusively practices one of the contemporary ethical systems, she would not deserve a patient's trust, because she has not taken on any obligation when she identifies with those systems. None of the contemporary ethical systems offer anything sufficient to justify that trust because the patient is merely a marginal factor in her ethical concerns under those systems. If the nurse enters into an informal discussion of the contemporary ethical system of her choice, this will not inspire trust. Quite contrary to this, if the discussion is with her patient, it might inspire anxiety.

> Being intertwined with other human beings, our life is characterized by encountering one another with natural trust. To trust is to lay oneself open to the other person. . . . Human beings should protect another's life when it is entrusted to them [as a nurse would with a patient]. (Fegran, Helseth, & Slettebo, 2006, p. 58)

A nurse takes on an obligation through an agreement that she makes when she professes that she is a professional, that she is a nurse. This agreement is the source of her obligation. Her obligation is guaranteed by her character.

A nurse's trustworthiness is revealed in her ability to deal with things rationally and responsibly as they arise. Just knowing that his nurse is a professional ordinarily will inspire a patient's feeling of confidence. This trust is a moral asset. It validates a nurse's pride in herself and her practice. A nurse makes a professional agreement to meet the obligations of the profession. A nurse should always be aware of the nature and the beneficiary of those obligations. A nurse takes on an obligation through an agreement that she makes when she professes that she is a professional, that she is a nurse. This agreement is the source of her obligation. Her obligation is guaranteed by her character.

## ETHICAL APPROACH OF PROFESSIONAL AND PATIENT

The philosopher Lao Tzu (604 BC) (Brown, 1938) has told us, "The longest journey begins with the first step." This is so obvious that we can see it for ourselves. We can hardly avoid seeing it. That said, it is so obvious that, without Lao Tzu, we might never have noticed the importance of it.

It is also obvious that we can take the first step of a journey in confusion. We may have brought the patient along. When we take the first step in confusion or act without thinking and with arrogant certainty, it is often in the wrong direction. If it is taken in the wrong direction, at the end of our journey we may find ourselves very far from our destination. If it is an ethical journey, we will probably be unaware of this and remain unaware of it. Our patient may not.

A series of actions taken in the pursuit of vital and fundamental goals may be regarded as an ethical journey. The possibility of arriving at an undesirable destination is very real for an ethical journey.

## PREPARING FOR THE ETHICAL JOURNEY

*To head in the right direction on any journey, the initial preparations are very important.*

To head in the right direction on any journey, the initial preparations are very important. The same is true when it comes to the direction of professional practice. These preparations are essential in the ethical decision making of any professional. To be certain of adequate preparation for an ethical journey, a number of conditions of the search, when practical, are desirable:

1. The details of the health care setting should be clearly perceived. It is also necessary to be aware of the authentically ethical aspects of a situation. These aspects are an integral part of the health care setting. They are not random occurrences. They are to be dealt with calmly, competently, and sequentially, not off-handedly and not inflexibly.
2. The essential qualities and exceptional circumstances of the ethical situation should be visualized. Bioethics calls for a patient's right to self-determination to be respected, but at times a patient's right to self-determination can be a fuzzy abstraction. It may become visible only in the most obvious circumstances.

    For example, consider a patient who is on her way to have a hysterectomy. As you are taking her to the operating room, she tells you that she hopes she can get pregnant after the operation. She very much wants to have a child. This situation requires the nurse to stop the surgery until the issues involved in this case are resolved. However, very few situations are as simple as this.

    A cloudy understanding of a patient's right to control his own situation is better than no ethical understanding at all. It is considerably better, however, and far more useful, if a nurse understands that a patient has a right to be protected against undesired or undesirable interaction of any sort. This illustrates a patient's right to control his own time and that to which he puts his effort.
3. The essential qualities of a situation are those qualities that can properly guide the nurse's ethical actions. They are like landmarks on a trip, guiding the traveler to her destination. The ethical aspects of a situation should be isolated. One should be able to draw general, but

tentative, conclusions that apply to very similar situations. No situation will be precisely the same, but without these general conclusions, a nurse has to face similar situations, one by one, without a basic understanding.

4. It is important to make decisions that have a beneficial effect into the future. It is of no importance to make decisions whose benefits cease the moment the actions are taken. Ethical actions do not have to occur in a disjointed series. They can be taken in ongoing integrated sequences, which is preferred.

5. Her decisions should be based on stable and permanent values, not on values that are temporary and changing. They should be relevant values, appropriate to a human being in the health care setting. These values should be the patient's values and appropriate to the specific patient at this current time. It is better, therefore, to see what these stable and permanent values are than to identify any transitory ones.

## THE NATURE OF ETHICAL ASPECTS

Take the sparsest situation imaginable. Imagine two lost people meeting in the middle of a wasteland. Not even in this situation is every aspect an ethical aspect. One person plans to follow the North Star and walk out of the wasteland. The other intends to build a fire and lay down debris spelling out "Help" in the hope that a passing airplane will see him.

Each person has come from different conditions of life. Each has different motivations. Each has different ways of going about things, and each will return to different conditions of life. Each has a unique set of abilities, strengths, and weaknesses. The way each has chosen to escape the wasteland is not an ethical aspect of the situation, and neither is the background from which each has come or the conditions of life to which each of them hope to return. Their health is not an ethical aspect, and neither is their knowledge or lack of knowledge.

Every ethical aspect of a situation arises in relation to aspects that are not, in themselves, ethical. The nonethical aspects of a situation determine what can be done. The ethical aspects, in relation to a purpose, determine what ought to be done, given what can be done.

Let's look at an example. Jane sees a young girl, Nancy, drowning. *Jane cannot swim.* There is a life preserver at hand. This establishes what Jane can do but not what Jane ought to do. Jane's ethical character, her natural empathy for other human beings, and her sense of beneficence determine what she ought to do. Let's go further and say that there is nothing at hand for Jane to throw to Nancy. Is Jane required to jeopardize her own life and jump in to try to save her? The answer has to be no. However, she is ethically required to do what she can do, such as using her cell phone to call 911, screaming so that another may hear, or doing whatever she can do short of putting her own life in severe jeopardy. No ethical system can demand that you lose your life to save another. Take

*The nonethical aspects of a situation determine what can be done. The ethical aspects, in relation to a purpose, determine what ought to be done, given what can be done.*

another example that probably has happened to some of you: A patient is being attacked by another person who happens to be a very large man. The nurse must get help, but she does not have to be the help.

Because ethics has to do with actions taken in the pursuit of vital (essential to preserving or enhancing life) and fundamental (essential to making a person's life what she wants her life to be) goals, rescuing Nancy is, at that time, Jane's only vital and fundamental goal—to act in honor of her own life by preserving Nancy's if possible. Sharing an affirmation of the value of life that their awareness implies highlights the ethical aspects of the situation for Jane and Nancy. Nancy's desire and efforts to survive are ethical aspects.

Suppose that when Nancy's peril arose, Jane had not been present and Nancy saved her own life by grabbing onto a log that came floating by. In doing this, she achieved a vital and fundamental goal. She saved her life. The floating log is obviously not an ethical aspect of this situation. Nancy's action is its only ethical aspect. Only those aspects of a situation that relate to human purposes and human virtues are ethical aspects of a situation.

To put it another way, the ethical aspects of a situation are determined by the human intentions that are set to operate in the situation. What is ethically relevant in any situation is determined by the purposes of the agents who can act in it. That something is relevant (of necessity) implies that it is important to some person in relation to a purpose. This is not to say that what one ought to do in any situation is simply relative to one's desires. To go from "I want X" to "Therefore, it is good (or right) that I do Y" is neither ethical nor rational. Justifiability is radically important to ethical decision making. To be the source of justifiable actions, one's desires must be justifiable in terms of their foreseeable consequences.

> To be the source of justifiable actions, one's desires must be justifiable in terms of their foreseeable consequences.

The most crucial step of the journey is for the nurse to discover the mapmaker, the authority that will guide the ethical journey, the authority that will guide nurse–patient interactions to its justifiable destination. The nurse needs to recognize the final authority.

## THE FINAL AUTHORITY

No two human beings are entirely different, so every nurse can feel a certain empathy with the human hopes and fears of all her patients. She has the basic resources necessary to learn through experience, and she can take ethical action through trial and error. However, this is the slowest possible way. Certain authorities advise that health care professionals adopt formalistic principles of ethics, but these are principles that are to be applied indiscriminately without regard to consequences. Other authorities would advise health care professionals to hold the convenience of others as their principle of ethical judgment. This principle is, at best, the principle of etiquette. Taken beyond the level of etiquette, it ignores the fact that health care professionals have knowledge and specific functions to perform. Trial and error, formalism, and convenience are not good choices to help the nurse to identify the final authority.

The only possibility is for a nurse as the agent of her patient to learn the requirements of the right action from a reliable authority on the subject. This leaves the problem of discovering an authority that is reliable. There is an authority who would advise health care professionals to begin from an objective awareness of what is going on in the health care setting. He would ask the professional nurse to exercise her time and effort in acting to help her patient to achieve a passage from his current condition to a more perfect condition. He would advise her to justify her actions on the basis of her professional agreement. This final authority, of course, must be the patient.

*This final authority, of course, must be the patient.*

## MUSINGS

No one ever did or said more to establish meaningful causal sequences in human relationships than the caveman "who gave it some thought."

There is a group of facts naturally tending to form a unique and intelligible context when nurse and patient come together. These facts establish a relationship between them through an interweaving of purposes and a meeting of the minds. A patient needs a nurse to provide him with the benefit of her professional skills. A nurse needs a patient in order to live her professional role. Their shared purposes take the form of an implicit agreement to interact and has this as its purpose, their self-directed interaction, the control by each of his or her time and effort into productive interactions in filling their needs.

The most basic link between people dictates that the first step of interaction shall be an agreement "not to obtain action . . . except through voluntary consent, objectively gained."

*A nurse is the agent of her patient, doing for her patient what he would do for himself if he were able.*

A nurse is the agent of her patient, doing for her patient what he would do for himself if he were able. That which nurses profess (i.e., that to which they agree) is beneficence. Their education, training, and experience fit them to exercise beneficence in the health care setting. The first ethical demand placed on nurses is that they accept the nature of human beings. The next ethical demand placed on them is that they recognize the nature, demands, and purposes of the health care setting. If a nurse is to act beneficently, she must know why she is doing what she is doing. These are the first steps of her ethical professional action. A nurse cannot act, let alone act beneficently, without this awareness. To know why she is doing what she is doing, a nurse must exercise judgment. Judgment is a precondition of beneficence. If a nurse does not know why her actions are beneficent, they are not beneficent. Beneficence begins in judgment.

*If a nurse is to act beneficently, she must know why she is doing what she is doing.*

This implies that it is impossible to function under a professional ethic without recognizing the patient as the center of ethical decision making and, therefore, as the final authority as to the direction of his ethical interactions. It requires the nurse to act as the agent of her patient until such time as he regains his own agency. A health care professional helps the patient in navigating through myriad facts by means of appropriate actions. However, a health care professional must never forget and may now and again remind her patient that the patient's life, health, and well-being set the destination.

*Note:* We do not use the term *advocacy* but instead use the term *agency*. An agent acts with the patient. An advocate acts for the patient, a subtle but vital difference.

## STUDY GUIDE

1. Does the fact that the patient is the final authority mean that any patient has a right to do anything and to make any type of demands on the nurse and other health care professionals? Support your answer.
2. Why must *rights* be a singular term, and how does this implicit agreement foster understanding?
3. What does the following statement mean: "Ethics pervades the practice of everyday life"?
4. Why is justification so important to bioethical decision making?
5. How does the rights agreement, the agreement not to aggress, foster interaction with patients?
6. What does it mean to be the agent of a patient?
7. What is the purpose of symphonology?
8. What is learned from the humorous caveman scenario?
9. In the scenario with Jane and Nancy, why does Jane have no ethical responsibility to go into the water to try to save Nancy when she cannot swim? (In the next chapter, you will learn about rational self-interest. You might want to come back to this dilemma at this time.)

## REFERENCES

Berbiglia, V. (2012). Editors' Column, Agency. *Self-Care, Dependent Care, & Nursing, 19*, 3–4.

Brown, B. (Ed.). (1938). *The wisdom of the Chinese*. Garden City, NY: Doubleday.

Churchill, L. R. (1989). Reviving a distinctive medical ethic. *Hastings Center Report, 19*(3), 28–30.

Dinc, L., & Gastmans, C. (2013). Trust in nurse-patient relationships: A literature review. *Nursing Ethics, 20*(5), 501–516.

Fegran, L., Helseth, S., & Slettebo, A. (2006). Nurses as moral practitioners encountering parents in neonatal intensive care units. *Nursing Ethics, 13*, 51–64.

Guido, G. W. (2013). *Legal and ethical issues in nursing* (5th ed.). Upper Saddle River, NJ: Prentice Hall.

Stanislavski, C. (1963). *An actor's handbook*. New York, NY: Theatre Arts Books.

van Hooft, S. (1990). Moral education for nursing decisions. *Journal of Advanced Nursing, 15*, 210–215.

# THREE

# THE NURSE–PATIENT AGREEMENT

## OBJECTIVES

- Examine the relevance and terms of the nurse–patient agreement.

- Discuss the purpose of the Code of Ethics for Nurses.

- Summarize the important lessons learned from the coconut scenario to nursing practice.

- Differentiate between dilemmas that can be resolved using probability and those that cannot.

- Distinguish rational self-interest from irrational self-interest.

- Cite reasons why the agreement with oneself is basic.

We all live in the same world. We all have the same world to understand and a human way of understanding it. We all are faced with the need to act to achieve happiness (a feeling of success with ourselves) and to avoid unhappiness (a sense of failing as humans). This involves the need to make decisions. Our lives are made better by making appropriate decisions. Our lives are also tremendously enhanced by agreements. Ethics is the science of making and acting on these agreements.

## THE NATURE OF AGREEMENTS

It is important to understand what constitutes an agreement before discussing all the nuances involved in the nurse–patient agreement. An agreement is a shared state of awareness on the basis of which interaction occurs. People engage in a variety of activities with one another. Together, two people might play volleyball, carry a plank, go out to dinner, hold hands at the movies, or even take a rocket to the moon. There are four possible reasons why they are interacting with each other as they are:

- Their behavior is directed by coercion. One person is pressuring the other to interact as they are, or both are being pressured by another person.
- Their behavior is directed by deception. One person is aware of what he or she is doing while the other has been misled into cooperating, or both have been misled by some other person.
- Their behavior is determined by evasion and elusion. They are not allowing themselves to be aware of information that is available that would reveal a better course of action that they could take.
- Their behavior is determined by an agreement. It is not forced, the result of hidden agendas, or the result of a conscious unawareness of any relevant factor. They are interacting and acting together by agreement. The terms of their agreement are clearly and completely understood by both parties.

Only this fourth reason of interacting and acting together is directed by objective and independent agreement and can be identified as a justifiable ethical interaction. Coercion and deception violate the rights of the person who is pressured, forced, or deceived. There is no justification for violating a person's rights. This right is the basic, fundamental interpersonal ethical concept. It is not possible to violate another person's rights and be a reasoning, ethical human individual. It is especially not possible to violate another person's rights and effectively and ethically satisfy the role of a nurse.

## RELATIONSHIP BETWEEN A NURSE AND PATIENT

The importance of the relationship between nurse and patient is well established. According to Dinc and Gastmans (2013), "The nurse-patient relationship is the cornerstone of nursing work" (p. 502). The relationship between the nurse and the patient is an implicit agreement. There is only one authority to whom a professional nurse can turn for advice, for motivating the relationship, and for providing care. The person of authority is the patient. Nurses can enhance their ability to be agents of their patients by examining their own agency and what it would mean to lose it (Houck & Bongiorno, 2006).

A health care professional practicing responsibly practices according to the purposes of her profession. If one is a responsible health care professional, then:

- One conscientiously acts as an agent. One acts with as keen an awareness and as firm a determination as one's patient would if he were able.

- One makes one's patient the reason for her being an agent and a professional. Therefore, the patient is the center of the nurse's attention and activity. This is defined by the nurse's professional agreement, and it defines her agency as a nurse.
- Interaction is guided by two objective standards: the skilled professional action of a nurse and the benefit of a patient. This is the justification for every change in action and interaction.
- Interaction is based on voluntary consent that is objectively gained. This ensures that neither party to the agreement will suffer a rights violation. It ensures that the agreement will be an agreement.

Although the patient is the source of authority and the focus of the nurse, families play an essential role as well. Lind, Nortvedt, Lorem, and Hevroy (2012) assert the importance of families' receiving "regular, honest, and responsible interactions" (p. 62) with their health care professionals. Family members are normally a good source of knowledge regarding the patient and should be included in treatment planning to the extent that it is beneficial to the patient and the patient is amenable to their involvement. Families are often the decision makers when the patient is unable to make decisions. The family becomes essential in the planning of care and can offer emotional support to the patient.

*Family members are normally a good source of knowledge regarding the patient and should be included in treatment planning to the extent that it is beneficial to the patient and the patient is amenable to their involvement.*

However, there are times when the family does not want to follow the wishes of the person or when members of the family disagree as to what should be done. This becomes a source of dissonance for the nurse and other health care professionals. Thinking about how and when to involve family members in care and decision making is an ethical consideration.

## CODES OF ETHICS

Both the International Council of Nurses (ICN) (see Appendix I) and the American Nurses Association (ANA) have established codes of ethics for nurses. The ANA code is in the process of being revised. See www.nursingworld.org/codeofethics for information on the ANA code.

The nurse is responsible and accountable for individual *nursing practice* and determines the ethical responsibilities of the nurse. The codes were established to give nurses guidelines for carrying out *nursing* responsibilities consistent with quality nursing care and to preserve the rights of all persons.

## AGREEMENT: THE FOUNDATION OF INTERACTION

The actions that a health care professional takes in her role as a professional always have an ethical aspect because they are always concerned with the vital and fundamental goals of health and life. As a professional, a nurse acts as an agent for her patients. The ethical aspects of

Every human relationship, whether it is a pitcher and catcher on a softball team, two people dancing, trapeze artists, or drivers getting directions, arises from an agreement. That agreement may be explicit or implicit.

this relationship are complex and are not always easy to identify. Every human relationship, whether it is a pitcher and catcher on a softball team, two people dancing, trapeze artists, or drivers getting directions, arises from an agreement. That agreement may be explicit or implicit. The expectations, roles, and directives may be clearly laid out in an explicit agreement, or they may be implied and embedded in the relationship itself in an implicit agreement. The relationship that arises between a professional nurse and patient is an implicit agreement. The principles by which a professional makes a decision are derived from the actual dynamics and directives of this agreement. The dynamics of the agreement are formed by the goals and values a patient seeks to attain, maintain, or regain during the course of the relationship. For the nurse, they are the goals and values that she agrees to help the patient realize and achieve. For the patient, they are the interactions and actions to achieve his purposes.

A patient, in becoming a patient, has a specific purpose and is forced by circumstances to take on a specific role. A professional, in becoming a professional, has a specific purpose and takes on a specific role. The professional nurse agrees to act for those who cannot act for themselves. Their purposes interface by design.

A patient, in becoming a patient, has a specific purpose and is forced by circumstances to take on a specific role. A professional, in becoming a professional, has a specific purpose and takes on a specific role. The professional nurse agrees to act for those who cannot act for themselves. Their purposes interface by design.

The purpose of a patient (regaining or maintaining the power of his agency) determines the role of a professional. A professional, in becoming a professional, becomes the agent of her patient. The nurse assists the patient in regaining the ability to take independent actions. The interrelationship between them is formed by the characteristics of an agent (one who acts for a patient) and the characteristics of a patient (one who lacks the power to act for himself). In the interaction between a professional and a patient, their roles structure the implicit agreement between them. They agree that, because the patient is a patient and the nurse is a professional, the professional agent will act as an agent for the patient and act on behalf of the patient to carry out the patient's values, goals, and purposes. The entire area of a professional's ethical action lies within these outlines of responsibility established by their implicit agreement.

That there is objective and voluntary consent between a health care professional and patient means that there is an interconnecting and interweaving of their purposes. Objective and voluntary consent never occurs outside of this interconnection. The agreement makes the nurse–patient relationship understandable and clear and thereby governs and directs the interaction. Effective interaction produces logical and understandable connecting sequences. The agreement also implies that a patient should not make any arbitrary, illogical, or frivolous demands on a health care professional, and a health care professional does not make any arbitrary, inattentive, or careless demands on a patient. Arbitrary demands, as well as coercion, do not have a place in a purposeful agreement or within a shared state of awareness in a relationship working toward shared purposes.

## THE NATURE AND FUNCTION OF THE AGREEMENT BETWEEN THE NURSE AND PATIENT

The professional nurse–patient relationship is based on an actual implicit agreement. A nurse is motivated to be a nurse. A patient is compelled to be a patient. *Nurse* and *patient* are defined in terms of the other. Their understanding of their common purpose—to interact and act in order to achieve the patient's values, goals, and purposes—is, in itself, an agreement to be a nurse and a patient. Their circumstances and viewpoints when they initiate interaction, the inferred passivity and suffering of the patient, and the nurse's inferred commitment to her profession combine to shape this implicit agreement between them.

This agreement is necessary to ensure dependability, trust, reliability, and commitment between them. The professional nurse–patient relationship requires this. The professionalism of the professional nurse necessarily involves being faithful to this agreement. The condition of the patient calls for this on the part of the patient as long as their relationship lasts. There is no commitment between two people who pass each other on the street simply because there is no common purpose between them and there is no motivation to form an agreement (except for a rights agreement requiring nonaggression). Between the professional nurse and patient, however, the case is very different and the agreement is essential.

Without the terms of an agreement:

- Their interaction is not based on a purpose.
- There is no solid basis for interaction between them.
- There is nothing to establish the parameters of trust.
- A nurse has no basis for a stable commitment to her patient.
- A patient has no objective reason to feel confident under a nurse's care.

Without an agreement between them, the professional nurse and her patient do not have an explicit understanding of their roles. The professional nurse and her patient will not understand their functioning in the relationship without an agreement between them, and reliably effective communication will not take place. Their agreement is what is implicitly understood and occurs before their interaction. The agreement makes each agent stronger, allows for interactions and discussions that will lead to knowledge that might have been missed by the other, and allows for improved outcomes and goal attainment.

*The agreement makes each agent stronger, allows for interactions and discussions that will lead to knowledge that might have been missed by the other, and allows for improved outcomes and goal attainment.*

To the extent that there is no explicit understanding of the roles established by their agreement, there is no foundation for their interaction. There is no way for them to structure their interaction. What action could a nurse take if she had no idea what the response of her patient would be? What actions could a patient expect a nurse to take if he had no certain knowledge that she was acting in her capacity as his nurse? Without a prior agreement, a nurse cannot be certain that her patient regards himself as her patient. Without this agreement, a patient cannot be sure that his nurse regards herself as his nurse. Nurses do what they do by agreement. An agreement produces expectations and commitments justifying those expectations.

The agreement between a nurse and a patient makes it possible for each to function. It also makes it necessary for each to apply ethical reasoning to his or her actions. Their agreement is the beginning and the principle of their ethical reasoning. Even when "a patient is not able to take part in the forming of an agreement or actively participate in it, it is an implicit agreement based on a high probability that, if the patient were able, it would be formed" (Husted & Husted, 2008).

> Even when "a patient is not able to take part in the forming of an agreement or actively participate in it, it is an implicit agreement based on a high probability that, if the patient were able, it would be formed" (Husted & Husted, 2008).

---

## DILEMMA 3.1: PATIENT'S CONFLICT ABOUT HER OWN CARE

Mrs. Baldwin is an 86-year-old widow who lives in a California retirement home. She is a gentle, sociable lady and likes to reminisce about her work doing make up for movie stars. She has no family locally but has one good friend nearby and a 101-year-old sister who lives on the East Coast. She is in the hospital for treatment of an infection, from which she is recovering. She also has chronic kidney failure and has been receiving dialysis for about 8 months. For at least the past 3 months, Mrs. Baldwin has told her doctors, her nurses, and her friend that she wants to stop the dialysis. She understands that her life depends on receiving it, but she declares that she hates the process and does not want to live this way. However, she continues to board the van that takes her to the dialysis center three times each week. She claims that every time she tells her doctor she wants to stop, he describes the risks of falls, fractures, and a miserable end. This frightens her (Colter, Ganzimi, & Cohen, 2000, p. 24). What is the nurse's responsibility in this case?

---

## THE DEVELOPMENT OF THE AGREEMENT

A health care professional does not approach each of her patients and declare that an agreement needs to be formed between the two of them, but an agreement is formed and does exists between each health care professional and each patient. As soon as a health care professional walks into a patient's care environment, an agreement is formed. "You are my patient. I will be your nurse." "You are my nurse. I will be your patient." Without being spoken, this agreement implicitly arises between them. The ethical aspects of the agreement are implied by this as well. "You are my patient. I will support your values, goals, purposes, and virtues (the strength of your character)." (Every virtue is a form of strength.) The nurse's strength and knowledge are available to the patient to support his recovery. The patient's implied response is: "You are my nurse. My virtues will interact with yours." Their initial interaction and discovery of each other in their current roles is sufficient to produce the agreement. They immediately recognize the facts that have brought them together. The agreement arises when a nurse, in effect, accepts a patient's invitation to be his nurse and a patient accepts a nurse's offer to be his nurse.

The agreement between the nurse and her patient is structured by the expectations and commitments of each of them. The nurse and patient both agree to satisfy the reasonable expectations of the other, and both agree to live up to their commitment to the other. The nurse is a professional; therefore, the nurse's agreement is necessarily stronger and more directive. The nurse's expectations and commitments establish the nature and characteristics of the agreement between a professional and her patient (Figure 3.1). This agreement formulates and conveys the expectations and the commitments of each person involved. It establishes the boundaries of a successful ethical interaction. The agreement establishes what each person has a right to expect from the other during all interactions. To follow through with the expectations and commitments involved with the agreement is right. To fail to live up to the agreement is wrong. Now and then a nurse or a patient will establish the relationship on the basis of bullying, coercion, hostility, intimidation, or aggression. This makes the existence of a purposeful agreement impossible. Such an arrangement is ethically intolerable, and a different arrangement needs to be made immediately.

> The agreement arises when a nurse, in effect, accepts a patient's invitation to be his nurse and a patient accepts a nurse's offer to be his nurse.

## AGREEMENTS AND INTERACTION

Interactions are complementary and balancing actions and reactions that occur between agents on the basis of an agreement. Interaction is possible only with an agreement between people about what each of them is going to do. An agreement between a nurse and a patient is a form of recognition between them about what each of them is going to do. It also involves recognition of the factual and ethical dimensions of their interaction. Wherever there is a connectable gap between the sequential causal and connecting chain and the purpose and desired end goals, it is frequently the result of a failure of one or both of them to recognize some aspect of the context created by their agreement. Once this recognition is achieved and addressed, the links of the chain can be reconnected.

An implicit agreement exists between a nurse and her patient and must exist for purpose and goal attainment. Without an agreement, professional interaction cannot begin. Their agreement requires that a nurse be willing to support her patient in any purpose to which he has a right and that is appropriate to his situation. A failure to do this is a failure to act as the agent of the patient.

> Their agreement requires that a nurse be willing to support her patient in any purpose to which he has a right and that is appropriate to his situation.

## MOTIVATIONS

A most intimate and personal ethical relationship emerges between a nurse and her patient. This relationship is formed on the side of the patient by the desire to regain independent functioning and self-agency. The loss of agency is a frightening experience. It can involve, to a degree, even the loss of self-image. It can be a very painful experience. It makes a patient dependent on others.

On the nurse's side, the relationship is formed by her response to her patient. Ideally, it will not be formed by any value of the patient's dependency on her but rather by her intolerance of her patient's misfortune and her concern for people and their well-being. This is the attitude that leads most people into a health care career.

At the same time, a nurse must be strong enough not to focus on her own emotions and not to inhibit her actions. She must not allow herself to be burned out by emotions or to resent her patient for being disabled.

Unfortunately, not every relationship between a nurse and her patient is structured in a healthy way. The motivations of each are sometimes deflected from their appropriate course. For example, a patient may handle his loss of agency and self-image—his state of dependence—in a way that the nurse finds challenging and even burdensome. The nurse's response to the patient may be resentment or apathy. The nurse may be motivated by an emotional intolerance, not of the patient's misfortune, but of the patient himself. When this occurs, it gives rise to form the breaking of an agreement. This motivation breaks the agreement the professional nurse originally made with herself when she began her career in health care.

A well-ordered nurse–patient relationship involves implied expectations and obligations accepted and agreed to by each person with a full understanding of the arrangements and directives. In each specific case, the expectations and obligations are somewhat determined by a number of contextual and situational factors. The leading factor is the condition of the patient and the way in which the ethical character-structures of nurse and patient engage and connect in their relationship or fail to engage and connect adequately. The quality of their relationship sets the outline of their interaction.

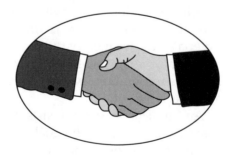

**FIGURE 3.1** The agreement.

## THE ROLE OF BENEVOLENCE

Benevolence is a psychological inclination to do good.

Benevolence is a psychological inclination to do good. Benevolence plays an important role in the nurse–patient relationship.

Anything that raises a person, an agent, or a patient to a state of greater perfection (a condition appropriate to survival and flourishing) is good in relation to this person. Of course, whatever reduces a person, an agent, or a patient to a condition in which the person cannot be his own agent and cannot survive and flourish as desired is bad. Benevolence motivates a nurse to act effectively as the agent of her patient. Her desire to do what is right, to do good, motivates her to guide and assist her patient in achieving a greater perfection. It generates caring and justice. Caring and justice are grounded in benevolence. Caring is benevolence expressed through emotions. Justice is benevolence expressed through reason.

To act with beneficence, a nurse must understand the agreement, her patient, and the patient's unique situations and circumstances; the nurse must also understand the reason she is acting as she is. The understanding between a nurse and her patient depends on this agreement and on what is and what needs to be understood between them regarding their roles and the interactions and actions between them. This is the dynamic basis of a professional, practice-based ethic. If a nurse is to do nothing that will bring about harm, is to do everything possible that will bring about good, and is to act on the basis of beneficence, then she must have an understanding of the agreement, know why she is doing what she is doing, and be capable of acting on the basis of this ethical understanding.

## AGREEMENTS AND COMMUNICATION

The biblical story of the Tower of Babel illustrates both the desirability and the necessity of communication and having an agreement on the success of interactions.

At one time, a universal language existed. A group of Babylonians, discontent with the way God was managing human affairs, decided to build a tower up to heaven, throw Him out, and run things the way they thought they should be run. When God observed this waste of time, He became perturbed, but also being amused, He took pity on them.

To frustrate the intentions of the builders of the Tower of Babel, God changed the language of each, creating a multitude of languages. This made it impossible for them to communicate, agree, and interact with one another. Work on the tower stopped, and eventually the tower collapsed (Gen 11:1–9).

The Bible asks this question: "How can two walk together lest they agree?" (Amos 3:3). If you think about this, you will see that two cannot walk *together* without agreeing that they will.

Builders cannot build a tower and two cannot walk together without communication and agreement between them. Two cannot interact to enhance each other's lives and overcome conflict when it arises without an agreement. The more closely this agreement is woven into the present context, the more effective the resulting interaction can be expected to be.

An unspoken but formal agreement is absolutely necessary between a health care professional and patient. Health care is not an understandable and entrusting activity without this agreement. If an activity is not purposeful and people cannot understand what they are doing and why they are doing it, the activity is ineffective and nonproductive.

*An unspoken but formal agreement is absolutely necessary between a health care professional and patient. Health care is not an understandable and entrusting activity without this agreement.*

## AGREEMENTS AND UNDERSTANDING

The motivating power of a firm agreement is well illustrated in the most famous ethical parable in the Western world: the story of Solomon and two mothers. King Solomon is traditionally thought of as the wisest man who ever lived. He was the king of Israel and served as judge in all disputes between the citizens of Israel.

One night, two women who shared a house each gave birth to a baby. One child died, but the other survived. When the mother with the living child was asleep, the other woman stole the surviving baby and gave the mother her deceased child. Needless to say, a conflict arose between these two women. They were brought before King Solomon so he could make a judgment on the case. After Solomon heard the case, he commanded one of his guards to cut the baby in half so that each woman could be given an equal half of the child. The woman whose child had died shortly after birth agreed to this arrangement quickly, but the living baby's mother instantly asked that the baby be spared and be given to the other woman (1 Kings, 3:16–28). Through this action, Solomon was able to determine who was the living baby's mother and he justly gave the child back to her.

Solomon made his famous decision on the basis of the nature and characteristics of an ethical agreement. Solomon knew that the agreement between a woman and a child who is not her own is typically not as strong as that between a mother and her own child. He knew that the woman who was not the child's mother might, out of envy and spite, agree to the death of the child. On the other hand, the agreement between a woman and a child that is her own will never permit her to agree to the death of her child to satisfy her resentment. Solomon's task was to achieve awareness of the true mother's identity. He was able to do this by discovering the power of the contextual interweavings and interconnections that motivate an agreement.

## THE NECESSITY OF COMMUNICATION AND UNDERSTANDING

### THE SECOND HUMOROUS VIGNETTE: THE COCONUT

One day, two inhabitants of a jungle village passed a coconut tree. As they passed, a coconut fell from the tree to the ground. An argument arose between them as to who had a right to possession of the coconut. Finally, in despair, they decided to do what seemed to be the only fair thing to do: They split the coconut in half. Each islander took one half of the coconut. They shook hands and then went their separate ways.

This appears to be the perfect arrangement. This appears to be the ideal resolution to this dilemma. This appears to be the way ethical decisions ought to be made and the way ethical interaction ought to take place.

In solving their dilemma, they faced a choice between fairness, which is an obvious standard of choice, and a calm and reasoned dialogue that might have led to a better understanding and a more perfect arrangement, given their circumstances. They concentrated their attention and discussion entirely upon the context of the situation and that desirable coconut lying on the ground. However, they communicated nothing to each other about the context of their personal knowledge or awareness of their needs and desires. When they reached their destinations, one villager scooped the fruit out of his coconut and threw it away. He needed a cup, and his only interest in his half was the shell that he could use to hold water. The other villager scooped out the fruit and threw away the shell. His family was hungry, and he only wanted the fruit. If they had communicated more adequately and had come to an agreement based on complete mutual understanding, one villager would have had twice the number of cups and the other twice as much fruit. They had served their own identified ethical principle of fairness completely but had served their own human needs very badly. This is how it is, all too often, in the health care setting as well. The more often actions are based on immediate, unquestioned assumptions, the more often the resulting action fails human welfare. The more time that is devoted to generalized ethical theorizing, the less time there is devoted to valuable human concerns.

Every agreement, to be effective, must be aimed toward a purpose and a final value to be attained through understanding and interaction. The more important this value and the clearer the perception of it, the more powerful the motivational pull it will have toward those working to attain it. Nurses often complain that they do not have enough time to achieve an understanding of their patients. This may be true. Time is rigid and difficult to stretch. But time is not what promotes understanding. Awareness is what provides for understanding. When one knows how and what to look for, awareness can easily be expanded and ultimately achieved.

Decision making based on imagination and distant memories without attention to the present context disrupts the ability to find awareness of the circumstances of the situation and to attain values and promote human wolfaro.

Decision making based on imagination and distant memories without attention to the present context disrupts the ability to find awareness of the circumstances of the situation and to attain values and promote human welfare. The only productive solutions to problems and dilemmas are solutions based on awareness of the present reality and circumstances. If the villagers had lifted their awareness to a higher plane, they would have discovered that understanding what we want is a function of desire. Understanding why we want what we want is a function of reason and a far better way of understanding.

A precondition to understanding a person is:

• Understanding a person's background and history and whether that person accepted or rebelled against these.
• Understanding the person's purposes.
• Understanding the person's agreements and unwillingness to form certain agreements.
• Understanding what the person is communicating.

## THE WAX TABLET EXERCISE

If people cannot understand what they are doing and why they are doing it, an ethically well-ordered health care system is impossible. When understanding another person is important and seems very difficult, there is a technique that may make understanding possible. This technique can be called the wax tablet.

Aristotle believed that the mind at birth possesses no knowledge before experience but is rather like a shaved wax tablet upon which experience will produce all knowledge.

To assist with the understanding of another person, one can use the following wax tablet exercise. Start by isolating yourself, and then try to make your mind as close to a wax tablet as possible. Now, take an imaginary razor and shave away everything that makes you who you are. Shave away any ideas you have picked up from your culture, any religious attitudes, and any attitudes that you hold because of your gender. Shave away your family circle—everything and anything that is familiar to you. Now, adopt your patient's cultural background, religion, gender, health condition, family background, and whatever peculiarities you have noted about him or her. Then ask yourself, as the patient, "What is my attitude and motivation in my present circumstance?" Almost invariably you will understand the patient.

## THE ROLE OF PURPOSE

Everyone struggles at times to understand other people. This usually happens when they have come together with others with whom they share no purpose or with whom they no longer share a purpose, or if it may happen if they, themselves, have no purpose. People without a common purpose cannot understand one another, and people without a purpose cannot understand themselves. People need a purpose.

People who have not come together for years enjoy reminding one another about purposes of the past. Through each other they reexperience times when they were most understandable to themselves. People who form an agreement to work together on a purpose almost immediately understand one another better than people trying to "figure each other out" while they carry on a conversation. The implications of how and why people form an agreement—in addition to what the agreements and purposes mean to them and the strength and weakness of their motivating ideas— reveal who they are while they are not thinking about it and trying to disguise their true selves.

## THE FALLACY OF ASSUMPTIONS

It is a mistake to use assumptions in ethical decision making, because there is no place for speculating and guessing. The resolution of an ethical dilemma cannot be justified by the fact that the decision maker assumes, with no adequate reason to believe, that it will produce the most desirable short- or long-term consequences and values. If it can be justified by an assumption that it will produce the most desirable outcome, then it can just as easily be defeated by an assumption that it will not. One assumption is as good as another. An assumption is a conclusion that is not based on the examination of considerations. Nothing can be justified by an assumption. An assumption cannot guide analysis, and it is a grave error if one does so in ethical decision making.

## PROBABILITY AND ETHICAL DECISION MAKING

That said, there are times when the nurse may not have a lot of information but still must take action.

To act purposefully and ethically when acting on behalf of a patient, a nurse must always act according to the evidence she has of the patient's values. That said, there are times when the nurse may not have a lot of information but still must take action.

Suppose a nurse, Sylvia, is stranded on a deserted island. A comatose stranger washes ashore. He has a hemorrhaging wound to the head and neck. Sylvia has no way of learning the name of the stranger, let alone his specific desires, purposes, or values. Even so, it is still possible for Sylvia to act according to a proper ethical standard. In this situation, she can use the element of purpose to arrive at justifiable decisions and actions.

Every nurse in a situation of this type can determine with little difficulty what most people would desire in this circumstance and what their purpose would be if they could act for themselves. Sylvia can see that the stranger is a human. This tells her all that she needs to know. It is perfectly reasonable for Sylvia to form her conclusion according to the purposes that most humans would hold. Whatever purposes the maximum number of persons would hold in this circumstance, this stranger would probably hold. When probability and reason are all you have, then you must act on the basis of what you have. There is no other ethically justifiable way of arriving at a decision. If a health care professional has virtually no evidence to go on, what little evidence is available must be relied on. This is how decisions should be made for those who cannot participate and for whom a nurse has no prior knowledge of what they would want.

> When probability and reason are all you have, then you must act on the basis of what you have. There is no other ethically justifiable way of arriving at a decision.

Suppose that the stranger were conscious. Sylvia can see that he is bleeding from the cut on his head and neck. Under these circumstances, Sylvia would probably act automatically, without stopping to ask permission. However, Sylvia might ask the injured person if he wants her to stop the bleeding. The odds are overwhelming that the stranger would reply that he did. Then she would know exactly what the context requires. Sylvia does not have all this evidence. She does, however, have all the evidence that she needs. She has enough evidence on which to make a reasoned judgment. In a circumstance of this type, the fact that it is reasoned is sufficient to justify the judgment.

In an emergency, a health care professional will almost automatically act for the purpose of saving lives. The justification for this is that the maximum number of people in the maximum number of circumstances would want their lives to be saved. Sylvia is justified by the fact that any individual person in the emergency would almost certainly want to be saved. That she will act according to her best judgment forms part of a nurse's implicit agreement with her patient. It forms part of her relationship to the rest of the world. It is a fundamental part of her role.

> In an emergency, a health care professional will almost automatically act for the purpose of saving lives. The justification for this is that the maximum number of people in the maximum number of circumstances would want their lives to be saved.

Suppose that the stranger for whom Sylvia acted were to claim that the decision she made was the wrong decision. Suppose he believes that a woman touching his head defiles him, and he declares that he would have preferred bleeding to death over being defiled. Sylvia still made the right ethical decision, because she made her decision on the basis of all the evidence available to her. She made the decision by reasoning from evidence that was available to her at the time of her action. If the stranger attempts to justify his claim that she acted wrongly against him, his claim has no merit.

If she did not make her decision according to her recognition of the evidence, then she would have acted without thinking. Her action was based on thinking, which made it predictable. Thinking limits the number of actions that could possibly be taken. If a person acts without thinking, then the ensuing action will be unpredictable. If Sylvia ought to have acted without thinking, she might have done anything at all.

A nurse can justify her ethical decisions and actions through the element of purpose. Purpose is a principle and a standard of all bioethical decision making; it is also the motivation. Every person is unique, but every person is a person and, as such, is ethically equal to every other person. Sometimes, a decision must be made on the basis of a person's sameness. All human beings have purpose. This, in itself, when necessary, justifies ethical action.

*Sometimes, a decision must be made on the basis of a person's sameness.*

The recognition of a patient's autonomy and the motivation of a nurse's beneficence do not necessarily lead to one exclusive and justifiable decision. This is because no rule, principle, or standard should by itself inspire a feeling of perfect confidence in any decision. One can be "certain" of the perfection of one's decision only if one ignores the context and makes a formalistic decision irrelevant to the situation. Whenever one makes a relevant judgment, not having absolute knowledge, one may make an imperfect decision. There is no context in which one has absolute knowledge. This is not a reason to ignore the context. It is a reason to develop the ability to function within a context, to content oneself with achieving what is objectively possible and desirable, and to ignore an ethical "perfection" that can be achieved only by going outside of the agreement and discarding professional relevance.

It is not the perfection of a decision but the reasoning that motivated it that justifies a decision. When both the reasoning for and the reasoning against a decision are equally valid, either decision is justifiable. However, the reason must not be tainted or corrupted by personal assumptions. No argument should be offered unless there is a distinct possibility that it is an argument that the patient might make.

## THE AGREEMENT ONE HAS WITH ONESELF

All interactions between a nurse and a patient need to begin with voluntary consent that is objectively gained. Voluntary consent, objectively and freely obtained from another person, can be established only by agreement. Interaction according to agreement and interaction according to coercion are not two different ways to reach the same objective. The course and every step in each of these directions are different. They are also two very diverse perspectives on human relationships and interaction. They are so different that they even change the character of the objectives. One is a value that agents achieve through reciprocity and mutual exchange. The other is a value that agents achieve through force and coercion. There are two bases for interaction: One holds the beneficiary of action, the patient, as an end in himself. The other holds the (apparent) beneficiary as a means to the ends of the nurse. The expectations established by an agreement and how they are pursued, whether through reciprocity or coercion, establish the nature of the context and the meaning of every motivation and every action.

This most basic link between people dictates that the first step of interaction shall be an agreement "not to gain action . . . except through voluntary consent, objectively gained," which is reciprocity.

This most basic link between people dictates that the first step of interaction shall be an agreement "not to gain action . . . except through voluntary consent, objectively gained," which is reciprocity. For effective nursing interventions and ethical interactions to take place between a nurse and patient, each must be open to the other. The best way for this to be achieved and sustained is through the establishment of mutually produced logical and understandable connecting sequences of interaction and action. The nurse–patient agreement is a schedule and plan for these sequences.

An objective agreement is any agreement in which both parties to the agreement are aware of the:

- Reason for the agreement.
- Terms of the agreement.
- Intentions of the other party to the agreement.

A nonobjective agreement is any agreement in which one or both parties lack awareness of these aspects of the agreement. A nonobjective agreement is a splintered, ineffective agreement. If it is a professional agreement, it will, predictably, fail the needs of the professional and the patient and the responsibilities of the profession.

Every nurse ought to examine her life, at least to the point where she comes to an agreement with herself that she will be a nurse.

Every nurse ought to examine her life, at least to the point where she comes to an agreement with herself that she will be a nurse. To the extent that a nurse has not made this agreement and a commitment to be a nurse, she resembles a patient more than what she would be if a nurse.

> A nurse who directs her long-term actions guided by her awareness of what is needed in order for her to keep that agreement embraces her profession. A nurse who is inspired by it [her professional agreement], and who is dedicated to it, is far less likely to experience burn-out.
>
> A nurse [who] tries to avoid taking those long-term actions that constitute her professional life breaks the agreement she made with herself to be a professional. She becomes indifferent. She undermines herself as a professional and as a person. If she has replaced her confidence and pride with indifference, she has done this because she abandoned herself when she abandoned her profession.
>
> If one is a nurse and is likely to continue to be a nurse, one ought to take the actions called for by the health care professions. At worst, this will make life far less boring. At best, it may restore one to the confident expectations and the pride that she began with at the beginning of her career.
>
> *Dedication to what one professes—acting on that which one affirms and believes—is sometimes difficult to do. Adversities and frustrations arise. And these attack one's desire and one's sense of self.* (Husted & Husted, 1999, p. 17)

To be a professional nurse means to face many challenges. Overcoming adversity and frustrations through dedication produces pride in oneself as a professional. A patient could not reasonably ask for more from his nurse—and should not find less.

## RATIONAL SELF-INTEREST

Few bioethics texts make the human values of those engaged in health care interaction the central focus of their concern. All give some attention to the values and well-being of patients. None hold the health care professional as a beneficiary of bioethical interaction. "Respect for the dignity of others is a familiar professional prescription and has a robust theoretical basis. Respect for one's own dignity is given less attention" (Gallagher, 2004, p. 587). This would be the focus of a rational self-interest ethic.

> It would be hard to argue that a nurse does not benefit from being a nurse. There are many wonderful benefits to being a professional nurse.

It would be hard to argue that a nurse does not benefit from being a nurse. There are many wonderful benefits to being a professional nurse. A rational self-interest ethic is practiced by an ethical agent, a professional nurse, with a view to enhance her life through interaction based on objective agreements and a trade of values from which the nurse benefits by achieving her personal desires. An agent's rational self-interest is defined in terms of her understanding of her individual character and nature against the background of what is needed for her personal development. It also requires a complete acceptance of the nature, motivations, and the self-interest of the nurse's "trading partners." Irrational self-interest is a contradiction in terms. Whatever is irrational cannot be to one's self-interest. Whatever decisions and actions truly serve one's self-interest cannot be irrational. Rational self-interest must begin in reason. The rationality of a nurse's choice of professions can be measured by the degree of satisfaction and fulfillment found in it.

> Irrational self-interest is a contradiction in terms. Whatever is irrational cannot be to one's self-interest.

A patient's rational self-interest is defined in terms of his understanding of his individual character and nature against the background of what is needed for his personal development. It also requires a complete acceptance of the nature and needs of his survival, healing, and flourishing. The reason for a rational self-interest ethic begins in its rejection of self-abandonment as the only possible approach to a profession. It equally rejects evasion, deception, and coercion as the basis of interaction. Rational interaction is conducted on the basis of objective understanding, self-respect, agreement, and fidelity. It cannot be conducted on the basis of unexamined emotions, self-doubt, or the desire to evade responsibility.

The functioning of a rational self-interest ethics is well formulated by William Shakespeare in these famous words:

> *This above all: to thine own self be true,*
> *And it must follow, as the night the day,*
> *Thou canst not then be false to any man.* (Hamlet, Act I, Scene I)

Shakespeare is correct and revealing in this quote. To be true to oneself, one must know oneself and respect oneself.

A nurse's rational self-interest is achieved through the competence of her professional activity. It is expressed by satisfaction in the practice of her profession, by confidence in her competence to act, in the pride she takes in herself and her professional activities, in her feelings of contentment, and, above all, in her pride in her ethical habits. All of this grows out of her professional actions and her assurance that these actions are appropriate to her profession. It arises from her skill at the practice that she does in the spirit of her profession. Every nurse begins her career with the decision that she will be a nurse. When she reaches this decision, she assumes that, in some way, her self-interest will be achieved through nursing.

A nurse's first ethical task is not to abandon who she is to become a cheerful nobody. The proper term for such activity would be *irrational self-disinterest*. This type of activity benefits no one. It benefits neither the nurse nor the patient. The idea that either an ethic must endorse self-abandonment and beneficence or self-interest and maleficence is wrong. The rational self-interest ethic described by Benedict Spinoza is a third alternative. It is the only alternative of the three that will produce an enduring beneficence. Self-abandonment will ultimately produce resentment toward patients. An irrational self-interest will produce a brutal unconcern for the welfare of others. A rational self-interest ethic will reveal itself in a commitment to the patient, sincere concern, benevolence, and pride.

> *The more each man seeks his own profit and endeavors to preserve himself, the more power does he possess to live according to the guidance of reason. But men most agree in nature when they live according to the guidance of reason. Therefore, men will be most profitable to one another when each man seeks most what is profitable to himself.*
> (Spinoza, Pt. 4, Prop. 35, Coro. 2)

A nurse's true self-interest is not served and, in fact, is lost the day she decides that her self-interest conflicts with that of her patients. A patient needs a rational agent to do for him what he would do for himself, simply because what he would do for himself needs to be rational. A patient needs a self-interested nurse (a nurse whose self-interest is fulfilled through nursing) because what he would do for himself needs to be self-interested.

## MUSINGS

Ethical realities are common experiences for all persons. They are not something accepted by mere convention, nor are they something brought into being by legislation. Everyone has desires and purposes. Everyone must act to achieve those desires and purposes.

## DILEMMA 3.2: THE DEMANDS OF AN AGREEMENT

You are taking care of a 5-year-old child, Jeffrey, who has a seizure disorder of unknown origin. He asks you to stay with him until his parents return from work. You know that this will be about 2 hours beyond your shift for which you will not get paid, but you agree to stay with him because he is so frightened. As you are giving report, your friends arrive from various floors to tell you that they have an early birthday surprise for you. They have purchased tickets to a concert that you desperately want to see. What should you do? How did you arrive at your decision?

Everyone faces the need to think before taking actions. There is an alternative to the need to think, but it is most undesirable. The alternative is that someone will suffer. These factors cannot exist without bringing the need for ethical thought—for "practical reason"—into existence.

That purpose and value are ethical phenomena pertaining to all people, that all people possess rights, and that all people possess ethical agency are not matters on which one decides. They are ethical realities already there for one to discover. Ethical realities are human realities, not because people have the power to choose them, but because they are part of human nature and part of the human situation. The supreme interpersonal reality is the network of agreements that makes human interaction possible.

> *For a nurse, as a professional, far and away the most important agreement—the agreement that must precede any agreement she can have with her patient—is the agreement she has made with herself. A nurse who practices her profession without dedicating herself to it, practices her profession without dedicating herself to herself.* (Husted & Husted, 1999, pp. 16–17)

The nurse–patient agreement is the court of last resort for justifying professional decisions. The more effectively a nurse meets the ethical agreement, the more effective she is as an ethical agent and as a professional. On the other hand, it is possible for the nurse to fulfill the agreement so ineffectively that she will hardly be a professional or an ethical agent at all.

The evolution and traditions of health care have produced certain definite expectations. These expectations form a bridge joining together the professional and the patient. When a patient enters the health care system, these expectations create an implicit agreement between the professional and the patient. The terms of the agreement are precisely the expectations defining the health care professions and the health care professional's commitment to her profession.

The appropriateness of the terms of their agreement depends on their human nature. More narrowly, it depends on the purpose of their interaction. Through necessity, nurses and patients interact under the terms of this agreement. Either the terms of their agreement guide their interaction or their behaviors are unintelligible. The agreement becomes a process in which two conscious beings create a resolution between them that then becomes their strategy for action. The agreement is foundational.

Agreement is shown in interaction. When the agreement is objective and sound, the nurse and patient benefit. When it is not, one or both suffer through it. When an agreement causes suffering, it is a flawed agreement. When it brings objective benefit, it is a sound agreement. An agreement can be analyzed by reference to the bioethical standards. The bioethical standards are in conflict with the forming of an irrational agreement.

If the desire behind an agreement is a rational, objective, noncoercive, and non-self-destructive desire, then the agreement, given the context, is the final "court of appeal" concerning interpersonal actions. The purposes of the patient and the nurse, as a nurse, are codified in the agreement. The ethical status of any decision, choice, or action is a function of the relationship of that decision, choice, or action to these purposes. The agreement, then, is the beginning of a nurse's ethical journey—and its principle. All ethical understanding, immediate and contextual, arises in the context of this agreement.

## STUDY GUIDE

1. Think about agreements that exist in physical things that enable you to function in your everyday life, such as wheels on a car, pen to paper, and a needle to skin. Some of these are not agreements involving people, but they are agreements nonetheless. Now try to think about things in your nursing world that agree and enable you to function.

2. Think about how you function as a nurse or as a student nurse (or any health care professional) within the context of an agreement. Does this agreement obligate you to perform in a certain way? If so, what are some of these ways?

3. What if there were no agreements? Would the health care environment take on a different function? What would happen?

4. What does it mean to have an agreement with yourself?

5. How does rational self-interest benefit you and your patient? You might want to go back to Chapter 2 and revisit the Jane and Nancy scenario where Nancy is drowning and apply rational self-interest to it.

6. What is learned from the humorous coconut scenario that can be applied to your practice?

7. Use this case for class discussion; the analysis of the case only appears in the instructor's manual. Note that the resolution rests within the realm of agreements and does not require the use of the bioethical standards.

## BENEVOLENT LIE VERSUS THE TRUTH

Hugh is dying. Lucy, his nurse, believes that his death is imminent. She remembers that Denise, his wife, had expressed a desire to be with her husband when he dies. Hugh and Denise had agreed to be with each other at the end so that the person who died first would not die alone. Lucy calls Denise to tell her of her husband's condition. It is a rather long time before Denise arrives at the hospital. Denise is blind and must find someone willing to drive her to the hospital. By the time she arrives, Hugh has died. Before Lucy takes her into her husband's room, Denise expresses how glad she is to have arrived before his death. She spends several minutes in the room with her husband. She does not know that he was already dead when she arrived. If Lucy tells Denise that her husband died before she arrived, she honors the *conventional* standard of objectivity (absolute truth-telling) but fails the test of beneficence. If Lucy tells her that she was with her husband while he was still alive, Lucy violates the standard of conventional objectivity but meets the test of beneficence and that of contextual objectivity. This poses a dilemma.

# REFERENCES

Colter, M., Ganzimi, L., & Cohen, L. M. (2000). Resolution and ambivalence/commentaries. *The Hasting Center Report, 30*(6), 24–25. Retrieved July 4, 2006, from ProQuest database.

Dinc, L,. & Gastmans, C. (2013). Trust in nurse-patient relationships: A literature review. *Nursing Ethics, 20*(5), 501-516.

Gallagher, A. (2004). Dignity and respect for dignity—two key health professional values: Implications for nursing practice. *Nursing Ethics, 11,* 587–599.

Houck, N. M., & Bongiorno, A. W. (2006, Fall/Winter). Innovations in the public policy education of nursing students. *Journal of the New York State Nurses Association,* pp. 4–9.

Husted, J. H., & Husted, G. L. (1999). Agreement: The origin of ethical action. *Critical Care Nursing, 22*(3), 12–18.

International Council of Nurses. (2012). The ICN code of ethics for nurses, copyright 2012 by International Council of Nurses.

Lind, R., Nortvedt, P., Lorem, G., & Hevroy, O. (2012). Family involvement in the end-of-life decisions of competent intensive care patients. *Nursing Ethics, 20*(1) 61–71.

Shakespeare, W. (1599). Hamlet, Act I, Scene, I.

Spinoza, B. (1675). *Ethics.* (Original work published 1675).

# FOUR

# THE BIOETHICAL STANDARDS AND THEIR ROLE AS PRECONDITIONS OF THE AGREEMENT

## OBJECTIVES

- Examine the nature of the bioethical standards.
- Discuss how each standard serves as a precondition to the agreement.
- Summarize how the aspects of fidelity relate to the nurse.
- Examine the classic virtues as related to the nurse–patient agreement.
- Examine the relationship of reciprocity to rational self-interest.

"There are certain individualized characteristics that every patient brings into the health care setting and retains by right. Any human characteristic—any virtue—that is necessary to his successful interaction, first as a human and then as a patient, is a resource that cannot, in any way, be justifiably violated" (Husted, Husted, & Scotto, 2013, p. 534). This is the nature of the bioethical standards. They are the principles that generate and construct the nurse–patient agreement. Traditionally, these standards are:

- Autonomy
- Freedom
- Objectivity
- Beneficence
- Fidelity

The health care system has developed in response to human needs and desires: the need and desire for life, health, and well-being; the human need to escape suffering; and the need to regain agency when agency has been impaired or lost. These desires and needs, and the purposes they inspire, are the source of the roles of everyone in the health care system. They determine the nature of the role filled by nurses, and they are the basis for the patient's seeking to recover the physical and emotional stability he had before the circumstances that brought him into the health care setting.

In the health care setting, the nurse and the patient know that the patient is there to regain his power of agency to take purposeful actions. A person's power of agency is his power or capacity to initiate and carry out actions directed toward goals. It includes his awareness of control over himself, his actions, and his circumstances. A patient comes into the health care setting to overcome a physical or psychological disability. He is there to regain his power to act, but no patient regards agency as his final purpose. His final purpose is the goals toward which he directs purposeful action. Agency enables an agent to realize purposes beyond the agency itself. For the health care system, agency is a goal in itself, but a patient is in the health care setting so that he will be able to return to the football field, the concert stage, or the factory floor. He is there in order to return to his family and to his life. If the nurse understands this agency from the patient's perspective, then the attitude they have toward each other is that of friends with a common purpose, that of making progress together.

> A person's power of agency is his power or capacity to initiate and carry out actions directed toward goals.

## THE BIOETHICAL STANDARDS AS VIRTUES AND RIGHTS

Previously we examined the nature of human rights and discarded the idea that human rights are a laundry list of things all humans should be granted. Rather, we found human rights to be an agreement between civilized humans to refrain from interfering in the life of another without permission. In examining the agreement that exists between the health care provider and the patient, we see that the agreement between a nurse and a patient not only makes it possible for each to function but also requires that each applies ethical reasoning to his or her actions. In this same way we will examine the bioethical standards to discover their individual essences.

> We found human rights to be an agreement between civilized humans to refrain from interfering in the life of another without permission.

## AUTONOMY

### Autonomy as Independent Uniqueness

Every ethical agent, every person, is autonomous. An autonomous agent is one with the right and the power to take actions and pursue goals according to personal desire and without obtaining prior permission.

Every autonomous agent has the right to enter into agreements or to refuse to enter into agreements unless it would violate an agreement already made.

One cannot make an agreement without being an autonomous agent. Every autonomous agent has the right to enter into agreements or to refuse to enter into agreements unless it would violate an agreement already made.

By nature, every human is autonomous. Everyone is, at least potentially, independent, self-directed, and unique. Every individual has a right to independence, self-direction, and uniqueness. Although this is a fundamental belief held by many, there are those who would deny or oppose it for reasons of their own. History is full of stories about people who deny the rights of others. Therefore, it is reasonable to redefine the term *autonomy* so that it signifies a visible and undeniable aspect of human character. In this way, we say that each unique independent and self-directed individual's differences serve as the basis on which autonomy is identified. The term *autonomy* signifies individual uniqueness. It is an integral, defining aspect of what a human person is, rather than a right we confer upon a person or allow a person to have. This makes it more useful analytically without losing its connotations of independence and self-directedness.

Although this is a fundamental belief held by many, there are those who would deny or oppose it for reasons of their own. History is full of stories about people who deny the rights of others

An ethical agent, a person, directs his efforts in ways determined by his unique individual nature. He is independently capable of expressing his character in unique actions, directed in highly personal directions. Autonomy, as a bioethical standard, refers to the uniqueness of an individual person. This uniqueness is the specific nature—the interwoven character structures—of that person.

Autonomy, as a bioethical standard, refers to the uniqueness of an individual person. This uniqueness is the specific nature—the interwoven character structures—of that person.

## Autonomy as Ethical Equality

Being a rational creature is the fundamental nature of every human person. We are all part of the same species—reasoning beings. It is our nature as living beings to be capable of thinking things over and moving about from place to place. This defines us. The needs of our human nature motivate us to the pursuit of life-sustaining goals. Our rationality assists and directs us to the pursuit of life-serving and fulfilling goals. Our autonomy, that is, our uniqueness, determines that for every individual these goals will be different. Our ability to reason, to choose, and to decide makes us free but responsible. This is how our uniqueness develops.

In ethical dignity, no ethical agent is identical to or superior to others of the same species.

Our ethical nature arises from our identity as members of the species. In ethical dignity, no ethical agent is identical to or superior to others of the same species. No ethical agent is identical or superior in ethical dignity to others of the same species. Every human being has an individual right to act on his or her unique and independent purposes and desires. No human being is more or less independent than another. No one has a right to override the purposes and desires of others. No one human being, nor any collection of human beings, has a right to alienate the self-directedness of another. This is so vital to bioethics that we will subject it to a rigorous analysis—an analysis conducted via introspection.

Reflect on your self-experience, and this is what you will find: You, as a human individual, are an organism who moves about from place to place under your own power. You guide your movements through thought—the ability to relate yourself to reality through the power of reason—and the inescapable need to choose and decide.

The choices you must make are, in many cases, the choices every human individual must make—to eat, to stay warm, to make survival choices. However, you make other choices that are based on meanings and reasons known only to you. Therefore, many choices you make are highly individualized—choices you make according to your purposes and the meanings you find in your lived world.

The rational human nature of an individual endows every person from birth with a striking potential. This potential is a matchless capacity for growth and development. This fact is the biological foundation of ethics. Only a living being with the power of reason can concern itself with vital and fundamental choices and decisions, a vital decision being one essentially related to the preservation or enhancement of life and a fundamental decision being one that arises as a result of an individual's own purposes.

Throughout the whole species of humankind, each person is different. Our differences begin to emerge when our development begins. This continues through the accumulation of our experiences and the mental and physical actions we take in relation to these experiences. Through the flourishing of our potential for development, we become who our nature and choices allow us to become. For each of us, who we become is unique. Throughout our lifetime, this uniqueness becomes more and more a part of us, and as we mature and become more active, we become more and more unique and complex. This is the experience and history of every human individual. Every person begins life as an individual different from all others, as each leaf in the forest is different from all others. Uniqueness increases throughout maturation and development.

The fact that each member of our species undergoes growth and development establishes three facts. These facts are vital to bioethical understanding.

1. You and every other person have a right to growth, development, and the pursuit of a destiny. Given your nature and the nature of all the people around you, it is an absurdity to believe that someone else has a right to determine your development or destiny or that you have a right to determine the development or destiny of another (Husted & Husted, 1997). When the cavemen formed the rights agreement many thousands of years ago, they made no special arrangements that anyone would be superior or inferior to another.
2. No two individuals will develop identically. You will be different from everyone else in the world. You and every other person will develop in your own time and circumstances according to your own experiences, decisions, and actions.

3. There is no rational, ethical basis for any person to refuse to accept the fact that another is unique in particular (nonaggressive) ways. There is no justification for you to refuse to accept the unique character structure of another—a patient most especially.

*In the right to be unique and to act from that uniqueness, every individual is the absolute ethical equal of every other.*

In the right to be unique and to act from that uniqueness, every individual is the absolute ethical equal of every other.

## THE RIGHT TO AUTONOMY

For these reasons, we define *autonomy* as independent uniqueness. An individual's right to autonomy is his or her right to be the unique rational being he or she is. This obviously includes the right to take independent and self-directed actions. Every bioethical standard is derived from the standard of autonomy. Autonomy is the ultimate standard of the rightness or wrongness of a nurse's ethical decisions. If a nurse is to be able to justify her decisions and actions, she must take account of the autonomy of her patient because she is the agent of her patient doing for her patient what he would do for himself if he were able. (Autonomy acts as the umbrella under which all of the standards fall. For example, how one views and uses his freedom is the result of who he is, his autonomy.)

*Every bioethical standard is derived from the standard of autonomy.*

The right to autonomy does not depend on the acceptance or permission of others. The right to be a unique person is nothing more than the right to be who one is. For any individual person, the right to be who one is means the right to exist. Quite often, a person's right to self-determination and independence, which is an implicit part of his right to be who he is, can be rationalized away by others. But his right to exist and to be who he is, ethically, in the nature of things is absolute and cannot be set aside. Ultimately, his right to self-determination and independence arises from his right to be who he is. His right to act as who he is is an aspect of his right to be who he is.

*For any individual person, the right to be who one is means the right to exist.*

## AUTONOMY AS A PRECONDITION OF AGREEMENT

The reason individuals make agreements and the terms of those agreements arise from who they are. The fact that people have different needs and values logically motivates their interactions. If they did not, they would have no reason to interact. Autonomy—the uniqueness of every person—is a precondition of the health care professional–patient agreement. That each individual is unique and independent is, in itself, an agreement that is implied and structures every other agreement.

For either professional or patient to violate the autonomy of the other is to act as if no agreement exists between them. This is, implicitly, to deny a necessary precondition of the existence of an agreement. If no agreement exists, then no stable and understandable relationship can exist between them. Their differences do not, as often is assumed, produce a basis for fear and distrust between them. Their differences extend into their goals and values and make trade desirable. The differences among people are the only reason they can be of benefit to one another.

Recognition of the right to autonomy involves a willingness not to interfere with another person's actions toward his or her goals. It involves recognition of the fact that a patient's purposes cannot be abridged on the grounds that the patient or his purposes are different from some personal or societal norm. A nurse has no right to attempt to frustrate a patient's purposes, no matter how much they differ from or clash with her own, nor does any health care professional have a right to enforce or to interfere with an obligation that a patient has chosen for himself.

## DILEMMA 4.1: COMPULSORY OBLIGATION TO OTHERS

Mabel has been diagnosed with cancer of the liver. She is 3 months pregnant with her first child. She and her husband, Mark, have been trying for a long time to have a child. Mabel's physician tells them that to treat her effectively, he will need to use radiation and chemotherapy. This will cause severe defects in the child or, more likely, an abortion. The physician recommends that treatment begin before the baby's due date. He suggests aborting the fetus and starting immediately. In his opinion, to wait until delivery would be detrimental, perhaps fatal to Mabel. But Mabel wants to wait until the child is delivered. How can her nurse, Sharen, best help Mabel?

A patient does not make a choice or decision in a vacuum. However, it is the health care professional's responsibility to remove as much coercion and undue influence as possible.

The notion of a compulsory obligation that a patient has to herself is ethically incomprehensible. Health care professionals should not compel anyone to do anything. A patient's autonomy is recognized through the recognition of his right to decide for himself. A patient does not make a choice or decision in a vacuum. However, it is the health care professional's responsibility to remove as much coercion and undue influence as possible. With Mabel's life at stake, indirection is not undue influence.

## FREEDOM

Freedom as a bioethical standard is self-directedness—an agent's capacity and consequent right to take actions based on the agent's own values and motivations. It is the power and right of an agent to control his time and effort.

Freedom as a bioethical standard is self-directedness—an agent's capacity and consequent right to take actions based on the agent's own values and motivations. It is the power and right of an agent to control his time and effort.

The standard of freedom involves single events as well as short or extended sequences of events, including those sequences that extend over a lifetime. One can possess freedom without making an agreement, but one cannot make an agreement without possessing freedom. Freedom is exercised in action. One can contemplate choices, consider possible alternatives, and imagine the outcomes. Freedom is evident when one takes action in pursuit of a goal.

Susan is walking down the street considering her future plans. Suddenly she is confronted by college posters on the one side and Air Force posters on the other. She stops to contemplate them. So far, Susan is passive. The posters are, so to speak, coming out and influencing Susan. Susan is taking no external action in relation to them. In the context of this experience, she remains passive.

Susan exercises her capacity for freedom and decides to enroll in college. She enters the admission's office and talks with a secretary there. She decides to fill out an application for admission. In these experiences, Susan is active. She has become an agent taking action toward a goal. This decision was an exercise of her freedom, not involving any agreement with any other person. It was a decision involving only an agreement with herself. Susan had the power and right to exercise agency or to refrain from engaging in action. Without the power and right to make a voluntary choice, there can be no agreement with herself or anyone else. Without agreement, there can be no ethical interaction. Freedom is presumed in any decision involving action taken toward goals.

## DILEMMA 4.2: FAMILY'S DESIRES OR PATIENT'S WISHES

Edgar has been in the hospital for almost 12 weeks. His prognosis is very poor, but the family remains insistent on the patient's remaining a full code, despite the physician's opinions on the poor prognosis and his present and future quality of life. Edgar has multiple medical problems, including metastatic cancer. He has been heard to say on a number of occasions, "I do not want to live." He now is semicomatose and cannot make his wants known. The family remains unrealistically optimistic.

When one person refuses to respect the rights of another, a meeting of the minds between them is impossible. The conflict between them leaves no room for an agreement. In the absence of an agreement, there is no basis between them for trust and ethically guided interaction.

## THE INTERWEAVING OF AUTONOMY AND FREEDOM

An agent possesses freedom in two senses:

1. In a biological sense, every agent possesses freedom in that he has the potential for taking independent actions determining the future course of his life.

2. In an ethical sense, every agent possesses freedom because there is nothing in human nature to justify one agent's right to interfere with the independent action of another. Whatever rights an individual possesses, he possesses by virtue of his human nature.

Every ethical agent possesses human nature. Therefore, every ethical agent possesses identical human rights. That one human is more human than another and therefore possesses "superior" rights is an absurdity. All ethical agents possess freedom equal to that of all other ethical agents and nothing more. An agent's existential freedom is enormously increased by her possession of rights, but it is limited by the fact that others also possess rights. Ethically, no agent has a right to violate the rights of others. In assuming rights for herself, she assumes that others also possess rights (Gewirth, 1978).

> All ethical agents possess freedom equal to that of all other ethical agents and nothing more.

Autonomy accrues to a patient by virtue of the fact that he has the power to pursue goals peculiar to his own unique desires. Freedom accrues to a patient by virtue of the fact that reasoning agents can and must plan and take actions directed toward future goals.

> One implication of freedom is the doctrine that nothing should be done to a patient without the patient's consent. It is a direct implication of the standard of autonomy.

One implication of freedom is the doctrine that nothing should be done to a patient without the patient's consent. It is a direct implication of the standard of autonomy. Autonomy permits a patient to be who he is. Freedom permits him to act for that which he perceives as his own benefit—to act on who he is. Under the standard of freedom, one may not interfere with a patient's purposes. One may not compel a patient to act or submit to the actions of others against his will.

Freedom is established by the very same line of reasoning as autonomy. To violate the standard of freedom is to violate the nature of an agent. It is particularly incongruous in a biomedical setting. The whole purpose of a biomedical setting is to enable a patient to regain agency, not to assist him in losing it. To work for a patient's agency while simultaneously violating it reveals a contradiction in one's actions. There is no such thing as an ethically justifiable contradiction. The agreement does not call for a patient to deliver whatever power of agency he possesses to a health care professional. A person's right to freedom is his right to the discretion of his will.

> A person's right to freedom is his right to the discretion of his will.

That an agent is autonomous—that he possesses desires, values, and purposes peculiar to himself—is the sole reason he requires a right to freedom. It is the reason why rational agents implicitly agree to respect these rights. At the same time, that an agent has a right to freedom means that he has a right to autonomy. Freedom is the ability to take unique and independent actions.

One can develop one's autonomy only if one enjoys the freedom provided by rights. Rights allow one to plan in terms of a lifetime. Rights allow one to relate oneself to reality abstractly, objectively, and proactively. One can enjoy the advantages of freedom if agents exercise goodwill. Rights turns aggression and coercion inside out and produces a demand for voluntary consent, objectively gained.

## FREEDOM AS A PRECONDITION OF AGREEMENT

Whenever two people reach an agreement, each implicitly assumes that the other possesses freedom—the power and the right to act toward individual goals, guided by his or her own awareness. This is a necessary precondition and a principle of the agreement. If a nurse remembers the necessary preconditions of an agreement, she has a powerful ethical resource. For, in the very nature of health care, every nurse has an agreement with every patient. Freedom is one of the necessary preconditions and principles of the nurse–patient agreement, as it is of every agreement.

A nurse should never forget that a patient has the right to free decision, choice, and action. To forget this is to forget that there is a nurse–patient agreement. If there were no nurse–patient agreement, there would be no nurse–patient relationship. If there were no nurse–patient relationship, the nurse would have no right to take any action in regard to the patient.

> If there were no nurse–patient agreement, there would be no nurse–patient relationship. If there were no nurse–patient relationship, the nurse would have no right to take any action in regard to the patient.

Freedom, as a standard, is a nurse's obligation to protect her patient from coerced action or undesired interaction. The whole world does not have a right to determine a patient's actions, nor does an individual. This is also implied by a patient's right to freedom. No one has a right to violate a patient's rights. Nor does any health care professional have a right to violate a third person's rights for the benefit of a patient.

A patient's right to freedom is one right that a nurse ought to be especially careful to protect. A violation of this right involves the unsupportable implication that the patient has no human rights. The worth and dignity of a health care professional rests in the fact that she deals with those who possess rights and human dignity. Freedom is the virtue that makes a patient's most basic actions possible. It is the source of those actions that a patient can carry to a successful conclusion. Therefore, it is the first action that a nurse ought to reinforce.

Demeaning the status of the patient involves demeaning the status of the health care professional herself. Protecting the freedom of a patient is precisely a recognition of his worth and human dignity. Protecting the worth and dignity of the patient is a professional's tribute to her own worth and dignity. "Personal control and autonomy are powerful components in terms of life satisfaction, survival, and how one defines one's role" (Rice, Beck, & Stevenson, 1997, p. 32). There can be no justification for denying this to a patient.

### DILEMMA 4.3: THE DEMANDS OF PROMISE KEEPING

A patient exercises his freedom by bringing himself into a health care setting. He comes into the hospital with a cardiac condition. While he is in the health care setting, he becomes quite friendly with his nurse. One day, he swears his nurse to secrecy. Then he informs her of a certain fact

*Continued*

regarding his condition. During the course of his treatment, the patient becomes incapable of making a decision. This poses a dilemma for his nurse around the standard of freedom. She has promised to maintain confidentiality in the matter he related to her, but the information the patient gave her is now needed by the physician to treat him effectively. What does she do?

## THOUGHT AND ACTION

Freedom is exercised in action. Actions can suffer from vices:

- The action of inertia—the absence of action when there is a call for action. Opportunities and responsibilities come and go, but the agent is passive in regard to them.
- Disoriented actions. The agent may anticipate the need for actions to be taken to meet future circumstances. Either these circumstances never arise, which was foreseeable, or he responds to circumstances that do arise without understanding what benefits they offer or what harms are latent in them.
- Compulsive actions—actions taken in response to pent-up nervous energy. The agent's actions provide no possible benefit other than a momentary release of feelings of anxiety.
- Compliant actions—actions spontaneously following any suggestion made by anyone for any reason are essentially flawed. No process of thought and analysis has gone into the person's motivation.
- Actions of an obstinate agent. This refers to the actions of one who will not be dissuaded from a course of action that is nonproductive or the failure to engage in a course of action that promises to be productive.

The standard of freedom involves not only physical actions but also mental actions. Freedom, when enacted without the influence of vice, is the virtue of a patient's actions. It is also the virtue of a nurse's actions when she is acting for a patient.

## OBJECTIVITY

As an intellectual capacity, objectivity is a person's ability to be aware of things as they are in themselves. As a physical capacity, objectivity is a person's ability to act on this awareness. One can objectively know what a chair is. One can recognize varied features of chairs and distinguish among different types of chairs. One can act on this knowledge when choosing a chair based on preference for a particular feature, such as the softness or the height. As a bioethical standard, objectivity is the ability to

*Objectivity is the ability to achieve and sustain the exercise of one's objective awareness.*

achieve and sustain the exercise of one's objective awareness. In relation to the standard of autonomy, it is a patient's right to be supported in the act of exercising and acting on objective awareness. A nurse will increase her patient's objective awareness. She will help her patient understand the facts about his condition: the cause, consequences, treatment alternatives, effects of the treatments, and intended outcomes.

It is logically impossible to have confidence in an agreement if one cannot have confidence in the understanding of the people making the agreement. Without confidence in understanding, one could not achieve certainty concerning the terms or even the existence of an agreement. An uncertain agreement—one in which no one can have any confidence—is, in fact, no agreement at all.

People can understand each other without entering into an agreement. The sun is bright. Paul reports to Marcy that the sun is bright. Paul has brought understanding to Marcy, but no agreement has been entered into between Paul and Marcy.

On the other hand, no one can enter into an agreement unless the parties to the agreement have reached a meeting of the minds. Harry and Bill agree to share the driving on a trip to Fort Lauderdale. Harry does not know how to drive. There cannot be a meeting of the minds. The agreement that Bill assumes to exist really does not exist. One can achieve objective awareness without entering into an agreement, but one cannot enter into an agreement unless one has achieved objective awareness.

When people communicate and interact on an abstract level, objective awareness is of the highest importance. If people do not communicate with each other objectively, their only recourse will be to give up communication and, with it, interaction. All the bioethical standards, in one way or another, involve objectivity. The standard of objectivity requires that a nurse accept the truth concerning the unique nature of her patient and of her patient's inalienable right to direct the course of his life. The standard of freedom indicates the need for objective awareness. It also assumes an emotional climate wherein the ability to act on objective awareness is not undermined.

## OBJECTIVITY AS THE PRECONDITION OF AGREEMENT

One person cannot make an agreement with another person without rightly expecting objectivity from that other person. There cannot be objectivity without a meeting of the minds. Each party to the agreement must have an informed knowledge of its terms. Without this knowledge, a person obviously cannot be party to an agreement. Each party to an agreement must be certain of the terms of the agreement. One can be certain of the terms of the agreement only if one has an assurance that one has access to its objective terms—the terms as they relate to reality. Therefore, objectivity is a standard—an ethical measure of an agreement. As a necessary precondition of an agreement, it is a bioethical principle.

## BENEFICENCE

*As to diseases, make a habit of two things—to help, or at least to do no harm.*
*—Hippocrates [460–377 BC], Epidemics, Book I, Sec. XI*

As a bioethical standard, beneficence is the power of an agent, and the necessity the person faces, to act to acquire the benefits desired and the needs his or her life requires.

The concept of beneficence refers to the fact that every agent acts to achieve benefits and to avoid harm. As a bioethical standard, beneficence is the power of an agent, and the necessity the person faces, to act to acquire the benefits desired and the needs his or her life requires.

> *In February 1985, [the] New Jersey appellate court ruled that a hospital had the right to dismiss a nurse who refused, for "moral, medical and philosophic" reasons, to administer kidney dialysis treatments to a terminally ill double amputee. Mrs. Warthen [the nurse] asked to be replaced, arguing that she could not submit the man to dialysis because he was dying and the procedure was causing additional complications. She . . . was fired. . . . The three-judge appellate panel agreed with the hospital. (Humphry & Wickett, 1986, p. 122)*

Mrs. Warthen was motivated to take her position by her understanding of beneficence and objectivity. Most health care professionals would agree that her stand was beneficent and objective. No doubt the hospital where Mrs. Warthen worked held the value of beneficence in high esteem, but the value of its beneficence was not very influential in this instance.

For a nurse to act with beneficence, she must rely on her objectivity—what is known about the situation. In most cases, empathy is also an important consideration. Empathy is the act of understanding, being aware of, being sensitive to, and vicariously experiencing the feelings, thoughts, and experience of another. The experience of empathy can be risky, because not all feelings, thoughts, and emotions are pleasant. Apathy, empathy's opposite, is a state in which there is no emotional recognition of the other. An apathetic attitude can serve to safeguard one's private feelings but can also prevent beneficent action.

### DILEMMA 4.4: DECEPTION OR TRUTH

Sixteen-year-old Robin is dying from lupus erythematosus. She is very fearful. Toward the end, she screams, over and over, "Don't let me die!" Robin's parents are called to the hospital, but before they arrive, Robin dies. They ask Robin's nurse if their daughter's death was peaceful. Robin's nurse dutifully relates all the details of Robin's death. Is the nurse's recitation of events ethically justified?

It is conceivable, but not very likely, that a person could act beneficently without making agreements. Under most circumstances, it is inconceivable that people without a sense of beneficence would make agreements. Under no circumstances should we make an agreement with such people. What possible purpose could be served by making an agreement with someone who had no intention of helping us attain a benefit that we desire? Although freedom is a standard of action, beneficence is a standard of quality of action. The attitude of the nurse toward the patient's autonomy, freedom, and objectivity should support and reinforce those standards in the patient. Beneficence is a consistent attitude of goodwill toward another or toward oneself. Beneficence is the practice of acting on the prompting of goodwill—the desire to benefit one with whom one empathizes.

Patients do not always find beneficence in a health care setting. The situation is far from perfect today. It is infinitely better than it once was, but it is cyclic and is slipping backward. Florence Nightingale (1991) was led by the conditions during her time to declare although that it is strange, it is necessary to enunciate as the very first requirement in a hospital that it should do the sick no harm. Nightingale was right. Whatever becomes fashionable, beneficence is, of necessity, an integral part of the nurse–patient agreement. A beneficent nurse acts with empathy for her patient—and without resentment or malice.

Although a patient entering a hospital makes a commitment to let the hospital function as a hospital, he has an absolute right to decline treatment and any form of abuse. "To force a patient to undergo treatment against his or her wishes . . . constitutes both a violation of autonomy, and the infliction of harm. In cases such as these, the autonomous patient determines what constitutes unwarranted suffering" (Fowler & Levine-Ariff, 1987, p. 193). Conflicts can arise concerning the demands of beneficence and the natural function of a health care setting. These are, in fact, the most common bioethical dilemmas, but in the final analysis, none is a genuine dilemma.

*Although freedom is a standard of action, beneficence is a standard of quality of action.*

*A beneficent nurse acts with empathy for her patient—and without resentment or malice.*

## BENEFICENCE AS A PRECONDITION OF AGREEMENT

Each individual person has a need to achieve good and avoid harm. Beneficence is a bioethical standard (and, more generally, a standard of ethical action) because humans are beings who can and do impede and injure one another. They also can and do agree on, and exercise, beneficence toward one another. The standard of beneficence arises when ethical agents have attained a sufficient degree of rationality to recognize the advantages of acting from benevolence. Beneficence is a precondition and principle of agreement.

Symphonology does not recognize nonmaleficence as a bioethical standard. The reasons are twofold: First, it is implied by beneficence. If one does harm, one has failed to act beneficently. If one acts beneficently, ipso facto, one will do no harm. Second, if 150 years after Florence Nightingale, a nurse must be counseled not to bring about harm or other evil consequences, it is futile to offer this person any ethical advice. This nurse has given up her profession and lost her pride—and, with it, her fidelity.

## FIDELITY

Fidelity, as a bioethical standard, is an individual's faithfulness to his or her autonomy. For a nurse, fidelity is commitment to the obligation she has accepted in her professional role.

Fidelity, as a bioethical standard, is an individual's faithfulness to his or her autonomy. For a nurse, fidelity is commitment to the obligation she has accepted in her professional role. A nurse lives her profession through fidelity. Fidelity is commitment to a promise. This is the promise to honor her agreement with her patient. A nurse's fidelity is not fidelity to an agreement. It is a commitment to her patient. More precisely, it is fidelity to her patient's life, health, and well-being. "Fidelity also implies an active concern for the well-being of those to whom a commitment exists" (Shirey, 2005, p. 61). Fidelity forms the foot of the agreement. Without fidelity to hold up the agreement, the agreement never was.

A nurse has an obligation to attend to her patient in the sense of providing care for him. She also has an obligation to attend to him in the sense of listening to him and counseling him. At the very least, she has an obligation to protect him from preventable harm.

Any person, including a nurse, has a right to speak against harm. This is an aspect of beneficence. When a nurse "blows the whistle" to protect a patient, she relies on something more central to their agreement than mere benevolence. Whistle-blowing is an aspect of fidelity.

For a patient, the demands of fidelity are quite different from those for the nurse. This is because the roles of nurse and patient are very different. A nurse's role, by definition, is much more active than a patient's.

If a patient fails to exercise fidelity to the agreement (e.g., if he fails to give the health professional information she needs in order to provide him with optimal treatment), he makes it impossible for his nurse to act effectively as his agent. Yet she is unaware that she does not have this information. She is unaware that, to this extent, she is unable to act as the agent of her patient. She is able to act more or less effectively in this, but a great deal of the context is not available to her. This is particularly harmful because she is not aware of this lack of understanding in her context.

This certainly does not mean that a patient has no moral obligation to exercise fidelity. If a nurse is to be the agent of a patient, the patient must cooperate in the exercise of this agency. This is an exercise of his responsibility to be faithful to his life, health, and well-being. This includes the avoidance of behavior that makes contradictory demands on her. For example:

• After surgery, a patient expects a nurse to protect him from pneumonia, but he refuses to cough and practice deep breathing postoperatively.

- A patient expects a physical therapist to help him become more mobile after a stroke, but he refuses to go to physical therapy.
- A patient expects a nurse to protect him from injury, but he refuses to get assistance before getting out of bed.

If a patient does not honor the terms implied by his agreement with his nurse, he violates this agreement. Worse still, he violates his own purposes. If a nurse does not honor the terms implied by her agreement with herself, she violates her purposes—she disconnects from her life.

Fidelity always involves an agreement. Therefore, it is not possible to practice fidelity without making agreements. It is also not possible to keep an agreement without practicing fidelity. An agreement made without the anticipation of fidelity is a logical impossibility. An agreement made without the anticipation of fidelity is to ethics what a square circle is to geometry.

However, in expecting fidelity from her patient, a nurse must always bear in mind the incapacities that his condition forces upon him. When she does not receive the cooperation of a patient, she must remember her commitment to her profession. Even when things cannot be done perfectly, she must do the best she can. This is her obligation to her profession, to her employer, and to herself.

> An agreement made without the anticipation of fidelity is a logical impossibility.
>
> In expecting fidelity from her patient, a nurse must always bear in mind the incapacities that his condition forces upon him. When she does not receive the cooperation of a patient, she must remember her commitment to her profession.

## FIDELITY AS A PRECONDITION OF AGREEMENT

> Agreements serve a purpose in human lives. This purpose is the benefit that people gain through cooperation.

Agreements serve a purpose in human lives. This purpose is the benefit that people gain through cooperation. Through cooperation, ethical agents are able to achieve good and to avoid harm. It contradicts the nature of an agreement that people would form an agreement and, within the confines of that agreement, refuse to do good or at least to do no harm to one another.

It is a very easy matter to see that no agreement between two people can be maintained if the standard of fidelity is not maintained. Fidelity is an outgrowth of the recognition of the other standards. To gain the benefits of interaction, individuals must be able to rely on each other. This reliance is made possible by the implicit and explicit understandings upon which their interaction is based. Fidelity is faithfulness to these understandings. It is an essential principle of agreement. Agreement would not be possible to imagine without fidelity.

> Fidelity is an outgrowth of the recognition of the other standards.

A denial of the relevance of any of the bioethical standards to the agreement cannot be logically justified. In one way or another, the denial would make a claim that, if it were true, would undermine all possibility of an agreement. To simplify the matter greatly, it is rather like someone's declaring in English, "I don't speak a word of English"; the very fact that this claim is made in English falsifies it.

If a nurse makes an agreement with a patient, she makes an agreement with a being who is autonomous, free, and so forth. If she interacts as if he were not autonomous, free, and so forth, to this extent she violates her agreement. To the extent that she violates her agreement, she refuses to act as a nurse. Her agreement and actions contradict each other. This is important. A nurse does not make any new ethical agreement after the nurse–patient agreement. Every ethical agreement is implied in this agreement.

## THE CLASSIC VIRTUES

The first virtue of a nurse, as a nurse, is fidelity to her patient. The first virtue of a patient, as a patient, is fidelity to himself.

The classic virtues—wisdom, courage, reciprocity, gratitude, integrity, pride, and justice—are not disregarded by bioethics. They are implied by the principle of fidelity to the nurse–patient agreement. Every virtue and every value involves fidelity, and without fidelity, nothing holds together. Fidelity is essential to a professional ethic. The contemporary ethical systems make fidelity impossible as will be shown in Chapter 6.

The virtue of **wisdom** requires a nurse to counsel and interact with her patient on the basis of a well-grounded knowledge. It calls on her to communicate with her patient. It requires her not to interact with her patient on the basis of unexamined beliefs, a lazy reliance on emotions, self-righteous rationalizations, or an unrealistic opinion of her ethical hunches.

The virtue of **courage** calls on a nurse to defend her own rights and never to violate the rights of her patient. It requires her to accept her own humanity and the humanity of her patient. It requires her to accept the uniqueness and the independence of the patient whose agent she is. Courage inspires independent action for the benefit of a patient. It is shown in her acceptance of a patient's desire even when this desire is not in line with social mores and customs (McFadden, 1996). "If [a nurse] chooses for her patient, she chooses for her profession. . . . This decision requires a certain kind of courage—a courage that . . . is indispensable to the development of a great nurse" (Husted & Husted, 1998, p. 53).

**Reciprocity** is a spontaneous exchange of values, especially when this practice is sustained over a period of time without any formal arrangements. The factor of surprise creates on both sides the most luxurious of the virtues: gratitude. **Gratitude** is the virtue that is the capstone of fidelity and all its aspects. The other aspects of fidelity are in different ways forms of reciprocity. An ounce of reciprocity is worth a pound of any other aspect of fidelity.

When a patient has expectations of the nurse and a nurse tacitly commits to a patient and the patient gives trust to the nurse, this is a stellar example of reciprocity. The expectations of a patient are a value to a dedicated nurse. If the nurse returns this value with the value of an implicit commitment— expressed in her attitude and in her actions—this begins a process of reciprocity. If the patient responds to his nurse with trust, this is the confirmation of reciprocity.

> **Reciprocity** is a spontaneous exchange of values, especially when this practice is sustained over a period of time without any formal arrangements.

## RECIPROCITY AND SELF-INTEREST

The possibilities for establishing a series of reciprocal-like trades perfectly illustrates the ethical nature and location of rational self-interest. Rational self-interest brings about successful reciprocal relationships. Both members must contribute value to the relationship; otherwise, the contributing member will withdraw for lack of value. The contributions of the members must be of equal value so that one member does not find himself impoverished by the interactions. Reciprocity based on rational self-interest provides members of a relationship with benefits they would have been unable to acquire on their own. The process of reciprocity over time enriches both, and each becomes known as a trustworthy trading partner.

In a bioethical context, **integrity** is a synonym for fidelity. Integrity is the name of the virtue that an agent practices when faithful to self, the external world, and the relationship between them.

**Pride,** as a virtue, inspires a nurse's commitment to herself to strive for professional excellence—to exercise fidelity toward her patient. Pride becomes a virtue when it motivates a nurse, through an agreement she has made with herself, to do nothing of which she need be ashamed, whatever others might think or do (Husted & Husted, 1999). It arises from the expectation she has of herself that she will not fail to act on her professional agreement and will do this as efficiently—as beneficently—as she can. Very few health care professionals, as patients, would want to be cared for by someone who took no pride in herself as a professional. If a nurse would not want this for herself, it follows that she ought not offer it to her patients.

The virtue of **justice** calls on a professional and patient to exchange values—to take meaning from, and give meaning to, their relationship. This makes justice in a health care context a type of friendship.

> To be a friend one must know how to suspend voluntarily his own perspective with its attendant needs and interests; he must know how to discover the principle that is the innermost being of the other; he must know how to use this principle to explore the personal world of the other; he must possess the discretion to will his friend's fulfillment without abrogating his friend's self-responsibility; and he must himself be capable of profound self-disclosure. . . . The will to friendship expresses the recognition that one is in oneself not the totality of goodness but rather an aspect—an aspect that in its actualization summons complementary aspects, willing their actualization together with its own. (Norton, 1976, p. 304)

In the context of professional nursing, the principle that Norton speaks of, "the principle that is the innermost being of the other," is a patient's fidelity to his health, well-being, and happiness. In the matter of the villagers and the coconut from Chapter 3, the principle was the needs and desires of each villager. By failing to "suspend voluntarily his own [narrow] perspective with its attendant needs and interests . . . to explore the personal world of the other," each, in being fair to himself and to the other, committed an unseen injustice against himself and the other.

The function of a professional ethic is to move the implicit professional–patient agreement from a necessary formality to a state of mutual trust—as would benefit friendship. A health care professional wills her patient's fulfillment without abrogating his self-responsibility. A patient appropriately responds with some level of gratitude. Gratitude is an incentive to friendship. Friendship is an incentive to achieving understanding, concern, and support. A professional appropriately acts with concern. Without this motivation, one cannot act as a professional. Without concern, one cannot be, in its true sense, a professional. Gratitude is the most reasonable response to friendship and concern. Gratitude is a form of justice and, for nurse and patient alike, the most pleasant of the virtues. A patient's freely given gratitude is health care's Olympic gold medal.

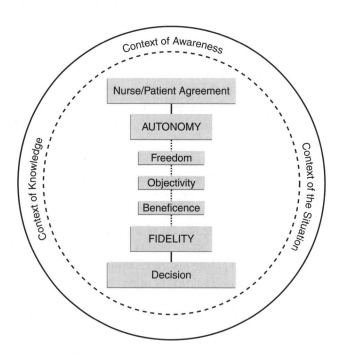

**FIGURE 4.1** Husteds' symphonological bioethical decision-making model I.

## MUSINGS

Whenever an agreement exists between two people, each has expectations and responsibilities as a result of that agreement. This is true of the professional–patient agreement, as it is true of every agreement. It is the expectation of a benefit that the person will receive that motivates him or her to take on the responsibilities of an agreement.

Every agreement is formed by the human character structures signified by bioethical standards. They are preconditions shaping any agreement. "Just as the bioethical standards are not to be considered as concrete directives, so too, they are not distinct entities. Each standard blends with the others as representative of the unique character of the individual" (Scotto, 2009, p. 591).

Fidelity to an agreement requires that each be aware of and respect the nature of the other. Without this awareness and respect, there is no reliable interaction. Fidelity to one's awareness is basic to agreement and interaction.

"Symphonology describes how the agreement, guided by the bioethical standards (BES) as preconditions and the inclusion of patient and family provides the ethical approach necessary for making ethical decisions, whether they are day to day activities, or an actual ethical dilemma" (Cutilli, 2009, p. 188).

Figure 4.1 is meant to be a guide for those using the theory of a practice-based, symphonological ethic. It gives a visual picture of the concepts and their approximate relationships. However, no diagram can convey the meanings, relationships, and use of the theory without an understanding of the theory itself. Note that except for context as context must surround everything, *autonomy* is in the largest print followed by *fidelity*.

## STUDY GUIDE

1. Define and discuss all the bioethical standards.
2. Think of ways in which you could assess your patient according to the bioethical standards.
3. What is the meaning of these standards as preconditions?
4. Does the agreement include them all, or could one or more be absent and there still be an agreement? Explain.
5. Give examples of reciprocity within the agreement.
6. Apply the idea of probability from Chapter 3 to Case 4.3 and 4.4.
7. Give examples of the classic virtues in action.
8. Examine what you surmise about the relationship of the concepts from looking at Figure 4.1.
9. Use this case for class discussion; the analysis of the case only appears in the instructor's manual.

## THE DEMANDS OF JUSTICE

The classic case of a conflict between autonomy and beneficence is the case of a comatose Jehovah's Witness who needs a blood transfusion. He has left no directions and has no family. His autonomy demands that, because he cannot explicitly communicate contrary wishes, it can be assumed that he would not want the transfusion. The standard of beneficence, on the other hand, demands that the professional act to bring about good. To allow a patient to die when he could have been saved is a very great failure to bring about good. Still, to give a patient a transfusion and save him, under these circumstances, might violate the standard of autonomy. If it were a child, how would this affect the resolution?

## REFERENCES

Cutilli, C. C. (2009). "Ethical considerations in patient and family education: Using the Symphonological approach." *Orthopaedic Nursing, 28*(4), 187–192.

Fowler, M. D. M., & Levine-Ariff, J. (1987). *Ethics at the bedside*. Philadelphia, PA: J. B. Lippincott.

Gewirth, A. (1978). *Reason and morality*. Chicago: The University of Chicago Press.

Humphry, D., & Wickett, A. (1986). *The right to die: Understanding euthanasia*. New York, NY: Harper and Row.

Husted, G. L., & Husted, J. H. (1997). Is cloning moral? *Nursing and Health Care, 18*, 168–169.

Husted, G. L., & Husted, J. H. (1998). The nurse as cynic—etiology and Rx. *Advanced Practice Nursing Quarterly, 4*(3), 51–53.

Husted, G. L., Husted, J. H., & Scotto, C. (2013). Ethics and the advanced practice nurse. In A. Joel (Ed.), *Advanced practice nursing* (3rd ed., pp. 522–543) Philadelphia, PA: FA Davis.

Husted, J. H., & Husted, G. L. (1999). Agreement: The origin of ethical action. *Critical Care Nursing, 22*(3), 12–18.

McFadden, E. A. (1996). Moral development and reproductive health decisions. *Journal of Obstetric, Gynecologic, & Neonatal Nursing, 25*, 507–512.

Nightingale, F. (1991). *As Miss Nightingale said . . . : Florence Nightingale through her sayings: A Victorian perspective*. (M. Baly, Ed.). London, England: Scutari Press.

Norton, D. L. (1976). *Personal destinies: A philosophy of ethical individualism*. Princeton, NJ: Princeton University Press.

Rice, V. H., Beck, C., & Stevenson, J. S. (1997). Ethical issues relative to autonomy and personal control in independent and cognitively impaired elders. *Nursing Outlook, 45*, 27–34.

Scotto, C. (2009). Symphonological bioethical theory. In A. M. Tomey & M. R. Alligood (Eds.), *Nursing theorists and their work* (7th ed., 560–579). St. Louis, MO: Mosby.

Shirey, M. R. (2005). Ethical climate in nursing practice: The leader's role. *Healthcare Law, Ethics, and Regulation, 7*, 59–67.

# FIVE

# THE NATURE OF THE ETHICAL CONTEXT

## OBJECTIVES

- Differentiate among the three aspects of the context.

- Illustrate the relationship of the agreement to the context.

- Determine the importance of interweaving the three aspects of the context to bioethical decision making.

- Examine what can be learned from the Queen of Hearts scenario.

- Explain the importance of intention.

- Apply the five rights to bioethical decision making.

*The world is given to us as a book. How strange we so seldom read it.*
— *Eugene Aben-Moha*

It is these virtues that place the agent, or the patient in the case of a health care setting, in a context that makes the context what it is in relation to the patient and that shape the patient's motivations and actions.

Context, including the environment and all the accompanying circumstances, is of absolute importance in any ethical situation. Actions that are ethically appropriate for a certain patient at a specific time may not be ethically appropriate to the same patient at a different time. Actions that are ethically appropriate for a certain patient at a specific time may not be appropriate for a different patient at this same specific time. The bioethical standards signify virtues that, working together, form and constitute the character of a rational being to the extent that the person is an ethical agent. It is these virtues that place the agent, or the patient in the case of a health care setting, in a context that makes the context what it is in relation to the patient and that shape the patient's motivations and actions.

71

Each virtue (the bioethical standards) shapes its own peculiar sort of motivation, and the interacting of the virtues produce the character and the nuances of an ethical agent's motivation in any specific circumstance. *Fidelity*, as a virtue, determines the strength or weakness of an agent's motivation. Fidelity is the virtue of an agent's decisions and agreements. *Beneficence* is the intensity of the person's motivation to pursue benefits and/or to defend against harm. Beneficence reveals the strength of the agent's self-interest and the appropriateness of the person's motivations. Beneficence is the virtue of the agent's practical and sensible reason. *Objectivity* is the virtue of maintaining an uncluttered awareness of one's circumstances and one's place in one's circumstances. The evidence of this is given in the competency of the person's action and whether he or she is motivated through a complete understanding. This virtue creates awareness. *Freedom* denotes an agent's interest in, and concern for, the value of his or her life and entire lifetime. Freedom is the virtue of the agent's rational self-interest. It is shown in the degree to which one is oriented appropriately to one's future and the reality of one's lived world. *Autonomy* is the person's unique character. The person's unique character is the interweaving and connecting of all these virtues. Nurses can, and ought to, use the bioethical standards as instruments of ethical analysis. A patient's virtues or vices will imply his motivations. His motivations will suggest his present intentions. His intentions will suggest his probable values, decisions, and actions. A nurse can encounter two problems in her use of the bioethical standards in her discovery of the character of her patient and in the meaning and tone of their relationship:

1. She can be uncertain as to her application of a bioethical standard.
2. She can feel a lesser or greater confidence in her application of a particular standard than is justified.

These problems arise because conflicts in the nurse's understanding of the appropriate application of the standards can occur. Any resolutions to conflicts that arise must come from the bioethical standards, because they must come from the nurse–patient agreement within a particular context. The nurse–patient agreement can be understood only in terms of the bioethical standards because they are the motivators and influences of the agreement.

In different ways the nurse and patient:

• Want self-awareness to clarify and retain the knowledge of who they are (she is a competent professional, and he is able to retain his competence).
• Look forward to their life span with confidence and anticipation (she is able to retain enthusiasm for her profession and knowledge that he will be able to continue to meet his responsibilities).

- Know that their ambitions and decisions are objectively justified (she will not have to defend her ambitions and desires against objective facts, and the objective facts do not threaten his ability to meet his obligations).
- Continue one's pursuit of benefit and successful avoidance of harm (she is continuing to enjoy the benefits of success and avoiding the drawback of failure, and he is continuing to be capable and is avoiding incapacity).
- Maintain fidelity to one's knowledge, one's motivations, and one's values (she is maintaining fidelity to herself and to her profession through fidelity to her patient, and he is maintaining fidelity to the value of his life).

## THE CONTEXT OF PRACTICE

> *In ethics everything is contextual; and the context of every action is unique and unduplicable, with the result that even a small difference between two situations may yield a difference in our moral verdict.* (Hospers, 1972, p. 63)

*What is and what is not justifiable entirely depends on the context.*

Driving 55 miles per hour in a 55-mile-per-hour zone is ordinarily quite justifiable. It is not justifiable if the road is covered with ice. What is and what is not justifiable entirely depends on the context. If one wants to drive safely from point A to point B, the condition of the road is a central factor one must consider in referring to the context to justify one's speed. (Note that context is vitally important to everyday decisions and actions.)

### DILEMMA 5.1: RIGHT TO CHOOSE AN UNHEALTHY LIFESTYLE

Martin is a home health nurse for the Visiting Nurses' Association. He has been caring for Frank for 9 months. Frank has severe chronic obstructive pulmonary disease (COPD). He is rushed into the hospital every 4 to 6 weeks for severe respiratory distress. Frank is a heavy smoker despite his condition. He is also nonadherent in other aspects of his care, such as diet. Martin is considering asking the physician to discontinue home visits because he has been unable to influence Frank's habits. What are the bioethical ramifications of stopping treatment in this case?

*No noncontextual system is relevant to practice, nor is any noncontextual system objectively justifiable.*

Ethical decision making in health care is specific to a changing context, because it is set in a practice venue. No noncontextual system is relevant to practice, nor is any noncontextual system objectively justifiable. A decision not justified within the context, one that is instead based on assumptions unrelated to the values or genuine well-being of a patient, cannot be an objectively justifiable decision for a specific patient in a specific context (Husted & Husted, 2004). This is as equally true in an ethical context as it is in the context of a nursing intervention.

If a system is to inspire relevant and justifiable actions, it must be adaptable to the context in which the action is to take place. Ethical actions are justified by considering ethical purposes, just as nursing actions are justified by considering nursing purposes. Each is justified by goals that serve life, health, and well-being. The context provides two resources. The first is a cognitive resource to increase understanding. It reveals what is to be done. The second is an ethical resource. It reveals why this is to be done, if there is anything that needs to be done. Without the context, there would be no way of knowing that there is something to be done.

By the same token, any change of mind and any differences in one's moral verdict ought to be traceable to changes in what one has previously identified as part of the context. Unless the new factor can be clearly identified as being contextually relevant, it is certain that the moral verdict has been reached through subjective and whimsical reasons. Ethical actions are actions taken in the pursuit of vital and fundamental goals. They are actions intended to make an important difference in a person's life. Ethical interactions and actions involve a purpose and an interplay between a person and a situation. This situation must either offer the person the possibility of achieving some value or it must threaten the loss of some value (Husted & Husted, 1993).

> The context provides two resources. The first is a cognitive resource to increase understanding. It reveals what is to be done. The second is an ethical resource. It reveals why this is to be done, if there is anything that needs to be done. Without the context, there would be no way of knowing that there is something to be done.

## DILEMMA 5.2: MAKING A DECISION AGAINST FACILITY POLICY

Mrs. Allison, a 46-year-old Australian woman, was admitted to Outback Hospital in critical condition. On report, Ron, Mrs. Allison's nurse, takes note of the fact that she has gotten worse on the 3–11 shift. He decides to make her the first patient he visits after report. He assesses Mrs. Allison and decides that, in his opinion (he considers himself an expert practitioner), she is extremely critical and needs to have more aggressive treatment done quickly. He is aware that his hospital does not have the means to give her the treatment she needs but that another urban hospital about 30 miles away does.

The policy at Outback is that an attending physician must sign a transfer order. The attending physician cannot be reached. Because Outback is a small, rural hospital, there are no interns or residents, and currently no physicians are at the hospital. It is around midnight. Ron would have tried to convince another physician to break policy and sign the transfer order because Mrs. Allison's condition is worsening, but this is not an option. Ron cannot convince anyone in nursing administration to risk going against the policy. What should he do?

## AGREEMENT AND CONTEXT

The agreement between nurse and patient must always take place within a context. The nurse–patient agreement establishes the fact of this relationship. The context establishes the nature and purposes of the relationship and actions that can and ought to be taken. No other actions are ethically justifiable and nothing can come from outside of this relationship.

*The context establishes the nature and purposes of the relationship and actions that can and ought to be taken.*

The center of a nurse's ethical context cannot be anything but herself and her individual patient. (This is not to say that the family is unimportant, but they are important only insofar as they desire what the patient wants and are willing to abide by the patient's wishes insofar as they are known. A strong loving family, however, is a tremendous asset to patients.) Her professional agreement cannot be with anyone but with her patient. The ethical limits of her professional context lie entirely within her professional agreement. Without the nurse–patient agreement, no bioethical context would ever arise, and the nurse and the patient's situation and interactions would be incoherent and meaningless. Only in the context of the agreement do they become clear and comprehensible. Only through an agreement does a nursing situation become a context. Only in proportion to the nurse and patient's dedication to the agreement is the nurse–patient situation a logical context. A nurse's professional practice is based on this agreement. When her ethical practice is based on this agreement and its practice, her ethical interactions are practice based.

*A strong loving family, however, is a tremendous asset to patients.*

Nursing, as an activity, has characteristics and essential qualities that make it unique. It is different from all other types of activity because it is oriented toward particular and specific purposes. It is characterized by specific interpersonal interactions. The character and quality of these interactions is determined by the characteristics, essential qualities, and purpose of nursing.

Within the interpersonal relationship of nurse and patient there is an interweaving of expectations and commitments. These expectations and commitments shape the characteristics of the relationship for both the nurse and patient. This complex of expectations and commitments between the nurse and patient forms an agreement between them. Each agrees to satisfy, to one extent or another, the expectations of the other. Both agree to live up to the commitments each has made to the other. Their agreement is the recognition by each of the expectations and commitments existing between them.

Interactions between people must be based on expectations and responsibilities that are known by each. The interweaving of their purposes and obligations forms the agreement that makes their interaction possible. When this agreement is abandoned, there is no pattern to their interactions. Without clear understandable patterns of interaction between the nurse and patient, nursing is not a specific exclusive activity.

## DILEMMA 5.3: EMBRYO OWNERSHIP

John and Peggy were married for several years and were not able to conceive. They visited a fertility clinic where Peggy was induced to produce many eggs. The eggs were then fertilized with John's sperm, and several eight-cell embryos were artificially produced in a glass test tube. Peggy then underwent surgery and was implanted with the embryos five different times. None of the attempts to have a child was successful.

John and Peggy began to have marital problems after a few years. The clinic had frozen 10 of the embryos made by John and Peggy during a happier time in their marriage. Peggy decided to keep the embryos to use in future procedures to try to have a baby. She believed that the embryos were her last chance at being a mother. John, however, decided never to have children with his ex-wife and wished to donate the embryos to research. Who owns the embryos ("The case of the embryos," 2000)?

## THE THIRD HUMOROUS VIGNETTE: THE QUEEN OF HEARTS

Imagine this scene: Your name is Alice. You are the Alice in Lewis Carroll's Wonderland. You work in a kitchen in Wonderland. The ethic of the kitchen is harsh, badly proportioned, and unjust. If you drop an egg and fail to report having dropped it, an unhappy child will go to bed hungry. So, if you drop an egg and want to prevent a child's unhappiness, you ought to report that you have dropped it. The last time one of the kitchen workers dropped an egg and reported it, the Queen of Hearts had her beheaded. You are in a perilous situation—one in which you ought to think very carefully before reporting the loss of an egg. Very seldom is the context of an ethical situation as clear-cut as this. However, in a very basic way, the context is relevant to every ethical decision and action. If you decide to report the fact that you dropped the egg, this will be an ethical decision. It may make a child very happy. It may also be the last ethical decision you will ever make. Imagine the character of a child who would be happy about your decision if he or she knew the particulars (the context) of it. If you decide not to report the fact that you dropped the egg, this will also be an ethical decision. Unlike many ethical decisions, it would be a contextual, well-proportioned, and rational decision.

## THE THREE ELEMENTS OF CONTEXT

A context is the interweaving of the relevant facts of a situation, one's awareness of these facts, and the knowledge one has of how to deal most effectively with these facts.

A context is the interweaving of the relevant facts of a situation (the facts that are necessary to act upon to bring about a desired result), one's awareness of these facts, and the knowledge one has of how to deal most effectively with these facts. A context consists of these three distinct but dynamically interrelated elements.

## CONTEXT OF THE SITUATION

The context of the situation is those aspects of the specific situation that are helpful in understanding it so that one can act effectively in it. The variables that a health care professional finds within her patient's situation form the context of the situation.

The context of the situation is those aspects of the specific situation that are helpful in understanding it so that one can act effectively in it. The variables that a health care professional finds within her patient's situation form the context of the situation. Every time a health care professional takes on the care of a patient, this action places her in a context. Factors such as the patient's history and physical findings, the physician's diagnosis, the patient's family situation, the laboratory results, the emotional state of the patient, and the age and sex, and so on, of the patient form the context of a health care situation. A nurse deals with this context every time she engages with a patient.

The interrelations among the patient's medical condition, individual circumstances, plans for the future, present motivations, and resources of character are aspects of his individual situation. How these relate to his central desires, his purposes, and his need to regain a position of agency are part of the context of the ethical situation. In an ethical context, agency is the power to initiate action and to sustain the actions necessary to successful living.

Her awareness of the context of the situation makes it possible for the health care professional to guide her actions according to what is implied by the situation in relation to her professional and ethical purposes. Without an awareness of the context of the situation, she has no reason to act and she cannot act on the basis of reason.

## THE CONTEXT OF KNOWLEDGE

The context of knowledge is an agent's preexisting knowledge relevant to the situation. A nurse brings with her a body of knowledge that enables her to approach each situation appropriately and effectively. This includes knowledge of factors that are usually found in similar situations, knowledge of potential individual peculiarities, and knowledge of factors that may influence the situation.

The context of knowledge is information brought into the situation and that which is found in the situation that aids in processing the information in order to make decisions. Each health care professional has her own body of knowledge to bring to the situation. The patient also has a body of knowledge about himself that is relevant to his care.

The context of knowledge is information brought into the situation and that which is found in the situation that aids in processing the information in order to make decisions. Each health care professional has her own body of knowledge to bring to the situation. The patient also has a body of knowledge about himself that is relevant to his care.

The fact that there is a situation accessible to the purposes of an agent is not enough for the existence of a context. She must be an agent whose knowledge enables her to recognize the presence and nature of the situation. In addition, she must have a desire to act within the situation. She must see it as either requiring action to prevent some undesirable consequence or as possessing aspects necessary to the accomplishment of a desirable goal. In ethical decision making, a context of knowledge is a body of previously acquired knowledge or knowledge gained in the situation. The value of that knowledge is achieved through applying this to the context of the situation and possession of one's present awareness.

## THE CONTEXT OF AWARENESS

An agent's context of awareness includes her awareness of those aspects of the situation that invite action. Her awareness of the possibilities for success in alternative courses of action is also part of her context of awareness.

An agent's context of awareness includes her awareness of those aspects of the situation that invite action. Her awareness of the possibilities for success in alternative courses of action is also part of her context of awareness. An agent's applying the context of her knowledge involves an awareness of changes in what is known, about changes in her context of knowledge, and an awareness of the emergence of new factors that may affect her purposes, that may offer new ways of realizing them, or that may offer new values worthy of pursuit.

The context of awareness forms a bridge between the context of knowledge and the context of the situation. This is what a nurse does, for instance, each time she makes a nursing diagnosis.

This awareness and knowledge on the part of an agent (nurse) presumes that she is able to organize the relevant aspects of the situation into an understandable form. The context of awareness forms a bridge between the context of knowledge and the context of the situation. This is what a nurse does, for instance, each time she makes a nursing diagnosis. For a nurse to maintain awareness of the context of the situation while she is acting requires her to maintain an awareness of the agreements and responsibilities that structure her ethical situation. It also means she needs to maintain an awareness of changes in those contextual factors that must shape her actions if she is to act effectively. A nurse who maintains these attitudes and abilities concerning the ethical aspects of her practice is holding to the standards of her practice.

Tina has promised to take a group of chronically ill pediatric patients to the zoo. Her purpose is to share their enjoyment. The children, their desires, and their handicaps form the essential context of the situation. While Tina is preparing for the trip, she discovers that Brucie, the sickest of the children, is scheduled for surgery the next day and will not be able to go on the trip. This change in the situation causes Tina to cancel the trip. She would not enjoy the trip knowing that Brucie could not come with them. She hopes the children would not want to go without Brucie and will be content to wait until later for the trip.

Tina maintained an awareness of the context. This enabled her to be aware of a change in the context and the influence this change had on her purpose. Then, however, Tina discovered another fact in the situation that changed the context for her again. She discovered that Brucie was afraid of animals and really did not want to go to the zoo. When Tina explained the situation to the children, she did not mention that Brucie was afraid of animals. Brucie was spared an embarrassing moment, and everyone had a wonderful time at the zoo.

Every decision that an agent makes, if she considers the context, must be made according to:

- Her knowledge.
- That which is relevant in the situation.
- Her awareness of what is relevant in the situation.

*Her knowledge enables her to be aware of what is relevant in the situation. That which is relevant in the situation enables her to apply her knowledge. Both enable her to act to accomplish her purposes.*

Her knowledge enables her to be aware of what is relevant in the situation. That which is relevant in the situation enables her to apply her knowledge. Both enable her to act to accomplish her purposes.

The context of the situation provides a nurse with an awareness that there is something to be done. Along with her knowledge of her patient's purposes, it provides her with an awareness of what is to be done. Keeping the context, or acknowledging and reviewing the context, is the way to maintain an awareness of the factors relevant to her ethical actions and any changes that occur in these factors. Keeping the context is the first order of ethical action. The context must shape a person's actions if she is to act effectively.

## THE INTERWEAVING OF THE THREE ELEMENTS OF THE CONTEXT

*The interweaving of a patient's purposes, a situation, a nurse's awareness of these purposes and the situation, and her knowledge gained from past experiences forms her context.*

Ethical purposes are justified by taking into consideration a patient's vital, fundamental, and, personal values. A patient's purposes are brought to the situation by the patient. The interweaving of a patient's purposes, a situation, a nurse's awareness of these purposes and the situation, and her knowledge gained from past experiences forms her context. The facts that are relevant to a purpose, to a nurse's decisions and actions, will be found in the situation. These facts, the considerations found in the context, this knowledge, and the nurse's purposive awareness, are interwoven in order to bring the context into existence (Table 5.1).

**The context of the situation is a context of discovery**. Through the context of the situation, an agent discovers whether something ought to be done, what ought to be done, and for whom it ought to be done. **The**

TABLE 5.1 THE THREE ELEMENTS OF CONTEXT

| Element | Description |
| --- | --- |
| The context of the situation | The situation as it is related to an agent's purposes and actions; those facts that can assist or can hinder her purposes and actions |
| The context of knowledge (brought to the situation) | The knowledge *relevant* to a situation that an agent brings to the situation |
| The context of awareness (of what is discovered in the situation and her knowledge) | The ideas that form the agent's awareness of the situation; awareness of the actions she might take and how the situation will assist or hinder her purposes and actions |

context of knowledge is a context of justification. Through the context of knowledge, an agent discovers why it should be done and how it should be done. The context of awareness is a context of engagement. Through the context of awareness, an agent actively enters a dilemma or situation to resolve it. The context of an ethical dilemma is the interweaving of three things: knowledge, situation, and awareness. An agent's preexisting knowledge is the general knowledge she brings to the situation, as opposed to the information she gains from her experience of the specific factors of the situation. Both of these aspects of the context of knowledge are essential. A nurse's recognition of a patient's right to make and act on decisions is part of her preexisting knowledge. Preexisting contextual knowledge is applicable to an ethical context, but it is known to the ethical agent before her experience in the current, specific context.

A context is very much like a sweater. All the strands making up a sweater are interwoven. Likewise, all the facts, realities, ideas, and beliefs making up a context are interwoven. The interweaving of a sweater is what keeps the strands together and makes it a sweater. Likewise, the interweaving of the strands of a context is what keeps it together and makes it a context. Efficient ethical decision making requires an interweaving of the context of the situation and the context of knowledge through the context of awareness in a way that leads to an appropriate insight and understanding.

On any given day, in order to decide whether to wear a coat to go outside, one must have a preexisting context of knowledge. One ought to know, in general, which weather conditions call for a coat. One ought to discover the context of the situation. One must determine what the actual weather conditions are outside at this time. One does this through a context of awareness. It is desirable for one to determine what changes in the weather are in store. Whether one will wear a coat is a dilemma. Knowing what weather conditions, in general, mandate the wearing of a coat is in one's context of knowledge. It is that part that one brings to the situation. The weather conditions, as they are outside

*Efficient ethical decision making requires an interweaving of the context of the situation and the context of knowledge through the context of awareness in a way that leads to an appropriate insight and understanding.*

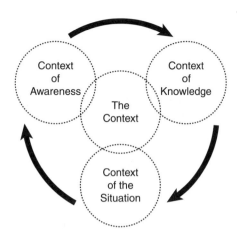

**FIGURE 5.1** The interweaving of contexts.

right now, are the context of this specific situation. One's awareness of these conditions is that part of one's knowledge that one acquires directly from the situation. One accomplishes this through the context of one's awareness.

Weaving the elements of the context together, the decision would be made like this:

- "It is now less than 40°F" (context of the situation).
- "Whenever the temperature is less than 40°F, I ought to wear a coat outdoors" (context of knowledge; what she brings to the situation).
- "Now I ought to wear a coat" (context of awareness; what one finds in the situation).

This decision is based on an interweaving of the context of the situation into the context of the agent's knowledge, by means of the context of awareness. It is a logically justifiable decision.

This decision is based on an interweaving of the context of the situation into the context of the agent's knowledge, by means of the context of awareness. It is a logically justifiable decision. This example was used only for the purpose of illustration, and it is not suggested that ethical analysis ought to be done this way. Doing so may narrow the context to the point where crucially relevant points are left out of consideration leading to a flawed decision.

## CONTEXTUAL CERTAINTY

While persons seek certainty in their decisions, "moral [ethical] certainty can provide [unwarranted] comfort for the ethical decision maker . . . and stifle dialogue and in-depth discussion of the [situation]" (Wurzbach, 1999, p. 287). Wurzbach goes on to say that when nurses "feel" too certain of their decisions, they tend not to question their own beliefs and actions, do not dialogue with themselves, and do not look for possible alternatives to their actions so that mistakes can be avoided.

## DILEMMA 5.4: SUSPECTED CHILD ABUSE

Doris brings Shawn, her 5-year-old son, into a clinic to be treated for injuries sustained through a fall. Alice, the nurse who treats Shawn, recognizes that his injuries are much more consistent with battering than with a fall. Beneficence seems to demand that Alice report her belief that Shawn is a battered child. She cannot do this, however, without creating an invasion of Doris's freedom. Whatever she does, she ought to do it only with full awareness.

The only possible ethical certainty a person can have in a biomedical setting is contextual certainty, which is limited to that particular time and specific circumstance. Certainty is only possible to the extent that:

- One has relevant facts available as evidence pointing toward a decision—the context of the situation.
- One has relevant knowledge to apply to these facts—a context of knowledge.
- One is presently aware of these facts and this knowledge—a context of awareness.

An attempt to avoid awareness of the situation, to ignore one's knowledge, or to escape into the blissful self-righteousness of a contemporary ethical system can replace the effort to understand and does not promote certainty. Irrelevance and evasion are not solutions to the problem of certainty. Certainty, like all cognition, should be arrived at contextually and objectively.

In the case of a certain state of affairs, either X is the case or X is not the case. In respect of our knowledge, there are three possibilities:

1. We are certain that X is the case.
2. We are in doubt (uncertain) as to whether X is the case.
3. We are certain that X is not the case.

For our thinking to be objective, it must be shaped by the affairs of which we are aware. It cannot be shaped by subjective factors, for example, desires. For it to be contextual, our thinking must be determined by all the factors relating to X of which we are aware, and nothing but these factors. If all our objective and contextual knowledge and awareness point to the fact that X is the case, then, in the context of our knowledge and awareness, we are objectively certain that X is the case. If all our objective and contextual knowledge and awareness point to the fact that X is not the case, then, in the context of our knowledge and awareness, we are objectively certain that X is not the case. If one part of our knowledge and awareness points to the fact that X is the case and another part points to the fact that X is not the case, then, in the context of our knowledge and awareness, we are objectively and contextually in a state of doubt.

> ## DILEMMA 5.5: RIGHT TO REFUSE DISFIGURING INTERVENTIONS
>
> Mrs. L. had cancer of the throat and needed extensive surgery, radiation, and chemotherapy. The surgery would require a temporary tracheotomy that the woman adamantly refused. Although the tracheotomy was thought to be a temporary airway solution to get her through the immediate postoperative period, it was also needed to lessen or prevent complications resulting from the radiation that would follow. She could not be convinced that it was necessary. This woman was young with school-age children, and her husband and surgeon were very concerned about the probable outcomes as a result of her decision. Therefore, they decided to go against Mrs. L.'s wishes and perform the tracheotomy (graduate nursing student, personal communication, 2007).

## REASONING TO AND REASONING FROM A DECISION

There is a habitual and routine way of thinking that keeps people from changing their ethical decisions and their actions. Rarely are people aware that they have formed such thinking patterns, nor are they aware of the negative outcomes and difficulties that can occur from these patterns. Many people have discovered that their personal tragedy was caused by this way of thinking. Others do not discover the problem with thinking this way, especially when it causes a patient's personal tragedy.

This way of thinking involves the difference between reasoning to a decision and reasoning from a decision. When reasoning to a decision, one starts with the objective reality of the health care setting and the patient's world. When reasoning from a decision, one starts from one's own subjectivity of present unquestioned beliefs and feelings.

*When reasoning to a decision, one starts with the objective reality of the health care setting and the patient's world. When reasoning from a decision, one starts from one's own subjectivity of present unquestioned beliefs and feelings.*

Asking, "As a nurse, what should my ethical attitude toward my profession be?" and "What can I learn from my patients?" are two examples of reasoning to a decision. Conversely, two examples of reasoning from a decision are asking, "As a nurse, how am I going to go about convincing my patients to do what is in their best interests?" and "What can my patients learn from me?"

The difference is in where one begins. If one begins with facts out there in the world, one can make a decision based on what one discovers out in the world. If one begins with the fact that the efficient practice of her profession calls for a specific and consistent ethical attitude and that it is her task to create it, she will be reasoning from the objective facts to a decision. This is beginning from an objective perspective.

If one begins with her feelings, the way things seem, or decisions that one made in the past, and one neglects to look at the specific facts present here and now, one will be reasoning from a decision that is already made and trying to rationalize that decision. This is beginning from a subjective perspective. If one begins here, one may never get out of the subjective perspective into the realities and essentials of the profession. If one begins and ends with what others call to her attention, one will never get to her own knowledge, and will never know anything. If one begins and ends with the person within the entire context, one will end by integrating what she learns in each ethical dilemma into her present knowledge.

## THE NECESSARY, THE SUFFICIENT, AND THE ETHICAL

A crucial aspect of ethical reality becomes apparent in the following scenario:

You take your son to a pediatrician. The pediatrician tells you, "Your son will have to have a nephrectomy." You ask the pediatrician, "If my son undergoes a nephrectomy, will this be sufficient for his recovery?" The pediatrician replies, "No, in all honesty, I cannot say that the operation alone will bring about his recovery. The operation, in itself, will not be sufficient to bring your son back to good health." You then ask the pediatrician, "Is this operation a necessary part of my son's recovery? Would it be possible to bring him back to health without the operation?" The pediatrician replies, "Well, yes. There are other ways to treat him that will bring about an optimal recovery. The nephrectomy is not a necessary mode of treatment. In fact, the nephrectomy is neither sufficient in itself to return your son to health nor necessary for his recovery." You breathe a sigh of relief, leave quickly with your son, and never visit this pediatrician again. If one thing is neither necessary nor sufficient to bring about a second thing, it has no significant causal relation to the second thing (Mill, 1843). If a nephrectomy is neither necessary nor sufficient to the recovery of your son, it is entirely useless and irrelevant in relation to your son's treatment and recovery.

If an ethical approach provides what is necessary and an agent wants to succeed at ethical interaction, then she should follow this approach. It is necessary to her ethical action, which means that her ethical interactions cannot succeed without it. If it is sufficient, it is more desirable (it alone will bring about the desired outcome). It includes all that is necessary, so the necessary is no longer a relevant consideration. It is superior to any other way of directing her actions; therefore, she should embrace and implement it in preference to a different approach.

If an ethical approach is both necessary and sufficient, an agent should embrace and implement it. Because it is necessary, she cannot succeed without it. Because it is sufficient, nothing else is necessary. If an ethical approach is neither necessary nor sufficient and if it will not enable an agent to succeed at ethical interaction, it is of no use to her, regardless of whether or not her ethical interaction can succeed without it. There is no reason for her to embrace it.

## DILEMMA 5.6: RIGHTS OF A HOMOSEXUAL PARTNER

Cal and Art are homosexual partners and have been living together for 10 years. Cal is in the final stages of AIDS. He has not made out a living will or durable power of attorney for health care. The family has said that they want everything possible done to keep him alive. Cal is now in a coma and cannot speak for himself. Art has told the physician and the family that this is not what Cal wanted. He told Art that he did not want heroic measures at the end. The family will not listen to Art and are trying to forbid him to come into the room. What is necessary and what is sufficient to make a justifiable ethical decision in this context?

## RELEVANCE OF THE BIOETHICAL CATEGORIES TO DECISION MAKING

*I am a man. Nothing human is alien to me.*
　　—Terence, 163 BC, *Heauton Timoroumenos [The Self Tormentor,* Act I]

Under most circumstances, it is impossible to attain perfect certainty in ethical decision making. However, to justify her decisions and actions, a nurse must attain the certainty that her decisions and actions have relevance to her patient's situation. To deal with the choices she must make, a nurse must develop a sensitivity to what is happening, and she must allow herself to discover that the ideas that pass through her mind are not automatically and reliably correct: "Any ethical analysis that does not take account of uncertainty will be inadequate to the concrete realities of clinical practice" (Beresford, 1991, p. 9).

According to Aristotle (McKeon, 1941), every virtue is a form of excellence at a basic function. A virtuous person is one who acts well on the basis of efficient thinking. A virtuous nurse is a nurse who is competent at nursing practice as a result of efficient thinking. The actions of a competent nurse can be justified, the competence behind them being the standard of their justification. Through the bioethical categories, the nurse's practice can be exceptionally justified. The right thing to do is that which one has agreed to do when one has agreed to do that which one's profession consists in and what this implies.

"Context is complex and comprehensive, dynamic, and interactive. Despite how tempting and how much easier it is to resort to the general, the abstract, and the theoretical, any form of bioethics that does not put moral [ethical] problems in their myriad contexts is, in many senses of the word, unreal" (Hoffmaster, 2004, p. 40).

A practice-based ethic must be different: It cannot assume that knowledge of the right thing to do is possible without the supporting knowledge of the other categories (Table 5.2). Without this knowledge of why, how, with whom, and how far action is to be taken, the right thing to do is isolated, out of context, and uncertain. It is this knowledge that forms knowledge of the right thing to do. Without this knowledge, there is no knowledge of the right thing to do. The five rights of bioethical analysis, taken from Aristotle's work, *The Categories,* in which he says that the excellence of humans is shown in doing (Cooke & Tredennick, 1938):

- The right thing (the product of close analysis and understanding),
- At the right time (when the greatest good can be accomplished),
- For the right reason (through an appropriate motive),
- For the right person (the person with whom one is interacting),
- In the right way (in a way that does good or at least no harm), and
- To the right extent (balanced and proportionate).

"The virtuous nurse cares for the patient, for his/her feelings, and his/her vulnerability, because she has learned to do the right things, at the right time, and for the right reasons" (Näsman, 2010, cited in Näsman, Nyström, & Eriksson, 2012).

## PURPOSE AND JUSTIFICATION

Both intention and effect are relevant to the quality of an ethical action. If one does not intend to do good but does so by accident, that person is not praiseworthy. Tschudin asserts: "People do not only have to do good but they also have to be good, that is they have to work and live out of personal and corporate values that are integral to how to deal with each other" (2013, p. 124). Intention is important—not sufficient, but

## TABLE 5.2  THE FIVE RIGHTS OF BIOETHICAL ANALYSIS

| Doing the Right Thing | How to Do the Right Thing |
| --- | --- |
| At the right time | When it is known to be the right thing and when the action will be most effective |
| For the right reason | With the knowledge of why this is the right thing to do |
| With the right person | When the person with whom one is interacting is the person with whom one ought to be interacting with and in relation to whom ethical actions can be known to be relevant and appropriate |
| In the right way | Knowing not only that is it the right thing to do but also that it is being done in a way designed to produce the greatest foreseeable benefit |
| To the right extent | With the appropriate expenditure of time and effort—neither deficiently nor excessively |

necessary. When a nurse is able to justify her thinking, she is not to blame for her actions. If she has done the best she can given the context of her knowledge, this is all that can be asked of her. When a nurse is unable to justify her thinking, her actions are not worth praise. If the good results that came from her actions were accidental, there is nothing in this for which she can be praised.

A nurse justifies her actions by describing how these actions would accomplish an ethical purpose. The purpose that justifies her actions is the subject of the agreement. Along with the purpose, there may also be an agreement on the actions that may or may not be taken.

For a decision or action to be justified, four conditions are necessary:

- The goal of the decision or action must be this predetermined purpose.
- There must be reason to believe that this decision or action will tend to bring about the accomplishment of its purpose.
- It must not be an action prohibited by the agreement.
- It must not be an action that would interfere with actions specified in the agreement.

In a health care setting, the bioethical agreement is an instrument by which both professional and patient can maximize the benefits of their relationship. Without the agreement, there would be no professional criteria on which to base ethical judgments. Each party to the agreement has ethical responsibilities according to the terms of the agreement and only according to these terms. The nature and terms of the agreement between nurse and patient are usually not made explicit and directly discussed or written down by the participants. However, the terms of this agreement are generally known and accepted.

## MUSING

If an ethical agent were to take actions without reference to the context, the actions would be irrelevant to the person's actions. One's actions would be meaningless and purposeless. **For this reason, a discussion of ethical issues in isolation from a context can never lead to a meaningful ethical decision.** Outside of the context, there is no way to differentiate between the relevant and the irrelevant. "The ethical quality of care practices can be improved by considering their contextual embeddedness" (Gastmans, 2011).

Furthermore, discussion of ethical issues outside of a specific context can be detrimental. Discussing issues in isolation from a context can lead a nurse or any agent to a predetermined conclusion. For this reason, discussions of ethical issues often serve not to strengthen and to expand a nurse's knowledge but to divert her attention from the patient's context. It is very easy to discuss issues such as organ transplantation, abortion, cloning, euthanasia, the use of fetal tissue, genetic engineering, treatment of anencephalic infants, and human experimentation, and so forth, and come away from the discussion with nothing to apply to a real-life dilemma.

The context of the situation is associated with an agent's purposes and actions and is composed of the facts that can assist or hinder her purposes and actions. A nurse's context of knowledge, including her awareness of relevant principles of judgment, enables her to recognize the context of the situation. Attention to the aspects of the situation that are relevant to her purposes through the context of her awareness makes it possible for an agent to relate her ethical actions to her ethical purposes.

Achieving awareness of the context means integrating that which is present in one's awareness of the circumstances into all of the relevant knowledge that one possesses. Achieving awareness of the context is a process of assimilating the context of the situation into a context of knowledge. Losing awareness of the context means ignoring relevant items of knowledge or relevant aspects of the situation. Failing to achieve awareness of the context is the worst possible way to begin a decision-making process. Not having awareness of the context makes it impossible to justify a decision or to act effectively.

When a nurse retains awareness of the bioethical context, she and her patient are most apt to gain the maximum benefit of ethical action. Success follows effective action. Effective action follows active awareness.

"The nurse functions both as a professional and as a human being within a variety of contexts. These contexts influence directly or indirectly the way in which the nurse performs caring tasks" (Gastmans, 1998, p. 236).

There is a group of facts naturally tending to form a unique and intelligible context when a nurse and patient come together. A patient needs a nurse to provide him with the benefit of her professional skills. A nurse needs a patient in order to live her professional role. These facts establish a relationship between them through a meeting of the minds. This meeting is a tacit agreement to interact and has this as its purpose—their interactive self-directedness—the control by each of their time and effort into intelligible causal sequences.

> Achieving awareness of the context means integrating that which is present in one's awareness of the circumstances into all of the relevant knowledge that one possesses. Achieving awareness of the context is a process of assimilating the context of the situation into a context of knowledge. Losing awareness of the context means ignoring relevant items of knowledge or relevant aspects of the situation.

## STUDY GUIDE

1. Give an example of how you have used context today in making a decision. It may not have been an ethical decision, but context is something we use every day and throughout our day.
2. Imagine to yourself a health care system devoid of any attention to the context. What would you see? Try to further imagine functioning in this system.
3. How does the interweaving of the three aspects of the context help guide your bioethical decision making? Are they all necessary?
4. What can be learned from the humorous vignette "The Queen of Hearts"?

5. What is the meaning of the Terrence quote?
6. Explain the difference between the necessary and the sufficient. Give an example of when something could be necessary but not sufficient or when something is sufficient in itself.
7. What is the relationship of the agreement to the context?
8. Use this case for class discussion; the analysis of the case only appears in the instructor's manual.

---

### RESPECTING THE LIVING WILL OR GOING AGAINST IT

Seven years ago, Beth and her husband's 2-year-old son was kidnapped. They have never found him alive or dead. Beth, age 42, is in the hospital dying of ovarian cancer. In all probability she will be sent home to die once the physician has controlled her pain. She is alert and able to get around, although she is weak. She has a living will, which states, among other things, that she does not want to be connected to any machines or to have cardiopulmonary resuscitation (CPR) performed. The physician has written a do not resuscitate (DNR) order. To better control her pain, the physician has ordered a new drug in addition to her morphine drip. You give the drug by intramuscular injection. Within minutes of receiving the drug, Beth has what you believe to be an anaphylactic reaction and goes into respiratory arrest. At the moment that Beth arrests, a colleague rushes in to say that they have just received a call from Beth's husband. The child has been found alive and well. You know your colleague to be entirely reliable. What should you do ethically?

---

## REFERENCES

Beresford, E. B. (1991). Uncertainty and the shaping of medical decision. *Hastings Center Report, 21*(4), 6–11.

The case of the embryos without parents. (2000). *Bioethics Case Study*. Retrieved October 24, 2006, from http://www.mhhe.com/biosci/genbio/olc_linked-content/bioethics_cases/g-bioe-04.htm

Cooke, H. P., & Tredennick, H. (1938). *The categories: On interpretation*. Cambridge, MA: Harvard University Press.

Gastmans, C. (1998). Challenges to nursing values in a changing nursing environment. *Nursing Ethics, 4*, 236–244.

Gastmans, C. Ethics of care.org/interview/ Sharing views on Good care, April 8, 2011.

Hoffmaster, B. (2004). 'Real' ethics for 'real' boys: Context and narrative. *The American Journal of Bioethics, 4*, 40–41.

Hospers, J. (1972). *Human conduct: Problems of ethics*. New York, NY: Harcourt Brace Jovanovich.

Husted, G. L., & Husted, J. H. (2004). Nursing ethics. In J. Daly, S. Speedy, D. Jackson, & V. Lambert (Eds.), *Professional nursing: Concepts, issues, and challenges* (pp. 174–191). New York, NY: Springer.

Husted, J. H., & Husted, G. L. (1993). Personal and impersonal values in bioethical decision making. *Journal of Home Health Care Practice, 4*(4), 49–64.

McKeon, R. (Ed.). (1941). *The basic works of Aristotle.* New York, NY: Random House.

Mill, J. S. (1843). *A system of logic.* London, England: Oxford Press.

Näsman, Y. (2010). *Habits of the heart, benevolence of the mind, and deeds of the hand— Virtue as a basic concept in caring science* (Dissertation ÅboAkademis förlag, Turku, Finland). (Cited in Näsman, Y., Nyström, L., & Eriksson, K. (2012). From values to virtue: The basis for quality of care. *International Journal For Human Caring, 16*(2), 50–56.)

Terence, 163 BC, *Heauton Timoroumenos (The Self Tormentor),* Act I.

Tschudin, V. (2013). Two decades of Nursing Ethics: Some thoughts on the changes. *Nursing Ethics, 20,* 123–126.

Wurzbach, M. E. (1999). Acute care nurses' experiences of moral certainty. *Advanced Nursing, 30,* 287–293.

# SIX

# CONTEMPORARY ETHICAL SYSTEMS

**OBJECTIVES**

- Compare and contrast the appropriateness of the ethical systems of deontology, utilitarianism, social/cultural relativism, and emotivism with regard to bioethics.

- Examine the purpose of an ethical system as it relates to health care.

- Consider the foundational concepts of commonly used ethical systems.

- Discuss the relationship of duty and justification.

- Explore the ethical practice of triage situations.

The function of an ethical code can be compared with the function of a travel agent. A vacation involves many decisions: the time of departure; the location, attractions, and accommodations; the cost; and more. Would any sensible person put his or her entire vacation into the hands of a travel agent, letting the agent decide the time of departure, the destination, the length of the stay, and so on? In that case, the traveler's desires would play no part in the planning of the vacation. No sensible person would agree to this arrangement, yet many otherwise intelligent people will make this arrangement with an ethical theory. They will turn their lives over to a random hodge-podge of notions that they have chosen or have had chosen for them. For many people the mandates of their ethical system may be in conflict with good judgment or a humane approach to human problems or anything resembling relevance. Nevertheless, the mandates of their ethical system are imperatives; they are essential obligations.

In our culture at this time, two broad theories of ethics are dominant: deontology and utilitarianism. If nursing and medical practice were to be patterned after the contemporary ethical systems, it would return practice to its nightmarish era of 1,000 years ago.

## DEONTOLOGY

According to deontology, right and wrong are the central ethical concepts. Ethical action consists of doing right; this is considered one's duty. To do one's duty is right. To shirk one's duty is wrong. The ethical agent has a duty to take the right action and to refrain from taking the wrong action. Beyond this, nothing is ethically relevant. The results of an action may be desired or deplored, but they have no ethical relevance.

The notion of duty as central to ethics arose with the Stoic philosophers about 300 BC, but its most powerful impetus was given by the German philosopher Immanuel Kant (1724–1804). The concept of duty is unrelated to our everyday concerns. Kant developed his duty ethic in response to the social subjectivism of David Hume (1711–1776). Hume argued that reason cannot be the only motivation for morality. He believed that feelings and passions are the true motivators of human action and, therefore, responsible for ethical action. This can be summarized by: "X is right" means society approves X. "X is wrong" means society disapproves of X (Hume, 1748/1955).

On the other hand, Kant believed that human experiences are structured by the mind, and that, on an abstract level, all human experience shares certain essential features. In this way there is a commonality of human thought so that "the good" (one's duty) can be, and is, innately known by all (Warburton, 2011). Kant held that the concept of duty is an innate idea. One is born knowing that he must do his duty and what his duty is (Kant, 1785/1964). This notion is also highly doubtful. In order to know the demands that duty laid upon him, a newborn would need to know of the relationships existing between himself and the world. To know this, he would need to know of the nature of the world. He would need to know this before even knowing that there is a world. This is impossible.

Kant offered the idea that we are born with a capacity to call on a spontaneous knowledge of our duty. Kant was confident that when a dilemma arises, we are presented with an awareness of our appropriate duty through a power of internal perception or intuition.

Deontology is a duty-based ethic that directs actions taken by the agent, while ignoring concern for rewards, happiness, or any resulting consequences (Hill & Zweig, 2003). Deontology is the theory that "action in conformance with formal rules of conduct, are obligatory regardless of their results" (Angeles, 1992).

Aside from assuming that all individuals have innate knowledge of right and wrong, a duty ethic is viciously circular. The right action is that action which one ought to take because one ought to take that action which is right. There is a logical drawback to this. It proves that which is doubtful (that people have duties) in terms of that which is even more doubtful (that people innately know what is right). It is like proving that the sun will rise at noon (a doubtful possibility) by declaring that Martians will cause this to happen (a much more doubtful possibility).

Deontology, as a bioethic, has not functioned well in the past. It is unsuited to be a bioethic in many ways. It calls for us to act on the rightness of an action and not consider the results. It assumes:

- That we know our duty—that which is right.
- That the duty most appropriate to a circumstance is known through a storehouse of innate ideas possessed by the mind before birth and to the onset of sense experience.
- That we possess a sort of intuitive "moral sense" which reveals to us the appropriate duty to be performed.
- That our duty is revealed to us by the interplay of our store of knowledge and our intuitive moral sense.

This requires that we are born knowing the nature of our ethical relationship to the world. This explains the doubtful (we have knowledge before we have experience of anything knowable), in terms of the impossible (we have the ability to use the logic necessary to interpret that which is presented by the moral sense), before we know anything.

Deontology is established by the fact that, supposedly, we do not know that it is not true. It would be impossible to offer positive evidence for this theory. The entire idea is a groundless assumption born in Kant's imagination. It is based on the secondary assumptions of the existence of innate ideas and of a faculty of intuition. These assumptions have nothing to recommend them other than the fact that they are assumed. Their denial would be equally reliable for it can be based on equally weighty (or weightless) assumptions.

In all cases, the duty that is chosen must be assumed to be the appropriate duty. If this assumption is trusted to be reliable, then an assumption that it is unreliable will be equally trustworthy for it has as much (and as little) to recommend it. However, the theory also calls for us to understand that duties are not chosen. They are given by insight and the moral sense. To choose a duty would be to violate the spirit of duty. Duties are given to be accepted.

## DUTY AND JUSTIFICATION

Deontology demands that right actions be taken without regard to conse-quences. A nurse cannot justify taking an action without concern for the effects it will produce. She should always be able to justify her action in terms of its foreseeable consequences. Could a nurse justify causing harm to a patient by saying, "I was doing my duty"? This would not suffice legally. It surely does not suffice ethically—not if *ethically* is understood in any practical or rational sense.

If the purpose of an ethical system is to serve human life—or the efficient functioning of a profession—then deontology is not an ethical system. It is the absence of an ethical system. Consider this: The original deontologists preached the rightness of duty in action. They saw that, for a person to blindly follow his or her duty, a certain mind-set had to be achieved. The permanent possession of this mind-set was the purpose of deontology—so that one would always carry out his or her duty. The Stoics called this phenomenon *apatheia*, which means apathy produced by living in the straitjacket of deontology. A modern name for it is *burnout*. Apathy demands indifference to pain or pleasure, health or illness, hap-piness or misery. The father of modern deontology, Immanuel Kant, sings the praises of apathy in the preface to *Groundwork for the Metaphysics of Morals* (1785/1964) in a section entitled "Virtue Necessarily Presupposes Apathy (Considered as Strength)."

The Stoics were inspired by the idea that the best thing about life is death. The best way to live is to grit your teeth and get it over with. To make this possible, they adopted a duty ethic in order to develop an indifference to the ebb and flow of fortune. Indifference is an undesir-able quality in a nurse. It is the opposite of what a nurse's state of mind ought to be, but one cannot consistently practice deontology without it. The practice of a duty ethic has never benefited patients or nursing—and certainly not individual nurses.

Nevertheless, many ethicists regard duty and morality as equiva-lent terms. They claim that ethics and deontology are identical. If this is true, then the only task of ethics is to list a person's duties, and, given intuitionism and the moral sense, this is unnecessary. The best a deon-tologist–ethicist can do is to give instructions to infallible abilities. "The idea that we are following rules when we act morally is a tired hangover from the days when the lives of people were controlled by religious and secular absolute rulers who accorded no respect or autonomy [indepen-dence] to ordinary people" (van Hooft, 1990, p. 211).

Nurses cannot escape taking the role of ethical agents. It is entirely unreasonable for a nurse to rely on an unfounded innate and prerational sense of duty. To do this, she must convince herself that she has an innate and prerational sense of duty. Innate knowledge is knowledge that is not learned from experience. This means that innate knowledge has no sup-porting evidence. It is knowledge that one has no reason to believe. An ethical nurse acts within the context of what is known.

---

*Deontology demands that right actions be taken without regard to consequences. A nurse cannot justify taking an action without concern for the effects it will produce*

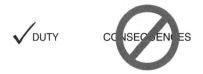

**FIGURE 6.1** Duty rules.

Deontology is entirely concerned with an agent's actions. It is unconcerned with consequences (Figure 6.1). It is also indifferent to the agent's intentions, except the agent's intention to do his or her duty. In principle, deontology demands indifference to individual autonomy. The recognition of autonomy would require that a nurse make choices appropriate to the uniqueness of her patient. Yet, in deontology, the demands of duty are imperative—they do not allow for choices to be made on the part of a nurse. Autonomous differences among patients call for a nurse to analyze each situation. A deontologist who analyzed contextual differences and made choices based on her analysis would have, perhaps unknowingly, abandoned deontology. A nurse who abandons her patient in order to pursue her duty has abandoned nursing.

---

### DILEMMA 6.1: DUTY OR SAVING A LIFE?

A nurse, Ralph, is hired to care for a wealthy man, Francis, on his estate. A prerequisite of Ralph's employment is that it will be his duty not to enter the swimming pool on the estate while Francis is using it. Francis fears that someone else in the swimming pool might contaminate it and transmit a fatal disease to him—a frail, vulnerable man. Francis is an extreme germophobe. One day, while sitting beside the pool, Ralph notices that Francis is foundering. He slips under water and does not resurface. Ralph immediately rises to go into the swimming pool and get Francis out. Then he remembers the ethical responsibility that his duty has placed upon him. So Ralph sits back down. Ralph resists the flood of ideas and emotions that rush through his mind. Within the constraints placed on him by duty, what can Ralph do? Granted, this is a silly case, but look at it on its own merits: It teaches one the difference of acting in the context or on one's duty.

---

While reading this section, any nurse might be tempted to think, "Ridiculous! Ethical decisions in health care are not made in this way." Yet, if you attend an Ethics Committee meeting (albeit not all), you will see deontological process is very commonly used. The details of a patient's situation will be reported in depth, and the first thing used to determine the best course of action is to consult the protocols, procedures, and standards of care for direction. Nurses routinely rely on deontological process when they refuse patient visitors because it is not visiting hours or the visitor is not a legal relative. Although visiting hours have been expanded in many places, the reality is that it is not universal. In addition, those areas that claim "open visiting" are often able to "close" visiting as it suits them. Of course, "closing" is meant to be in the best interest of the patient—but often is about other things. When there are semiprivate rooms involved, what is good for one patient may not be good for the other, so a nurse can choose to be legalistic—instead of working on a more creative solution. Patients in pain are forced to wait until "it is time." Disruptive patients, those who are being disrespectful or threating, may be treated according to the specific protocol of the policy: loss of privileges, isolation, or other sanctions, rather than taking the time to address the source of the behavior.

Policies are necessary but they are not perfect and should act only as more of a framework than anything else. Institutional or unit policies are often used to respond to patients' or significant others' needs. Anytime a nurse resorts to following a policy rather than finding a solution to a problem, she is choosing a deontological path, choosing duty in direct opposition to human and professional values.

Case 5.5 is an example of a husband and surgeon doing their duty for the best interest of the patient in direct opposition to what the patient stated she wanted.

> I think that nurses assume the **duty mind-set** when they do not have time to think out of the box or when they are not in touch with their patients. I think the biggest issue today for nurses is relationships and the impact that these have on doing their duty. The power relationships of more senior peers, physicians, and other leadership personnel have a huge influence on the choices that nurses make. They may not call a particularly challenging physician at night even though a patient has a need (the nurse may minimize the need to avoid a nasty interchange). They also may respect a physician highly and therefore not want to challenge an order or a procedure that the physician wants to perform. There is an unwritten policy in every hospital that I have worked in that the physician is the captain of the ship and what they say, goes. Mentoring nurses in managing that relationship is extremely important but takes quite awhile to accomplish. In the meantime you have one rule (duty) driven nurse. (Personal communication, Nurse Administrator, 2014)

## UTILITARIANISM

The idea of modern utilitarianism was first introduced by Jeremy Bentham (1748–1832) and brought to its full development by John Stuart Mill (1806–1873). The central ethical concepts of utilitarianism are good and evil. It is the doctrine that an ethical agent's responsibility is to bring about "the greatest good for the greatest number."

Utilitarianism was inspired by determinism. Determinism is the doctrine that every human action is a response to a prior event. This prior event originates outside of the person who is acting without volition in a predetermined way. The determinist holds that deciding and choosing are illusions. Determinists describe the feeling of being able to control one's thoughts and actions as a kind of dream. Psychological hedonism is a form of determinism. It is the doctrine that every action of an agent is a response to the experience or the expectation of pleasure or pain. It holds that one acts only to seek pleasure and to avoid pain and holds that one cannot act otherwise because this tendency is inborn.

Utilitarians claim that people cannot escape holding pleasure to be the good. Their next step was to argue for the necessity of the principle that approves or disapproves of every action whatsoever according to the tendency that it appears to have to augment or to diminish the happiness of the party whose interest is in question (Bentham, 1879/1962). That is, an action is determined to be good or to be bad based on whether it increases the happiness/pleasure of an individual. This led to the idea that the good of two persons is better than the good of one; the good of three is better than the good of two, and so on. The greatest possible good, then, would be the good of everyone, or the good of the greatest possible number. This good, they declared, ought to be the goal of every ethical agent.

> An action is determined to be good or to be bad based on whether it increases the happiness/pleasure of an individual.

Early opponents were quick to point out flaws in this reasoning. Thomas Carlyle (1795–1881) called utilitarianism a "pig philosophy." He noted that in every conceivable way, a symphony by Beethoven was a greater good than the victory of a pig wrestler. In fact, Beethoven's creativity, from every point of view, seems a greater good than the victories of a large number of pig wrestlers (Trail, 1896).

In response to this, utilitarians amended their principle to read "The greatest (or highest) good of the greatest number." This reasoning ignores four relevant facts:

1. Let us grant that a person, through psychological necessity, holds his own pleasure to be an end in itself. This fact, in itself, gives him no reason, logical or otherwise, to concern himself with the good of others. A person might hold his good to be of value to him not because it is a good, but because it is his good. His own good might be uniquely valued by him. Utilitarianism holds that the good of one agent is freely interchangeable with the good of another. In this manner, personal good loses its motivational relevance.

   Let us imagine someone for whom this is the case. Joe is very excited about going to a rock concert. Sally tells him that she is also going. Now, Joe is no longer excited. If Sally is going, it does not matter to Joe whether he goes as long as someone goes. Joe regards values as interchangeable. Psychologically, this does not make sense, but it is utilitarianism's view of human nature.

2. It is difficult to see how a nurse could justify actions by reference to "the greatest good for the greatest number." Her primary responsibility is to her individual patient. Her patient, in turn, has a right

to choose his own goals and the consequences he seeks. He has a right to choose highly individualistic goals based solely on his own desires.

Utilitarianism not only directs us to consider the results of an action when making moral judgments but also holds that we should look only to results. Considerations of one's feelings or convictions are seen as irrelevant to the question "What is the right thing to do?" (Arras & Hunt cited in Arras & Rhoden, 1989, p. 8). A nurse in pursuit of "the greatest good of the greatest number" would have no time to attend to her individual patients. Nor would the patients have any right to expect individualized nursing treatment from her. Being a nurse would not allow her to take ethical action. It would be a wall between her and the possibility of ethical action.

3. Utilitarianism collapses into deontology. This has finally been recognized even by utilitarians. To address this flaw, a distinction was drawn between *rule utilitarianism* and *act utilitarianism*. Rule utilitarians claim that an agent has a duty to obey certain rules. These are the rules best adapted to bring about the greatest good for the greatest number. Act utilitarians declare that the value of an action is determined by its goal. This simply means that an agent has a duty to aim for a specific goal. He or she has a duty to act to bring about the greatest good for the greatest number. Utilitarians cannot escape deontology.

4. Justice is the most highly honored interpersonal virtue of our society. It is the goal of our entire legal system. Ironically, utilitarianism is a prescription for injustice.

> *One such limitation [of utilitarianism as an ethical theory] is the violation of personal autonomy . . . its inherent potential for discrimination, the possibility that what is perceived as "good" for the majority may be bad for the minority.* (Franklin, 1988, p. 35)

In fact, it is somewhat worse than that.

> *Utilitarianism . . . has fallen into bad odor, and particularly when it comes to a defense of individual rights and personal liberties . . . suppose . . . the general welfare of the community, or the greatest happiness of the greatest number, might conceivably be furthered or increased by the sacrifice of the liberty, or the well-being, or even the life of a single individual . . . [Would not this sacrifice be] . . . the moral consequence of anyone's adhering strictly to Utilitarian principles.* (Veatch, 1985, pp. 30–31)

Utilitarianism requires an agent to do that action which brings about the greatest balance of good over evil in the universe as a whole . . . to maximize the good of all humans . . . to consider all of the available alternatives and perform that act which will maximize the good of all affected parties

Nevertheless, utilitarianism is today's dominant ethical trend. Many nursing ethics textbooks recommend it as a tool for ethical decision making. However, utilitarianism requires an agent to do that action which brings about the greatest balance of good over evil in the universe as a whole . . . to maximize the good of all humans . . .

to consider all of the available alternatives and perform that act which will maximize the good of all affected parties (McConnell, 1982, p. 14).

This is utilitarianism. Does it not seem unreasonable to expect a nurse to know:

- What action will bring about "the greatest balance of good over evil in the universe as a whole"?
- What the nature of "the greatest balance of good over evil in the universe as a whole" might look like?
- How one might "maximize the good of all humans"?
- The precise number of "all of the available alternatives"?
- Precisely that "act that will maximize the good of all affected parties"?

Suppose that, by some miracle, the nurse could know all this. Even then, how could utilitarianism be justified in a health care system that places a high value on the individual's rights and autonomy? "No action is, in itself, ethically good or bad. Utilitarians hold that the only factors that make actions good or bad are the outcomes, or end results, that are derived from them" (Burkhardt & Nathaniel, 2002, p. 28). Utilitarianism is a theory in which the ends justify the means (Gibson, 1993). The utilitarian's ethical advice consists of emotionally charged, high-flying, and empty phrases urging the pursuit of the impossible. It is an impractical approach to the practical science.

## DILEMMA 6.2: IMPLIED CONSENT OR VIOLATION OF ONE'S RIGHTS?

A John Doe came in with a massive subdural hematoma. He had surgery and was not doing well. The police helped to identify him but were unable to locate next of kin. The following night, he progressed to brain death. Donor network was notified per protocol. The patient could not express his wishes and there was no family, not even a friend or girlfriend, to tell the team what he would want. In the morning the donor coordinator had a meeting with the MDs and the hospital attorney to document that everything had been done to try to locate his family and that the patient was an excellent candidate for organ donation. They proceeded to take him to the operating room (OR) and harvest his organs. Were there any rights violations involved in doing this?

## TELISHMENT

*Telishment* is a term coined by John Rawls, a philosopher who focused on justice. Telishment derives from the words *telos,* the end or the purpose of a process meant to achieve a goal (Angeles, 1992), and *-ment,* as in *punishment.* This term is used to criticize utilitarianism.

## DILEMMA 6.3: TELISHMENT

Utilityville is a village run on utilitarian principles. Periodically, the town fathers randomly choose someone to serve the community. They put this person in chains in the public square and torture him to death. They inflict a punishment on this innocent person similar to but milder than that which they would inflict on a habitual criminal.

The death of this unfortunate benefactor serves the community in two ways:

1. Once they witness the gruesome fate of an entirely innocent person, potential criminals can imagine, in bloodcurdling detail, the horrible fate awaiting the guilty. This leads a number of potential criminals away from a life of crime and a horrible death by torture. This, in itself, brings about "the greatest good for the greatest number."
2. Many people who would otherwise be victims of crime are saved from this fate by the death of the village benefactor.

The town fathers have found a very effective way to bring about "the greatest good for the greatest number." They save potential victims by making actual victims. However, this violates any rational conception of justice. There is nothing in utilitarianism to prevent any crime by a greater number against a lesser number or against an individual. Individual justice is necessary to a civilized human existence and to objectively justifiable ethical action. Nothing in the principle of utility establishes or protects the principle of individual justice (Sarikonda-Woitas & Robinson, 2002).

Societies based on individual rights, nonaggression, and interaction through agreement flourish far better than utilitarian societies. It is clear that utilitarianism is not necessary to rational, ethical interaction. As an ethical approach, utilitarianism neither is sufficient in itself nor is a necessary addition to other approaches to bring about justifiable ethical action.

No health care setting should be a Utilityville. Utility undermines a professional's ethical awareness by directing her away from the objectives of her profession. Under utilitarianism, reciprocity, cooperation, trust, and respect for individual rights have no ethical import because none of these serves utility. It is interesting to consider here the radical difference if the principle of utility—each serving the greatest good of the others—had been replaced with the principle of reciprocity. This would be the greatest good, by the greatest number, for the greatest number.

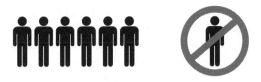

**FIGURE 6.2** Numbers rule.

## TRIAGE

Triage is not a contemporary ethical system. It is an objectively justifiable ethical practice. A triage situation comes to mind as the scene of disaster, a major fire, a train wreck, or some emergency situation. With the exception of paramedics and emergency room personnel, few health care professionals normally face situations as tense and confusing as these. Yet, every nurse's shift has elements in common with triage situations. Patients constantly enter and leave the health care setting. The conditions and the needs of patients are constantly changing. A nurse's professional actions are best approached with triage elements in mind. An efficient nurse must be able to meet the ethical demands of the profession with a consistent mind-set and awareness appropriate to the unpredictable.

Every triage situation, from the most catastrophic to the everyday, calls for ethical balance and proportion. Even in situations that are not so complex or demanding as a catastrophic situation, the health care setting itself is a continual triage situation. Every time a professional enters the health care setting, some patients, or one patient, will have needs greater than others. A nurse masters the problem of ethical balance and proportion as she learns to identify these patients. The mastery of this art (ethical balance and proportion) can be seen in an analysis of a hypothetical situation.

Arletta and Francine share a home that is burning down, and some of their possessions have been left inside. Arletta is upset because her wedding dress has been left behind. Francine is distressed to realize that her dog is trapped in the house. Bill, a firefighter, has an opportunity to act beneficently in this situation. He is able to help either Francine or Arletta, but not both. In and of themselves, neither Arletta nor Francine is intrinsically more deserving than the other. How can Bill make the best decision?

There is no doubt that some possessions are more important than others. So all possible possessions can be in effect, evaluated and numbered by Bill. He can rate them from 1 to 10 according to their importance: Suppose class 1 possessions are those that are least in importance and class 10 possessions are those that are most important. A class 3 possession will not be prized by the person who holds it as much as a class 8 possession will be prized. In a triage situation, the benefactor analyzes the situation in this way: Bill will ask himself, "If Arletta and Francine were not two persons but only one, what would be the best thing for me to do?" He knows very well that Arletta and Francine are not one person, but in this situation, in order for him to make the best decision, he will think of them as if they were. He will act as if they were one person with two possessions. He will rescue the possession that would be the more highly rated by this person.

If Bill can bring just one thing from the burning building, he will bring out Francine's dog rather than Arletta's wedding dress. He will judge that, if Francine and Arletta were one person, this person would rate her dog at least an 8, whereas she would rate her wedding dress perhaps a 3.

Although it is one person's dog and another person's wedding dress, Bill would still rescue Francine's dog for the same reason. He judges Francine's dog, Tippy, a living thing, to be an 8 to Francine; he judges Arletta's wedding dress to be a 3 to Arletta. He will rescue Tippy because this is what is called for in the triage situation. The triage situation is an ethical situation where all the potential beneficiaries become one person. The professional commitment is not to an individual but to everyone involved taken as one person so that the most appropriate beneficiary can be discovered.

In a triage situation, there is another consideration in addition to the value of a benefit. We have been assuming that there is an equal probability of Bill's being able to salvage either Tippy or Arletta's dress. We have assumed that the risk to Bill is equal in both cases. The likelihood of a benefactor being able to bring about different benefits and the risks involved must also be weighed. If Bill could easily salvage Arletta's wedding dress but the probability of his rescuing Francine's dog was very low and/or the peril to him was very high, then it might be more reasonable for him to salvage Arletta's wedding dress.

Suppose there had been three persons living in the home and each one, including Francine and Arletta, had wedding dresses hanging in the same closet. Triage-type thinking would still bring out Tippy. George, a utilitarian, would multiply $3 \times 3$, which is 9. Nine is a higher number than 8. Therefore, George would save the wedding dresses, leaving Tippy behind to perish.

In a triage situation, a health care professional must sort out all the possible benefits to everyone involved in the situation—wounded soldiers on a battlefield, people injured in an airline disaster, people trapped in a burning building—regardless of whose benefits they are. She cannot make her decision according to the normal professional–patient agreement. Therefore, she must make it according to the benefits that she can bring about without encountering significant danger.

If a nurse on a battlefield finds a soldier with a broken arm and a sprained ankle, she will attend to the arm first. If she finds two soldiers, one with a broken arm and one with a sprained ankle, she will attend to the one with the broken arm for the same reason. This is the most critical benefit she can bring about in this situation.

After an airline disaster, a nurse might treat the severe bleeding of a person with a broken back before immobilizing him. His bleeding presents a greater threat to his life than does his back. There is something she can do for his bleeding and little she can do for his back. In addition, his bleeding presents a greater threat to his life than does his back. If she found two survivors, one with severe bleeding and the other with a broken back, she would attend to the one with the severe bleeding for the same reason that she would attend to an individual person's bleeding before attending to his back.

According to the triage analysis, a health care professional ought to choose her beneficiary according to:

- The importance of the benefit.
- The probability of her being able to bring about the benefit.
- The risks, if any, she will encounter.

In a triage situation, she ought to regard every possible beneficiary as one person. Then she ought to direct her actions according to the most rational desires of this one person. This is what an objective reading of the situation calls for her to do. According to her education, training, and experience, a nurse would recognize this action as having the greatest objective value. As members of the human race, patients in a triage situation would recognize this action as having the greatest objective value.

The analogy between the triage situation and the professional's everyday circumstances is obvious. If the benefit to one patient is rated a 6 and the benefit to another patient is rated a 7, and providing the first patient's benefit would interfere with the second patient's benefit, the professional should act for the benefit of the second patient first. When it is possible to benefit everyone, then everyone ought to be benefited. When this is not possible, then those individuals who can be brought the greatest benefit ought to be the beneficiaries of a nurse's actions. To analyze a triage situation, the nurse considers every potential beneficiary as being one person. In the context of a triage situation, the nurse ought to bring about the greatest benefit. She ought to do this because this is what the rational desire of this one person would want her to do. Nurses face triage-type situations frequently in their practice as there can be competing needs and nurses, unfortunately, have to make decisions regarding this.

## SOCIAL/CULTURAL RELATIVISM

Ethical relativism is the view that the rightness of an action and the goodness of an object depend on, or consist of, the attitudes taken toward it by some individuals or groups (Runes, 1983). No individual or group has superiority over another. Different cultures espouse

Human rights do not
exist according to a
relativist.

different moral values; therefore, there are no universal moral values shared by every human society. Human rights do not exist according to a relativist.

Beginning in fifth century Greece, relativism was rarely employed until the 19th and 20th centuries. At that time, the historical context made "social" relativism appear reasonable. This was due to several things: a new awareness of cultural diversity, the diminishing importance of religion in modernized cultures, the questioning of colonialism and its inference of moral superiority over the occupied societies, and growing skepticism toward any form of moral objectivism, given the difficulty of proving value judgments the same way one proves factual claims (Harré & Krausz, 1996).

At any time, the values of a society may shift. As a society adopts a value, it may be because it is the simplest way to solve a problem, or for no reason at all. There is no method to determine whether a value chosen by a society is good.

If, at a certain time, a society decides that kidnapping is evil, is kidnapping evil because of the nature of kidnapping or because the society decides that it is evil? Or, if a society believes that human sacrifice is good, is it good because society believes it is good or is it good because of its intrinsic nature that sacrifice is good?

We must be able to recognize the good before we can know that this is where the sentiments of the society lead us. If we know that that which society approves is evil, then we ought to reject relativism. If we know that that which society approves is good, then the approval of society is unnecessary. If we do not know, then there is no virtue in following society. We may as well follow a fortune-teller or a magician. The sentiments of society are equally superfluous.

---

### DILEMMA 6.4: RIGHT TO ONE'S OWN BODY

Fauzuja Kassindja is 17. She is facing an arranged marriage and female circumcision (usually done between the ages of 4 and 12 but in her country it is done along with the marriage celebration). She does not want this. She was able to flee her country and come to America to ask for asylum. This brought public attention in the United States to this practice. Was she wrong in wanting to go against the practices of her country? Should she have been granted asylum? (Althaus, 1997)

---

Concern with what the society feels is not a way to understand anything except to understand what the society approves or what the society feels or intuits. From knowing what the society feels, one could never become aware of the significance and importance of the society's feelings. Worse than this, one might never become aware of the insignificance or the harms caused by acting on the feelings of society.

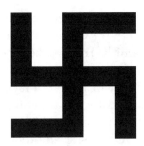

**FIGURE 6.3** Society rules.

No argument for social or cultural relativism or any type of relativism as an objectively justifiable bioethical guide can succeed. The argument would have to begin by assuming that individuals, alone or together, are incapable of judging what is good or evil in relation to them. Otherwise, there would be no need for an external guide. Then the values and feelings of society are set up as the standards of ethical judgment. It is assumed by the relativist that the sentiments of society are reliable ethical principles. This implies the following:

- The society or culture or religion is capable of judging what the individual cannot, what is ultimately good or evil in relation to the individual.
- The individual is capable of discovering that the ethical judgment of the society is valid, and that of the individual is not.

In order to do this, the individual must be capable of recognizing the validity of an ethical judgment in order to judge the judgment of society. And, if the individual is capable of this, she has no need of guidance by the sentiments of society.

There is no way of knowing if the society is the source of our awareness of the good unless we have an independent knowledge of the good. If we have independent knowledge of the good, then we have no need for guidance by the sentiments of the society.

> There is no way of knowing if the society is the source of our awareness of the good unless we have an independent knowledge of the good.

## EMOTIVISM

> Emotivism arises from two ideas: (a) ethical nonnaturalism—ethical judgments are not based on factual evidence, and (b) noncognitivism—because ethical judgments are not based on factual evidence, they cannot be described as true or false.

Emotivism is the theory that value terms are grounded in emotional attitudes. According to emotivist theory, ethical terms express nothing but attitudes of approval or disapproval. Emotivism arises from two ideas: (a) ethical nonnaturalism—ethical judgments are not based on factual evidence, and (b) noncognitivism—because ethical judgments are not based on factual evidence, they cannot be described as true or false. Emotivism has nothing whatever to recommend it, but we include it here because it is in general practice.

A. J. Ayer (1910–1989) was the ethicist who proposed to legitimize the system of emotivism. Emotivism holds that moral judgments express only positive or negative feelings. Therefore, if someone says, "It was wrong for you to steal money," this statement says no more than, "You stole money." Adding that the action was wrong does not say anything more about it. The speaker is only exhibiting moral disapproval. It is the same as if he said, "You stole money," using a tone of horror or displaying an angry or horrified facial expression. The tone or facial expression does not add any meaning to the statement, but it expresses the speaker's feelings about it (Ayer, 1936).

*Emotivism holds that there are no objective moral truths; therefore, moral statements are meaningless except as an expression of the speaker's feelings*

Like relativism, emotivism holds that there are no objective moral truths; therefore, moral statements are meaningless except as an expression of the speaker's feelings. In emotivism a moral statement is not literally a statement about the speaker's feelings on the topic, but it expresses those feelings with emotive force. Expressing feelings about a moral issue may influence another person's thoughts and conduct. Emotivism is focused on the way in which people use language and holds that a moral judgment expresses only the attitude of the speaker. It's like shouting "Hurray!" or making a face and saying, "Ugh." That's why this theory is called emotivism, because it's based on the emotive effect of moral language.

How did such thinking come about? Some emotivists base their view on logical positivism, which holds that any genuine truth claim must be capable of being tested by sense experience or logical processes derived from sense experience. Empirical evidence is the only way something can be known. Because moral judgments cannot be tested by sense experience, they cannot establish genuine truth claims. So moral judgments only express feelings. Thus, logical positivism leads to emotivism.

## DILEMMA 6.5: NURSE'S CONFLICTED EMOTIONS

Evelyn, a nurse, always has a feeling directing her as to what she ought to do. But these feelings are always accompanied by the feeling that she ought not do what she feels she ought to do. She has been misled by her feelings many times in the past. She has not blamed her feelings but herself for the shortcomings of her ethical decision making. How can she correct the flaws in her character that cause these unfortunate errors in judgments?

Stevenson (cited in Soames, 2006) promoted the idea that the purpose of ethical or moral judgments is to create influence. Moral judgments are not meant to clarify facts or reality, but instead are used to change or intensify the feelings of others. The speaker is not just expressing emotions, but he is also trying to have an effect on others (Soames, 2006). However, there is more to ethics than just the expression of an attitude or an attempt to influence behavior. Ethical practice needs a better explanation and foundation for shared standards of morality than emotivism can provide.

Emotivism, in presenting itself as ethical analysis, is an abandonment of concern for ethical understanding. If a nurse needs an ethic, she needs an objective ethic. If she needs a nonobjective ethic, then she needs no ethic at all. "Nurses and nursing are at the center of issues of tremendous and long-lasting impact . . . nurses cannot afford to limit their actions [through nonobjective behavior]" (Milstead, 2015, in press).

## DILEMMA 6.6: BENEVOLENCE OR PATERNALISM?

Harold has a gangrenous leg. Harold's physician wants to perform an amputation in order to save Harold's life. Harold refuses the surgery. His physician tells him, "No one could possibly want this," and gets a court order declaring Harold incompetent. The court order permits the physician to perform the surgery. Harold's physician tells herself that she has acted benevolently.

The contemporary ethical systems quickly drive ethical agents to their feelings as standards of ethical judgment. Emotivism claims that, in disputes about basic moral principles, we cannot appeal to reason but only to emotion. This method leads to debates in which each side, unable to resort to reason, simply tries to manipulate the feelings of the other side. Emotivism as an applied theory refers to the practice of making ethical decisions on the basis of emotional responses to dilemmas. Despite what ethical agents profess, making emotivism decisions on the basis of out-of-context emotional responses is, far and away, the most widely practiced way of making ethical decisions. Nurses will recognize this type of conflict quite frequently in clinical practice.

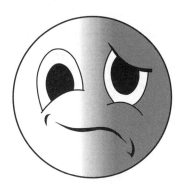

**FIGURE 6.4** Emotions rule.

To ask, "What do I feel ought to be done?" rather than "What ought to be done?" is to miss the ethical demands of a circumstance entirely. How does one become conditioned to the point where an ethical dilemma does not draw out one's attention to it but instead drives one's attention back into oneself?

## MUSINGS

None of the contemporary ethical systems will do any harm unless they are taken seriously. Ethics is not a mere adornment to human life. It is the science of a successful human life. This has been obvious since humanity first began to consider ethical ideas. It has always been obvious in itself but not always obvious to the people who might benefit from ethical understanding. For various reasons, ethics, although given much lip service, is seldom taken seriously. The alternatives to clearly and objectively defined ethical ideas lead not toward but away from successful living. Ethical ideas appropriate to the health science professions can enhance professional practice and a professional's life enormously.

Deontology cannot offer a logical argument in its own support when actions based on duty are correct, irrespective of their consequences (Pieper, 2008.) Therefore, it cannot justify itself. (The spirit of formalism—rigorous or excessive adherence to recognized forms—in deontology is captured in the Latin maxim: "One should tell the truth though the heavens fall.") One has a duty to accept deontology is not a justification of deontology.

Utilitarianism might also avail itself of formalism. If, in a certain country, there were many rich people and very few poor ones, a Robin Hood who robbed from the poor to give to the rich would be practicing a utilitarian formalism. When the end justifies the means and supports the greatest good for the greatest number, with no regard for the individual, the theory is not a useful theory for bioethics (Pieper, 2008). If relativism can be discovered to be the source of ethical awareness, then the nature of ethical awareness can be discovered. If the nature of ethical awareness can be discovered, relativism is extraneous. Most ethicists reject the theory of ethical relativism. Some claim that although the moral practices of society may differ, the fundamental moral principles underlying these practices do not (Velasquez, Ander, Shanks, & Meyer, 2014). Emotivism, in presenting itself as ethical analysis, is an abandonment of concern for ethical understanding. If a nurse needs an ethic, she needs an objective ethic. If she needs a nonobjective ethic, then she needs no ethic at all. ". . . beliefs that are closely connected to emotions are busy serving subjective needs in ways that may interfere with perceiving situations realistically" (Halpern, 2012, p. 112). How can a theory that keeps us away from objectively perceiving the context be justified for a bioethical theory?

Animals act to avoid various perils to which they are vulnerable. As rational animals we (sometimes) use our powers of reason to initiate actions to oppose the loss of our well-being. One of the ways we can do this is through ethical awareness, extending the time frame of our actions and making them more intelligible. Another is by establishing health care systems whose focus is benefit and individual rights. The motivation for each of these systems is a reasoned desire to escape the consequences of various aspects of our vulnerability.

When these systems—for example, deontology, utilitarianism, and so forth—are dominant in a health care setting, they expose patients to a virulent and entirely unnecessary form of vulnerability.

*Note: Cultural competence* is not to be confused with *relativism,* although some use the terms interchangeably. Cultural competence for the profession of nursing and all health care professionals relates to being sensitive to, and respectful of, the clients' values and traditions that make up their culture (de Chesnay, Hart, & Brannan, 2012). "Cultural competence is the ongoing process in which the health care provider continuously strives to achieve the ability to effectively work within the cultural context of the client (individual, family, community)" (Montenery, Jones, Perry, Ross, & Zoucha, 2013, p. e56).

> When these systems—for example, deontology, utilitarianism, and so forth—are dominant in a health care setting, they expose patients to a virulent and entirely unnecessary form of vulnerability.

## STUDY GUIDE

1. Discuss each of the systems: deontology, utilitarianism, emotivism, and relativism. Would any of these give you a sense of pride in what you are doing or enable you to think that you have done the best thing in the context for this person?
2. Think about the consequences to patients if a nurse took seriously each of these standards.
3. Discuss one of the cases in the book or from your own practice from each of these systems. Note that you may reach a similar conclusion, at times, with that of symphonology, but the process of analysis is entirely different. Thus, you may reach an appropriate decision by default.
4. Sometimes, when little children are very angry and they cannot express their anger, rather than holding it back they will slap or punch their own faces to express their frustration. How is this similar to adopting emotivism as one's ethical decision-making system?
5. What CES (or CESs) does Dilemma 6.6 illustrate?
6. Use this case for class discussion; the analysis of the case only appears in the instructor's manual.

## KEEPING A PATIENT'S CONFIDENCE OR TELLING THE FAMILY

Harry is in the hospital. He is dying. Harry's very large family is unaware of the fact that he is dying. He does not want his family to know. Harry's son has been discharged from the army and is returning home. The family intends to surprise Harry with his son's return when he arrives home. What should be done?

# REFERENCES

Althaus, F. A. (1997). Female circumcision: Rite of passage or violation of rights? *International Family Planning Perspectives, 23*(3). Retrieved June 4, 2007, from http://www.guttmacher.org/pubs/journals/2313097.html

Angeles, P. A. (1992). *Dictionary of philosophy* (2nd. ed.). New York, NY: Harper Collins.

Arras, J., & Rhoden, N. (Eds.). (1989). *Ethical issues in modern medicine* (3rd ed.). Mountain View, CA: Mayfield.

Ayer, A. J. (1936). *Language, truth, and logic.* London: Gollancz.

Bentham, J. (1962). *The works of Jeremy Bentham.* (J. Bowring, Ed.). New York, NY: Russell & Russell. (Original work published 1879)

Burkhardt, M. A., & Nathaniel, A. K. (2002). *Ethics and issues in contemporary nursing* (2nd ed.). Albany, NY: Delmar.

de Chesnay, M., Hart, P., & Brannan, J. (2012). Cultural competence and resilience. In M. de Chesnay & B. A. Anderson (Eds.), *Caring for the vulnerable: Perspectives in nursing theory, practice, and research* (3rd ed., pp. 29–41). Burlington, MA: Jones & Bartlett.

Franklin, C. (1988). Commentary on case study. *Hastings Center Report, 18*(6), 35–36.

Gibson, C. H. (1993). Underpinnings of ethical reasoning in nursing. *Journal of Advanced Nursing, 18,* 20–27.

Harré, R., & Krausz, M. (1996). *Varieties of relativism.* Oxford, England: Blackwell.

Halpern, J. (2012). When concertized emotion-belief complexes derail decision-making capacity. *Bioethics, 26,* 108–116.

Hill, T. E., & Zweig, A. (Eds.). (2003). *Immanuel Kant: Groundwork for metaphysics of morals.* New York, NY: Oxford University Press.

Hume, D. (1955). *Enquiry concerning the principles of morals.* New York, NY: Handel. (Original work published in London, 1748)

Kant, I. (1964). *Groundwork for the metaphysics of morals* (J. H. Paton, Trans.). New York, NY: Harper & Row. (Original work published 1785)

McConnell, T. C. (1982). *Moral issues in health care.* Monterey, CA: Wadsworth.

Milstead, J. (2015, in press). *Health policy and politics: A nurses' guide.* Sudbury, MA: Jones and Bartlett.

Montenery, S., Jones, A., Perry, N., Ross, D., & Zoucha, R., (2013). Cultural competence in nursing faculty: A journey, not a destination. *Journal of Professional Nursing, 29*(6), 51–57.

Pieper, P. (2008). Ethical perspectives of children's assent for research participation: Deontology and utilitarianism. *Pediatric Nursing, 34,* 319–323.

Runes, D. D. (Ed.). (1983). *Dictionary of philosophy*. New York, NY: Philosophical Library.

Sarikonda-Woitas, C., & Robinson, J. (2002). Ethical health care policy: Nursing's voice in allocation. *Nursing Administration Quarterly, 26*, 72–80.

Soames, S. (2006). Analytic philosophy in America, in Misak, *The Oxford Handbook of American Philosophy*. New York, NY: Oxford University Press.

Trail, H. N. (Ed.). (1896). *The centenary edition of Carlyle's work*. New York, NY: Oxford.

van Hooft, S. (1990). Moral education for nursing decisions. *Journal of Advanced Nursing, 15*, 210–215.

Veatch, H. B. (1985). *Human rights: Fact or fancy?* Baton Rouge, LA: Louisiana State University Press.

Velasquez, Andre, Shanks, &. Meyer. (nd). Ethical relativism. http://www/scu.edu/ethics/practicing/decisions/ethicalrelativism.html

Warburton. N. (2011). Rose-tinted reality: Immanuel Kant. *A little history of philosophy*. Yale University Press.

# SEVEN

# NURSING PRACTICE INTERSECTIONS: LEGAL DECISION MAKING WITHIN A SYMPHONOLOGICAL ETHICAL PERSPECTIVE

Suzanne Edgett Collins, JD, PhD, MPH, RN

## OBJECTIVES

- Describe the elements of caring advocacy (symphonological agency) as one foundation for integrated ethical-legal decision making in professional nursing practice.

- Recognize that compliance with the legal boundaries of nursing care is a necessary antecedent for the practice of the profession.

- Give examples of two nursing decision-making challenges at the intersection of ethics and law.

- Discuss the ethical and legal consequences of nurse rule-bending behavior.

- Identify strategies to facilitate integrated ethical-legal nursing decision making.

## CARING ADVOCACY (AGENCY) AS A FOUNDATIONAL FRAMEWORK FOR ETHICAL-LEGAL DECISION MAKING IN NURSING

Caring is one of the core values of nursing. It is part of the social contract between the profession of nursing and the public that nursing serves as articulated in *Nursing's Social Policy Statement* (American Nurses Association [ANA], 2003). Professional caring advocacy occurs in the presence of unequal relationships. Thus, the nurse (or any health care provider, for that matter) is providing essential support for the vulnerable patient who is dependent on the nurse's power and superior knowledge. This vulnerability, in a time of acute need, creates an unavoidable trust by the patient for the nurse; therefore, nurses are bound to adhere to a high standard of moral conduct in their professional caring.

> This vulnerability, in a time of acute need, creates an unavoidable trust by the patient for the nurse; therefore, nurses are bound to adhere to a high standard of moral conduct in their professional caring.

Caring theory is a subset of a branch of ethics that examines unequal relationships based on the premise that most people therein are not equally autonomous or free to make choices. Caring theory is also based on the premise that human caring is necessary for human survival. It is through being cared for that human beings are able to attain or retain their agency and thrive. The ethics of care emphasizes responsiveness and responsibility in unequal relationships.

Noddings (1984) discerned that there appears to be a kind of caring that is natural and accessible to all human beings and is built on relationships. Caring, as an ethic, consists of two forms. Natural caring, such as mother for child, is the enabling sentiment that allows for the development of ethical caring. Individuals learn to care for others based on being cared for themselves and, for the vast majority of the population, this is true. Ethical caring is a feeling of "I must" even in the presence of conflicting feelings that "I don't want to do this thing that I must." Through being cared for and experiencing what caring for someone takes, nurses learn to combine the feeling of "I must" with a commitment "to do."

The nurse–patient relationship is inherently unequal. The nurse has the power; the nurse is the one fully clothed and well, able to come and go, able to exercise free will within certain professional practice legal constraints. The patient is dependent on the nurse for even the most basic items: water, food, medicine, and safety. The nurse has the knowledge; the nurse has pertinent, clinical experiential expertise and understanding of the environment (the hospital or other care setting). The patient is a compromised stranger in this system and therefore quite vulnerable. The patient has no choice but to trust the nurse—this is called an unavoidable trust because in order for the patient to receive the care, the patient must trust the nurse to deliver it, analogous to the environment of agreement in symphonology.

Care orientation focuses on the moral vision of not turning away from someone in need; it values attention and response to the needs of others, and it abhors detachment or abandonment. In developing a personal ethic of care, a nurse traverses three stages, stages 1 and 2 leading to the culmination of caring in stage 3 (Gilligan, 1982). Stage

1—caring for self—relates to self-survival. This stage ends when the person matures and begins to realize that this approach is selfish and there is a need for interconnectedness and relationships with others. Then the second stage of development begins. Stage 2—caring for others—is the stage when the person realizes that caring relationships encompass great responsibility to be attentive and responsive to others' needs and to not hurt others. When this understanding reaches the point of self-sacrifice to the exclusion of self-care, a transition occurs that leads to the third stage in an attempt to bring balance into the relationship between caring for self and caring for others. Stage 3—caring for self and for others—is the highest level, when balance is gained in realizing that the responsibility in a caring relationship means harmoniously caring for both self and for others. Care morally binds nurses to the patients for whom they care, thereby creating a high moral standard of responsibility on the part of nurses. Ethical-legal decision making in professional nursing requires the nurse to engage in stage 3 caring. The nurse must fulfil the patient's agency requirements mandated by the agreement to promote the patient's rights while remaining self-protected by engaging in nursing practice within legal boundaries.

## ADVOCACY AS AN EXPRESSION OF AGENCY

Patient advocacy, as an expression of symphonological agency, is speaking or acting on a patient's behalf to protect the patient's rights and help the patient obtain desired information and services.

Patient advocacy, as an expression of symphonological agency, is speaking or acting on a patient's behalf to protect the patient's rights and help the patient obtain desired information and services. Patient advocacy is fundamental to nursing. *Nursing's Social Policy Statement* (ANA, 2003, p. 6) includes advocacy in its definition of nursing as "the protection, promotion, and optimization of health and abilities, prevention of illness and injury, alleviation of suffering through the diagnosis and treatment of human response, and advocacy in the care of individuals, families, communities, and populations." Advocacy in nursing professes its theoretical basis in nursing ethics. ANA's *Code of Ethics for Nurses* (2001, p. 9, provision 2) includes language relating to patient advocacy: "The nurse's primary commitment is to the patient, whether an individual, family, group, or community." The corresponding interpretive statement emphasizes the "primacy of the patient's interests . . . " in that the commitment of the nurse, even in a persistent unresolved conflict, remains to the patient (ANA, 2001, pp. 9–10).

Two critical ethical questions (Chinn & Kramer, 2011, p. 88) for all nursing acts are, "Is this right?" and "Is this responsible?" Ethical frameworks provide the analytical tools for nurses to apply the core values of nursing so that nurses are able to answer these questions. Many ethical frameworks have been developed over centuries; this chapter will explore the symphonological approach within the constraints of legal realities from which practicing nurses may not escape. Nurses are able to decide right and wrong because they are beings of intellect who are rational and have the ability to appreciate the potential consequences of their proposed actions. Good human acts have certain qualities: good ends, good means, and good circumstances to achieve the good end. The nurse, in acting on behalf of the patient, in an ethical sense, becomes a moral actor, yet remains bound to the legalities of practice so is also a legal actor. Not only must the nurse moral-legal actor perform the right, good, and valued action but also the nurse must perform it from the proper motivation with an understanding of the potential ethical-legal consequences of the action.

> The nurse, in acting on behalf of the patient, in an ethical sense, becomes a moral actor, yet remains bound to the legalities of practice so is also a legal actor.

Nurses have a responsibility to become consciously aware and maintain awareness of their ethical-legal decision making processes and how they might be improved. ANA's *Code of Ethics for Nurses* (2001) states that "The nurse owes the same duties to self as to others, including the responsibility to preserve integrity and safety, to maintain competence, and to continue personal and professional growth" (p. 18, provision 5). The interpretive statements for this section include moral and professional growth and development to preserve integrity and wholeness of character (ANA, 2001, pp. 18–20.) Values clarification is a practical approach to developing this personal insight. It is the iterative process of becoming more conscious of, and being able to articulate in a logical way, what the nurse believes is an ethical-legal response. It is an ongoing reflective process that helps a nurse mature as an ethical-legal agent by examining the circumstances and rationale for decisions, and how decision making might improve in the future. Chinn and Kramer (2011) identify the integrated expression of the ethical pattern of knowing as ". . . moral comportment" (p. 7). As health care providers, nurses participate as the patients' agents in many decisions on behalf of the vulnerable patients under their care. Developing insight into personal values, in conjunction with professional legal mandates, will improve nurses' abilities to demonstrate moral comportment as ethical-legal agents for patients.

## CARING ADVOCACY: THE HEART OF THE MATTER

Relationships between nurse and patient are necessarily unequal, with the professional nurse having greater power than the patient in need of the nurse's services. This creates a heightened ethically responsible relationship in that the patient is forced to trust in the nurse's ability to competently minister to the patient's needs. From this arises the concept of caring advocacy that permeates all that nurses do. Nurses are morally bound to high standards in these unequal, unavoidable trust relationships and must learn to caringly advocate for their vulnerable patients, as well as for themselves in maintenance of legal scope of practice and standard of care, in order to attain the essential self-other care balance. The usefulness of the symphonological approach is apparent, because this approach respects the unavoidable trust inherent in the initiation and effective maintenance of the agreements: nurse–self, nurse–patient, and nurse–society.

> The usefulness of the symphonological approach is apparent, because this approach respects the unavoidable trust inherent in the initiation and effective maintenance of the agreements: nurse–self, nurse–patient, and nurse–society.

## LEGAL REALITY: COMPLIANCE WITH THE LEGAL BOUNDARIES OF NURSING CARE IS A NECESSARY ANTECEDENT FOR THE AUTHORIZED PRACTICE OF THE PROFESSION

Professional nursing is a very highly regulated profession. Specific regulations vary from state to state and country to country. Yet the idea of professional nursing care is global, as is the idea of governmental oversight to protect the public that professional nurses serve. The myriad laws, codes, regulations, policies, and protocols at multiple levels that regulate the practice of professional nursing are complex and can be duplicative or inconsistent, ambiguous or prescriptive. In many cases, nurses are held to legal standards of practice for which they have no actual knowledge. For simplicity's sake, hereinafter, these will be collectively referred to as **rule sets.** Figure 7.1 provides a superficial but necessary overview to the interactive enormity of the rule sets operational in professional nursing and into which nurses must integrate as ethical-legal agents.

Five rule sets commonly operational in professional nursing in the United States are depicted in Figure 7.1 in the first level as

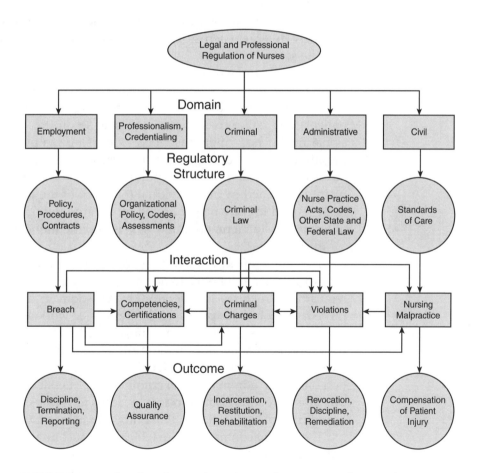

**FIGURE 7.1** Legal and professional regulation of nurses. © Collins & Mikos (2005).

domains: employment, professionalism/credentialing, criminal, administrative, and civil. Many additional categories of rule sets exist, however, and the practicing professional nurse is mandated by licensure to comply with all of them. Each of the five domains portrayed is then characterized by its regulatory structure, interactions with other domains, and outcomes.

The administrative domain is of great importance for the nurse, as that is the domain in which professional education, clinical experiential training, and initial and continued licensure for practice lie. The primary mission of the regulatory structures in this domain is to protect the public that nurses serve from unsafe or incompetent practice. State nurse practice acts and the associated state administrative codes are examples of the regulatory structures in this domain. These rule sets establish the scope of practice, which are the boundaries of a nurse's practice—what nurses can do, and the standards of care, which are the necessities of practice—what nurses must do. Within this domain are the legal definitions of what constitutes professional nursing practice, what constitutes breaches of professional nursing responsibility (unprofessional practice), and the disciplinary or remedial processes for discovering and preventing further acts of unprofessional, unsafe, or incompetent practice on the part of a nursing professional. Unprofessional practice is widely divergent across jurisdictions and may also incorporate external rule sets.

> These rule sets establish the scope of practice, which are the boundaries of a nurse's practice—what nurses can do, and the standards of care, which are the necessities of practice—what nurses must do.

The civil domain encompasses many categories of rule sets that relate to encounters between nurses as individuals or agents of other entities and those with whom they are professionally engaged, such as patients and colleagues. A common rule set in this category is professional negligence, often described as nursing malpractice. Whereas in the administrative domain described earlier, the legal complaint is initiated by the state to protect the public, in the civil domain, the legal complaint is initiated by an individual (or agent of the individual) who has been proved to have been harmed by the nursing professional's breach of her professional practice and who is seeking monetary compensation for the harm.

The employment domain is probably the one with which the nurse is most familiar secondary to actually engaging in the environment. The regulatory structures for the employment domain include policies and procedures, job descriptions, and contracts or work agreements, all with which the nurse is expected to comply in order to remain employed. Any breach of these obligations may result in discipline or termination. What many nurses do not realize is that the employer may itself have an obligation under the administrative, criminal, or professionalism/credentialing domains to report certain types of breaches to various authorities, triggering additional legal action in those other domains.

The criminal domain, one in which the state brings an action against an individual or entity, is one that most nurses do not consider. The regulatory structures comprise the vast and ever-changing criminal codes related to a culpable degree of professional negligence, participation to any degree in the fraudulent allocation of government funds, and personal behaviors that do not withstand the scrutiny of the boards of nursing as to the perceptions of contribution to the inability to engage in professional practice (driving under the influence [DUI], using illicit drugs, or engaging in violence, theft, or inappropriate sexual relationships). The criminal domain outcomes are incarceration, restitution, or rehabilitation, all in an effort to promote protection of the public at large.

The fifth domain is professionalism/credentialing. The regulatory structures for this domain are organizational policies, codes, and assessments. Through competency assessments and certifications, the outcome for this domain is the enhancement of quality assurance in health care delivery by nurses.

Now consider the interactions among the domains. Nursing legal life, like any life, does not occur in a vacuum. Many legal actions have an equal or professionally greater reaction in another domain. The interaction level of Figure 7.1 explains some of the most common interactions. Because nursing malpractice (civil domain) requires a harm to be directly related to a breach of professional nursing practice, a formal report may be generated to the administrative body that monitors nursing practice, triggering a licensure investigation (administrative action). If an employer disciplines a nurse employee for a breach of professional practice as dictated by the work agreement or institutional policies and procedures, the employer may be legally required to report it to the appropriate administrative agency, which will then take action against the nurse's license, and to the credentialing agency, which may take a revocation action against the nurse's advanced credentials, and to any law enforcement agencies, if a law has been broken, who will then institute criminal charges against the nurse. The breach of the employment contract or policy/procedures may become evidence in the nursing malpractice action. So conceivably, and actually, just one poorly reasoned act by a nurse may become the fodder for regulatory actions in all five common domains. Nurses are themselves vulnerable by their general lack of understanding about their own contexts of knowledge, situation, and awareness.

> Nurses are themselves vulnerable by their general lack of understanding about their own contexts of knowledge, situation, and awareness.

## INTERSECTIONS = CHALLENGES + RESPONSES

Nurses may then sometimes, even unknowingly, be conflicted in fulfilling their perceived roles as caring advocates by legal constraints that sculpt their professional practices in any particular jurisdiction. The professional and legal regulation of nurses binds nurses to certain rule sets (see discussion regarding ethical individualism in Chapter 2). It is true, as explained earlier in this textbook, that these rule sets are derived from rights; however, although the law is dynamic, it changes slowly in response to societal inputs. Therefore, the required compliance with legal boundaries may provide troublesome challenges to the nurse as a caring advocate. Consider Table 7.1.

> The required compliance with legal boundaries may provide troublesome challenges to the nurse as a caring advocate.

**TABLE 7.1** ETHICAL-LEGAL DECISION MAKING

| Nature/Perception of Nursing Act | Legal According to the Rule Sets at the Time | Illegal According to the Rule Sets at the Time |
| --- | --- | --- |
| Moral to "Good" "Ethical" | Easy and congruent decision | Hard incongruent decision |
| Immoral to "Bad" "Unethical" | Hard incongruent decision | Easy and congruent decision |

For the most part, nurses do not have trouble with the easy decisions. Those are straightforward and comfortable. Those are the kind of decisions that are ethically and legally coherent and result in comfort, and a feeling of "this is right" to all those involved.

In the case of the ethical-legal decision, contexts—knowledge, awareness, and situation—are clear and relevant, and views through all bioethical standards "lenses" present an integrated comprehensive application/fulfillment of the patient–nurse agreement. The patient's wishes are honored, the family or significant others are in accord and express gratitude; the nurse feels deeply gratified for sustaining fidelity to the patient and to self, in that the perception of the act as legal is realized. For example, consider a patient with end-stage amyotrophic lateral sclerosis (ALS) as he approaches the end of life. He is cognitively aware and expresses decisional capacity on his own terms, with family concurrence, and opts for terminal sedation, a legal procedure in the jurisdiction, in the presence of his loving family. The procedure will occur in a health care facility that has embraced the philosophy of facilitating terminal patients' end-of-life choices and that has hired willing staff accordingly. The patient is also supported by his third-party payer and his community church. In this scenario, the decision to administer the terminal sedation is easy and comfortable. The nurse was able to honor all agreements: nurse–self, nurse–society, and nurse–patient.

For the opposite of this scenario, the illegal and immoral decision, consider the eugenics sterilization movement in the United States in the 1900s (Currell & Cogdell, 2006), based on the premise that the human population should define and direct its own evolution. Therefore, many women who were deemed as being mentally insufficient, of poor economic means, or of inferior "character" were sterilized without consent as a "public good" (Currell & Cogdell, 2006). In this case of ethical-legal decision making, contexts—knowledge, awareness, and situation—are immature and irrelevant, and views through all bioethical standards "lenses" present unilateral comprehensive application/fulfillment of only the care providers' sentiment. The patient's wishes are not considered, the family or significant others are not consulted; it is impossible for the nurse to sustain fidelity to the patient, nor would that have ever been considered. One could argue that was the past, not the present. However, history

*In the case of the ethical-legal decision, contexts—knowledge, awareness, and situation—are clear and relevant, and views through all bioethical standards "lenses" present an integrated comprehensive application/fulfillment of the patient–nurse agreement.*

provides valid lessons for the present, especially when considering the current use of genetic information in health care allocation and outcomes decision making (see case study "Savior Sibling").

Unfortunately, all the intricate interactions of this scenario, a constructed positive hypothetical, hardly ever synchronously occur. The hard decisions are the ones that are not coherent, are uncomfortable to all involved, and ultimately may have negative consequences to nurse and patient (see Chapter 9, "Moral Distress"). Therefore, examination through hypothetical analysis of the two categories of hard decisions within a context of symphonology will promote reflective values clarification and experiential testing to refine/enhance the nurse's ability to honor the agreements: nurse–self, nurse–society, and nurse–patient.[1]

## THE LEGAL BUT IMMORAL DECISION—SUBTLY COERCED HARVESTING OF BIOLOGICAL MATERIAL

Popular literature and entertainment venues as well as factual case examples have explored the concept of the creation of a "savior sibling" (Rivard, 2013), through the use of embryonic preimplantation genetic selection/diagnosis, to provide a near perfect match of blood and tissue donations to an older sibling (Picoult, 2004). A hypothetical composite scenario loosely based on these reports follows.

## SAVIOR SIBLING

Mark (age 14), the oldest child of the Smith family, was diagnosed with a type of cancer that research has reported to be responsive to the use of tissue compatible infusion of cells and other biological materials to prolong life and in rare cases, effect a cure. The Smith family, in an effort to save Mark, undergoes preimplantation genetic selection of an embryo, from many embryos conceived in vitro, to effect the birth of a tissue compatible donor for Mark. The procedures were successful, and Matthew was born, accepted into this family, and loved for his unique presence in the family (see the Ayala case in Chapter 12 for another perspective) and for the lifesaving tissue/cells that he can donate to his older brother. From the moment of birth, biological material was harvested from Matthew for the benefit of Mark. At first, the harvesting procedures were not too painful and of little to moderate burden to Matthew; however, over the years, greater demands for tissue/cells resulted in frequent hospitalizations, painful pharmaceutically enhanced tissue/cell donations,

---

[1]The case scenarios reflect the author's own bioethical standard lenses: autonomy/uniqueness, freedom/self-directedness, objectivity, beneficence, and fidelity. Readers must develop their own rational interpretations.

and psychological trauma to Matthew, secondary to his internalized perception of being responsible for the well-being of Mark and the continued cohesion and survival of his family. Matthew, now a near teenager (age 12), has been donating tissue/cells for his entire life. Mark now needs a living donor liver transplant. Matthew tearfully confides in his nurse the night before the planned surgical procedure. Matthew's parents consented to the planned surgery; both Mark and Matthew also assented at the time of the family meeting with the surgeon. Mathew cries to his nurse that he does not want to have an operation and lose "a big chunk of his body." He is afraid that by saying no he will "kill" his beloved older brother and that his mother and father will cease to love him.

## SYMPHONOLOGICAL ANALYSIS

Appropriate nursing management of this situation first involves careful symphonological analysis, viewing the situation through the lenses of the bioethical standards as depicted in Table 7.2. This situation examines the agreement between the nurse and patient in congruence with the agreement between the nurse and society.

Absent evidence of the inability to make decisions in the best interest of the child, parents generally have the power to make decisions on behalf of an unemancipated minor who is younger than 14 years of age. In addition, certain members of the health care team may focus their decision making based on the utilitarian perspective of maximizing the benefit for the "most," in this case the family as a whole, but specifically on Mark's life, while minimizing the burden to the "few," in this case Matthew, who will likely suffer no permanent physical harm from the living donor liver transplant. This course of action, although perhaps sound from a purely medical risk/benefit analysis, negates Matthew's rights, psychological health, and presents a decisional crossroad for the nurse in both caring and advocacy. Figure 7.2 algorithmically captures a resonable conflict resolution pathway for the nurse at an ethical-legal decisional crossroad. If the parents are unwilling or unable to openly acknowledge Matthew's feelings, other support persons, such as the physician, the nursing chain of command, social worker, risk manager, the ethics committee of the hospital, or an independent court-appointed guardian ad litem, should be consulted. If the legal disagreement with the ethical analysis cannot be resolved, judicial intervention may ultimately be required. However, it is clear from the ethical analysis, the nurse is on notice that Matthew's rights may be in jeopardy and that the validity of his assent has been challenged. Ethical and legal principles are likely to be violated, if the nurse remains silent. To demonstrate moral comportment and professional practice within the legal standards of care, the nurse must intervene.

**TABLE 7.2** ETHICAL-LEGAL RESPONSE TO SAVIOR SIBLING

| Bioethical Standard | Ethical-Legal Agent Response |
| --- | --- |
| Autonomy | Although Matthew is not legally of age to make his own health care decisions, the contexts of knowledge, situation, and awareness suggest that Matthew is mature beyond his years and thoroughly understands the medical implications of his decision for himself and for Mark. His independent uniqueness and ethical equality demand that his feelings in this matter be seriously considered. Notice of the rescinding of his assent must be communicated to the health care team. |
| Freedom | Matthew has previously experienced multiple tissue/cell donations to his older brother, and he is now probably quite capable of understanding the immediate and possibly long-term consequences to both himself and Mark. His evolving freedom has allowed him to progressively self-direct his earlier choices to donate as he has matured from infant to adolescent, and also self-direct his present reluctance to undergo this major invasive surgical donation. Matthew should be able to control his time and effort. His declaration to the nurse may represent his heartfelt attempt as a legally unemancipated child to assert his choice and defy what he may perceive as unintentional, or even subtle intentional coercion on the part of his parents or older brother. |
| Objectivity | Matthew's objectivity is based on his prior experience of being a donor and the associated internal and external environmental conditions surrounding his past donation experiences and his brother's illness. At 12, he may not have sufficient understanding of the medical or psychological technicalities of long-term risks/benefits to himself, his brother, and his family, but assuredly he does understand that he will undergo major invasive surgery, not for his medical benefit, but for someone else's. |
| Beneficence | Matthew knows that he was specially conceived to provide benefit to the family unit in general, but specifically to his older brother. As he matures into an autonomous adult, he is beginning to see his benefit/life needs as separate from his family's benefit/needs. The nurse is therefore morally compelled to bring the ambivalence stated by Matthew to the attention of those who can intervene on Matthew's behalf. |
| Fidelity | The nurse has been entrusted with information that alerts the nurse to the potential failures of the preconditions to Matthew's agreement with the health care team, and that may present legal challenges to the voluntary nature of Matthew's concurrence to the procedure. The nurse's agreement with Matthew demands intervention on behalf of Matthew's rights. The nurse may be the sole caring advocate/agent for Matthew capable of this intervention purely on Matthew's behalf. |

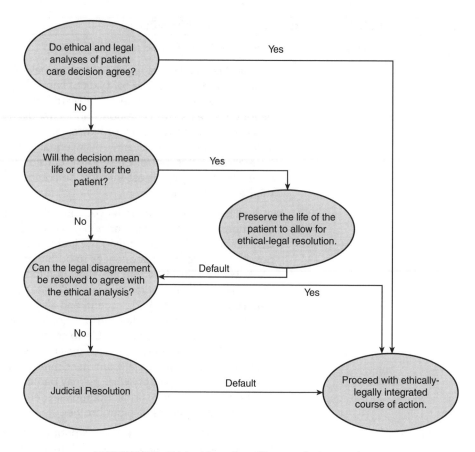

**FIGURE 7.2** Ethical-legal conflict resolution pathway.

## THE ILLEGAL BUT MORAL DECISION—RULE BENDING FOR THE GOOD OF THE PATIENT OR UNIT

True narratives from licensure defense practices help provide an introductory, reality-based framework for understanding the concept of rule bending (breaching established rule sets in multiple domains) for good purposes.

A nurse was unable to keep a patient calm and free from self-inflicted injury. This experienced nurse recognized that the patient was suffering from acute alcohol withdrawal and needed a higher dosage of medication but was unable to convince the physician. The nurse felt thwarted in multiple attempts to care for the patient. The nurse covertly administered a higher dosage of medication than was ordered, thus calming the patient and diminishing the risk of self-inflicted injury. The physician found out about this and made a complaint resulting in licensure disciplinary action for exceeding the scope of practice (Collins, 2003).

A large number of nurses in a long-term care facility collusively devised a way to borrow and return controlled medications for their

The nurses in these scenarios engaged in reasoned, intentional rule-bending behavior to solve the immediate care problems and to provide the care that they, as agents for the patients, reasonably believed was paramount. Negative licensure consequences for the nurses were the unfortunate result.

patients' pain relief needs when outside pharmacy services failed to deliver them in a timely manner, a system failure work-around that continued for a long period of time. The patients' pains were relieved; however, state surveyors were not impressed by this creative but illegal solution to the drug supply problem, and licensure disciplinary actions for violation of drug dispensing regulations and scope of practice were instituted against the nurses (Collins & Mikos, 2008).

The nurses in these scenarios engaged in reasoned, intentional rule-bending behavior to solve the immediate care problems and to provide the care that they, as agents for the patients, reasonably believed was paramount. Negative licensure consequences for the nurses were the unfortunate result.

## WHAT IS NURSE RULE BENDING?

Rule bending has existed as a concept in nursing practice anecdotally and more subjectively for a number of years. It is a sensitive topic, one that is not often addressed in the "polite society" of the nursing profession's assessment of its own social behaviors and is infrequently found in the scholarly literature (Collins, 2012). The tolerance for rule bending seems closely related to the nurse's evolving understanding of what constitutes real harm to a patient (Collins, 2001). Rule bending can become a socialized behavior on a unit as in the second scenario. Noncompliance with the rules was accepted by the nurses working in the long-term care unit, and as time went on, the members of the unit no longer saw the action as a violation of the rules. This phenomenon is identified as the normalization of deviance in which individuals, teams, and organizations repeatedly drift away from what is an acceptable standard of performance until the drift becomes the norm (Vaughan, 2005).

Rule-bending behaviors can be traced historically through select nursing literature. As early as 1984, Benner noted that nurses learn through experience what can be safely added to or omitted from physicians' orders, as in the first scenario. She noted that "nurses must use discretion . . . and are expected to assess what they should do to provide the best possible care for the patient . . . even though this may involve risks for them [the nurses]" (pp. 139–140). Hutchinson, in her seminal 1990 qualitative study of responsible subversion, first described the behavior of rule bending among nurses. According to Hutchinson, nurses' knowledge, experience, and ideology are necessary preconditions for rule bending. Nurses proceed through four stages in deciding to bend the rules: evaluating, predicting, subverting [rule bending], and covering. This is the covert process that nurses use to achieve patient or unit workflow benefit when they feel trapped by the rules and/or lack of response from those in a position to help solve the problem. Hutchinson (1990) reported that nurses perceived their values of patient advocacy conflicted with those of the system. By bending the

Nurses proceed through four stages in deciding to bend the rules: evaluating, predicting, subverting [rule bending], and covering.

rules, nurses were better able to obtain their goals of caring for patients. These nurses' acts were responsibly done for good intent, and therefore justifiable in these nurses' perceptions.

Rule bending encompasses a general societal understanding that it is sometimes acceptable and perhaps even tacitly encouraged to bend the rules to "get the job done." Galperin (2003) discussed the concept of constructive workplace deviance, which is purposeful employee behavior enacted for reasons thought to be innovative by the employee. This behavior violates workplace organizational norms. Previous studies (Collins, 2001; Hutchinson, 1990) suggest that nurse rule benders sometimes intentionally violate nursing practice standards/rule sets but generally do so with good motive such as for the benefit or good of the patient or the workflow in the particular nursing unit. Rule bending occurs when there is system–nurse conflict that the nurse believes impedes the goals of nursing care. These rule-bending nurses consider themselves to be caring and responsible. Rule bending requires a higher level of expertise to manage successfully and therefore may be more frequently practiced by experienced nurses who can evaluate the risks of such behavior, rather than by novices. Successful rule bending seems to be self-propagating, and socially, although covertly, approved as a quick fix to a persistent work goal achievement problem over which the nurse perceives no control or ability to remedy. Nurses acknowledge that rule bending can lead to negative professional consequences because it generally involves violating the professional standards of care (necessities of practice) or exceeding the scope of practice (boundaries of practice) to solve the problem and provide good benefit. Unfortunately, if the rule-bending behavior is rejected by others, the outcomes can be devastating for the nurse(s), as depicted in the two scenarios.

> Rule bending occurs when there is system–nurse conflict that the nurse believes impedes the goals of nursing care.

## SYMPHONOLOGICAL ANALYSIS

Appropriate nursing management of this situation first involves careful symphonological analysis, viewing the situation through the lenses of the bioethical standards as depicted in Table 7.3. This situation examines the agreement between nurse and self in congruence with the agreement between the nurse and society.

Rule bending presents a dichotomous ethical-legal conflict. Rule bending is expressly forbidden in all rule sets but is sometimes tacitly accepted and culturally approved, individually by nurses, and consensually by nursing units. The professional nurse's agreement with society mandates compliance with the rules sets established to protect the public. A nurse caught in a failure to do so, even if the failure to do so was for good motive, sadly has little room for defense against a charge of unprofessional practice.

> Rule bending presents a dichotomous ethical-legal conflict. Rule bending is expressly forbidden in all rule sets but is sometimes tacitly accepted and culturally approved, individually by nurses, and consensually by nursing units.

**TABLE 7.3** ETHICAL-LEGAL RESPONSE TO RULE BENDING

| Bioethical Standard | Ethical-Legal Agent Response |
| --- | --- |
| Autonomy | The unique character structure of a nurse is essential to nurse identity, encompassing independent self-direction. Caring and advocacy, as described earlier, comprise the heart of this identity and focus on the patient or on the care unit in which the patient resides. The nurse's responsibilities as a caring advocate are to honor the agreement to competently care, and to be respectful of the unequal relationships, power discrepancies, and unavoidable trust inherent in professional nursing practice. Rule-bending nurses generally engage in this behavior to preserve their caring advocate identities. |
| Freedom | The self-directedness and right to take long-term actions based on the nurse's own caring advocacy values and patient/unit benefit motivations, when thwarted in attempts to meet patient care goals. Nurses perceived their values of patient agency conflicted with those of the system. By bending the rules, nurses were better able to obtain their goals of caring for patients. These nurses' acts were responsibly done for good intent, and therefore justifiable and beneficial in the nurses' perceptions. |
| Objectivity | The nurse's ability to be aware of things as they objectively are and to sustain the exercise of objective awareness. Rule bending is employed to achieve patient or unit workflow benefit when nurses feel trapped by the rules and/or lack of response from those in a position to help solve the problem. |
| Beneficence | The right to act to acquire benefits perceived as necessary. The rule-bending nurse makes patient care and management decisions based on knowledge, experience, caring advocacy ideology, and harm risk benefit analysis for the good of the patient and the good of the unit in which the patient resides. |
| Fidelity | The nurse's commitment to the obligation accepted in the professional role. Nurses acknowledge that rule bending can lead to negative professional consequences because it generally involves violating the professional standards of care (necessities of practice) or exceeding the scope of practice (boundaries of practice) to reasonably solve the problem and provide good benefit. The unfortunate reality is if the rule-bending behavior is rejected by others, the outcomes can be devastating for the nurse(s) and their professional identities. |

## STRATEGIES TO FACILITATE INTEGRATED ETHICAL-LEGAL NURSING DECISION MAKING

The adage "knowledge is power" is central to strategy development for integrated ethical legal decision making in nursing as well as to understanding the associated legal risks. Compliance with rule sets relevant to professional nursing practice is essential and pertinent to the nurse agreement with self. The professional nurse's "career toolbox" should include the following to promote integrated ethical and legal conduct and decision making.

- Knowledge of current jurisdiction nurse practice laws and rules to include:
  - Key role-related definitions (NP, RN, LP, NA)
  - Standards of care for each category of nursing provider
  - Scope of practice for each category of nursing provider
  - Conditions for initial and continuing licensure
  - Jurisdiction specific practice parameters
  - Grounds for discipline
  - Disciplinary process
- Knowledge and application of ethical decision making frameworks including but not limited to practice-based ethical approaches such as symphonology
  - Personal values clarification
  - Ethical-legal conflict simulation
  - Development of rapidly available ethical resources
- Development/enhancement of caring advocacy skills
  - Assertiveness training
  - Personal malpractice insurance (includes coverage for licensure disciplinary defense of unprofessional practice—the most common regulatory nursing legal action)
  - Conscientious reflection on ethical-legal agency and decision making to validate and refine practice

## MUSINGS

Caring advocacy, or in theoretical terminology, symphonological agency, provides a foundation for both ethical and legal decision making in professional nursing practice. However, compliance with the legal boundaries of nursing care is a necessary antecedent for professional nursing practice. Nurses may find themselves at a decisional crossroad when a proposed caring action may be interpreted as immoral and legal or, conversely, as moral and illegal. Clarification of these intersections, in consideration of the concepts of symphonology, through explanatory narrative, hypothetical case application, and algorithmic representations may assist nurses in the maturation and refinement of decision-making processes within this theoretical framework. Strategies to facilitate integrated ethical-legal nursing decision making will provide a means for incorporation of core ethical and legal concepts into professional nursing practice resulting in enhanced moral and legal comportment.

## STUDY GUIDE

1. The three essential elements of a caring advocacy perspective are (a) the vulnerability of the patient, (b) the unequal relationship between the nurse and the patient, and (c) the resultant unavoidable trust. Consider a recent patient care experience and operationalize these elements.
2. Describe and reflect upon how the five common domains of nurse regulation (Figure 7.1) affect your personal professional practice. Provide examples of rule sets in each category with which you have had experience.
3. Consider the breadth of your professional practice in conjunction with Table 7.1. Identify an example that would fit into each category. Describe how you managed the conflict and whether the results were congruent with the patient's perceived desires.
4. Contemplate the decisional pathway in Figure 7.2. Apply this pathway to an ethical-legal decisional conflict in your clinical experience.
5. Explain what strategies to facilitate ethical-legal decision making would work best for you at this particular stage of your professional career.

## REFERENCES

American Nurses Association. (2001). *Code of ethics for nurses with interpretive statements*. Washington, DC: Author.

American Nurses Association. (2003). *Nursing's social policy statement*. Washington, DC: Author.

Benner, P. (1984). *From novice to expert*. Menlo Park, CA: Addison Wesley.

Chinn, P. L., & Kramer, M. K. (2011). *Integrated knowledge development in nursing* (8th ed.). St. Louis, MO: Elsevier Mosby.

Collins, S. E. (2001). *Knowing nursing error: Understanding nursing error through nurses' error experiences.* (Doctoral dissertation, University of South Florida). UMI Dissertation Services/ProQuest Company. 3041099.

Collins, S. E. (2003). Legally speaking: The trouble with bending the rules. *RN Magazine, 66 (7)*, 69–72.

Collins, S. E. (2012). Rule bending by nurses: Environmental and personal drivers. *Journal of Nursing Law*, 15(1): 14-26.

Collins, S. E., & Mikos, C.A. (2008). Evolving taxonomy of nurse practice act violators. *Journal of Nursing Law*, 12(2); 85–91.

Currell, S., & Cogdell, C. (2006). *Popular eugenics: national efficiency and American mass culture in the 1930s*. Athens: OH: Ohio University Press.

Galperin, B. L. (2003). Can workplace deviance be constructive? In A. Sagie, S. Stashevsky, & M. Koslowsky (Eds.), *Misbehavior and dysfunctional attitudes in organizations* (pp. 154–170). New York, NY: Palgrave Macmillan.

Gilligan, C. (1982). *In a different voice*. Cambridge, MA: Harvard University Press.

Hutchinson, S.A. (1990).Responsible subversion: A study of rule bending among nurses. *Scholarly Inquiry for Nursing Practice*, 4(1), 3–17.

Noddings, N. (1984) Caring. In V. Held (Ed.) (1995) *Justice and care: Essential readings in feminist ethics*. pp. 7-30. Boulder, CO: Westview Press.

Picoult, J. (2004). *My sister's keeper*. New York, NY: Simon & Schuster Pocket Books.

Rivard, L. (June 11, 2013). Case study in savior siblings. *Scitable*. Retrieved on 6-20-14fromhttp://www.nature.com/scitable/forums/genetics-generation/case-study-in-savior-siblings-104229158

Vaughan, D. (2005). The normalization of deviance: Signals of danger, situated action and risk. In H. Montgomey, R. Lipshitz, & B. Brehmer (Eds.), *How professionals make decisions* (pp. 255–276). Mahwah, NJ: Lawrence Erlbaum.

# EIGHT

# PRACTICE-BASED ETHICS AND THE BIOETHICAL STANDARDS AS LENSES

## OBJECTIVES

- Discuss the nature of the bioethical standards as "properties of ethical agents."

- Interpret the nature of a practice-based ethics.

- Summarize the meaning of the unbroken chain to nursing practice.

- Describe the practice milieu.

- Examine the use of the bioethical standards as the lens through which a nurse can assess a patient.

- Illustrate the results of "out of focus" nursing practice.

In the objective relationship between the mind of a person and the reality known by the person, there are three kinds of "things."

- There are "things" in the world outside of the mind that exist whether any mind is aware of them or not.
- There are "things" in the mind that do not exist outside of the mind, but there is still something in the world outside of the mind that serves as a foundation to that which is in the mind.
- There are "things" in the mind that have no counterpart in the world outside of the mind.

The first kind of "thing" really exists in the world. This includes such things as this chair, that tree, the gust of wind blowing that newspaper, those hills in the distance, and so on. Whether or not anyone is seeing them or touching them, these things actually exist in the world outside of consciousness.

The second kind of "thing" does not exist out in reality, but something exists out in reality that serves as the basis of this thing existing in the mind. For instance, furniture exists in the mind. Outside of the mind there is no such thing as furniture. For its own use, the mind observes these four chairs, this table, that sofa, this bookcase and groups them all together according to what they have in common, under the concept "furniture." The chairs, table, sofa, and bookcase all exist in the real world apart from the mind. However, in addition to the four chairs, table, sofa, and book, there is no eighth thing—furniture—existing out in the real world.

The third kind of "thing" exists only in the mind. This includes such things as leprechauns, the tooth fairy, square circles, unicorns, and so on. These things exist in the mind in the sense that they can be imagined. But there are no leprechauns, tooth fairies, square circles, or unicorns in the real world outside of the mind.

Furniture does not exist in reality apart from the mind as do chairs, trees, wind gusts, and hills. However, unlike leprechauns, tooth fairies, square circles, and unicorns, furniture does not exist in the mind without a reference to reality. The existence of furniture in the mind has a foundation in the chairs, tables, sofas, bookcases, and so forth, that exist in the real world.

The bioethical standards are not a kind of thing in the world. They are not independently existing realities. Their existence depends on independently existing things. They have a certain kinship to various qualities or properties of things in the world; as colors and shapes are properties of entities, the standards are properties of ethical agents.

> The bioethical standards are not a kind of thing in the world. They are not independently existing realities. Their existence depends on independently existing things

- There is no such thing as autonomy out in the world; there are only autonomous agents. Agents have this in common: They are all unique.
- There is no such thing as freedom out in the world; there are agents who possess or lack freedom.
- There is no such thing as objectivity out in the world apart from knowers who know what is objective.
- There is no such thing as beneficence out in the world; there are only agents who do good and fail to do good.
- There is no such thing as fidelity out in the world; there are only agents who uphold or fail to uphold the terms of their agreements.

The bioethical standards are things that exist in the mind and have a foundation in reality. They are the characteristics of human individuals; they are the virtues of human individuals. All people possess these characteristics individually. Individuals are autonomous. They act freely.

They have a need for objectivity, freedom, and beneficence. They make agreements, and they are faithful to these agreements. It is these characteristics of human individuals that keep a health care professional's awareness of the bioethical standards tied to reality out in the world—the reality of her patients.

For a health care professional to function on an ethical level, there must be something tying her awareness to the people of whom she is aware. This something consists of the bioethical standards. Everyone is autonomous. Everyone is free. The standards pertain to everyone—to humans as human. Recognition of these characteristics is the focus and foundation of ethical practice.

---

### DILEMMA 8.1: WHAT IS TO BE DONE WHEN INTRAFAMILY COERCION IS SUSPECTED?

Rick works as a copyeditor. He is a 27-year-old homosexual with a long history of kidney disease. Three years ago, he tested positive for HIV, but he has been symptom free and his T-cell count has been greater than 400 cells/mm$^3$. Ten months ago, he suffered kidney failure, but since then, he has been doing well on dialysis. He now wants to receive a kidney transplant from his 49-year-old mother, Mrs. Raymond. He has been very insistent that she donate a kidney for him, and she now agrees to the procedure. She knows that he is HIV positive. The psychiatrist, who evaluated both Rick and his mother, reports that both are extremely guarded in their communication and that their relationship seems complex and troubled. The case comes to the ethics committee. Should the mother's consent be accepted as a free and autonomous choice? (Rhodes, 1992, pp. 75–76)

---

## PRACTICE-BASED

> Through a process of analysis and induction, symphonology, the study of agreements, was born. It had nursing practice as its model

Through a process of analysis and induction, symphonology, the study of agreements, was born. It had nursing practice as its model. It is a practice-based ethical theory because it was based on and derived from nursing practice. It is applicable to practice in any health care setting, with any patient population, and with all health care professionals. It enables health care professionals to make decisions that are contextually justifiable.

Nursing practice is ethical; it violates no one's rights and breaks no agreement implied by rights; it is humanly desirable (that is, its reason-for-being is to benefit human individuals); therefore, it provides excellent criteria for an ethical system, for these are the criteria of an excellent ethical system. No rights violations are built into the nature of nursing practice. The purpose of this practice is to increase the power of patients to take independent actions. It is humanly desirable. It serves human life. At its best, it can provide matchless criteria for an ethical system. Symphonology, a practice-based ethical system, is one whose fundamental definitions of human purpose, benefit, desire, right, good, justifiable, and so on are the same definitions that guide competent nursing practice. For practice, and for a practice-based ethical system, four things happen simultaneously: The patient becomes a partner in his care, he is recognized as an ethical equal, the nurse becomes his agent, and the context becomes the standard of judgment.

> For practice, and for a practice-based ethical system, four things happen simultaneously: The patient becomes a partner in his care, he is recognized as an ethical equal, the nurse becomes his agent, and the context becomes the standard of judgment.

A practice-based system of ethical decision making is a context-based system. It is one that inspires objectively justifiable actions. If a system is context based and the context is fundamental rather than merely superficial, then it is practice based. A practice-based system of ethical decision making is context based on two levels:

- It is a response to the needs that brought the patient into the health care setting.
- It is an integral part of professional practice, modeled on professional practice.

Awareness of the ethical situation is the foundation of a relevant practice-based ethic. Unless the causal processes forming the context of the situation are perceived, no relevant ethical action is possible. Nursing provides the ideal milieu for the perception of these processes.

Adhering to a practice-based ethic, a nurse can attain a very high degree of competence or excellence. A practice-based ethic, like nursing practice itself, is based on agreement. In each case, agreement produces competence.

The aim of clinical practice is to heal, nurture, and strengthen a patient's:

- Ability to control his immediate time and effort.
- Ability to pursue benefits and to avoid harms.
- Ability to deal with his circumstances.
- Ability to live his life span successfully.
- Commitment to himself and his life.

The aim of a practice-based ethic is the same—to heal, nurture, and strengthen the person. The aim of a practice-based ethic is to create these causal sequences that lead to a common goal. The promise of a practice-based ethic is that the causal sequences that are established in the health care setting promote excellence and are meaningful, and that they can be continued by a patient after discharge and by a nurse throughout her lifetime.

**Intelligible** (*that which is understandable*) means that sequences are clear and arise from the context of awareness and a system of abstract health care knowledge. The nurse and the patient understand the present context and recognize a common desired outcome. *Causal* means that sequences are initiated and controlled by the actions of an agent or

> The nurse and the patient understand the present context and recognize a common desired outcome.

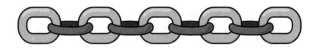

**FIGURE 8.1** Intelligible causal sequences.

The nurse and the patient bring about a result by volitional efforts.

directed to an agent's purposes by her time and effort; volitional efforts purposefully link past events and future events. The nurse and the patient bring about a result by volitional efforts. *Sequences* are a series of future events intelligibly and causally linked to a series of past events. *The result evolves from causal actions.*

An agreement sets up a sequential causal and connecting chain of actions between nurse and patient, and the purposes and goals they desire to achieve together. An agreement creates a context for their interaction. Wherever there is a connectable gap between the sequential causal and connecting chain and the purpose and desired end goals, the gap is frequently the result of a failure of one of them or both to recognize some aspect of the context created by their agreement. Once this recognition is achieved, the links of the chain can be reconnected.

## THE MILIEU

The milieu is the health care arena taken as a learning device.

The milieu is the health care arena taken as a learning device. Everything is there to be observed and understood—the nurse as agent, the patient, the values, the actions and direction of the actions, their progress or regress, the foreseeable consequences. All are there to be observed by a nurse and to be continued or to be changed.

The modern health care setting has evolved over centuries in response to societal development and advances in science. The health care milieu is a practice environment where events can be predicted, actions can be controlled, and intelligible causal sequences can arise from volitional action based on contextual awareness.

The milieu can provide guidance and be replicated. The intelligibility indicates that what occurs is based on shared contextual awareness. Causality indicates the connection between what is and what will be. Directed sequences substantiate predictability. The milieu makes it possible to control an intelligible progression—in practice and in ethical interaction.

The agent–patient context enables the nurse to maintain that which is ideal in the health care arena. It is an ever-present illustration of intelligible causal sequences. It establishes intelligible causal sequences to return her patient to a condition of autonomous optimism and stability. "When a nurse, as an ethical agent, learns how to identify the various parts of an ethical context and their interrelations, she has developed a significant practical skill. When she is able to understand the individual human values that make each context what it is, she has developed a . . . [valuable] skill and competency" (Husted & Husted, 2004, p. 646).

If a machine were invented that could accomplish this and effectively act on this understanding, its value should be immediately recognizable, and it would be worth a very high price.

## THE ANALYTIC PROCESS

The bioethical standards as ethical lenses can serve as:

- Aspects of human nature.
- A blueprint of the nature of human nature.
- A description of what it is for a patient to experience himself as human.
- Objects of awareness through which each person is able to come to an understanding of the internal being of others.
- Critical indicators of ethical thinking and of everything preconditional of ethical states (e.g., ethical decision/agreement/interaction/justice).
- Basic motivators of ethical agreement and interaction.
- Instruments to evaluate one's ethical decision-making process.
- Principles of human action.

Every bioethical dilemma is unique. Every patient's circumstances are unique. Every patient is unique. Uniqueness is not threatened by dilemmas, but patients are. The ways they are threatened and the ways out of their dilemmas are shaped by uniqueness, thus, the *importance* of uniqueness.

A health care professional's first task, in order that she might understand her patient's dilemma, is to understand her patient. The direct and relevant way to do this is to study her patient's fundamental virtues—his character structures as described in the bioethical standards. This journey begins with the least complex character structure—freedom. Freedom, more than any other character structure, is revealed to a health care professional very near to the perceptual level. It requires a minimum of analysis to detect the presence or absence and the nature of her patient's freedom. What actions does he initiate? What predictable changes can be brought about by these actions?

From there, analysis proceeds through the character structures as they become more complex, more abstract—further from the perceptual level and more in need of analysis. Finally, analysis arrives at the virtue that includes or fails to include, all the others—the patient's self-created autonomy.

In using the standards as lenses into the character of another, one proceeds most quickly and efficiently through these steps:

- Freedom: The actions chosen and exhibited by the patient.
- Beneficence: The extent to which his time and effort is self-consciously devoted to the pursuit of benefit and/or to the avoidance of harm.

*This journey begins with the least complex character structure—freedom.*

*From there, analysis proceeds through the character structures as they become more complex, more abstract—further from the perceptual level and more in need of analysis.*

What benefits does he consider worthy of attention? What possible harms occupy his concern? Why, and to what extent, does he consider, rightly or wrongly, changes beneficial or harmful? Why, and to what extent, is he engaged with the purposes of the health care setting?

- Objectivity: The degree to which he is in cognitive contact with himself, his thought processes and motives, and the clarity of his cognitive contact with his circumstances. Do his evaluations and actions reveal that he is in an objective cognitive contact with his context? Are his motives and efforts well or inefficiently directed?
- Fidelity: The degree to which he is concerned for the needs of his life, health, and well-being; the extent to which he is faithful to who he is; if he is still the autonomous person he was. Does he know himself as well now, after the onset of his disability, as he did before the onset of his disability? Do his actions and his lifestyle still reflect who he is, or do they reflect the power of external forces working through him? Does he still have an interest in the values he held before the onset of his disability?
- Autonomy: The extent to which he has retained his independent uniqueness by keeping his virtues interwoven.

Autonomy is remarkably complex, but it is the goal one ought to keep in mind when moving through the process of analysis from freedom to fidelity.

Autonomy is remarkably complex, but it is the goal one ought to keep in mind when moving through the process of analysis from freedom to fidelity. Even if a health care professional never gets beyond the point where she can foresee how her patient will, generally, exercise his time and effort in action, his freedom, her understanding of her patient will already be above average.

---

### DILEMMA 8.2: FAMILY DISPUTE OVER DONATING A CHILD'S ORGANS

Kim, a 19-year-old, is brain-dead as the result of severe head trauma she suffered in a Jet Ski accident. Her mother indicates that Kim had always said, "I'd donate my organs to help someone else live." Her father, who remains extremely distraught, refuses to even talk about the issue. Both look to you for support. What would you do? (Haddad, 2002)

---

## NURTURE

To nurture is the commitment and objective of nursing. It is the motivation for a nurse's making the agreement with herself that she would become a nurse. In most cases, when she made this agreement with herself, it was a decision to be an excellent nurse and to nurse virtuously (with excellence). The development of her efficacy, her power to produce a desired result or effect in the practice of nursing is also the realization

If her agreement with herself was to be a nurse and to nurse excellently, then the nurse ought to do this primarily for her own sake and for her own benefit.

of her rational self-interest. If her agreement with herself was to be a nurse and to nurse excellently, then she ought to do this primarily for her own sake and for her own benefit. In this way, the motivations of her actions will provide the maximum benefit for herself and ultimately for her patient. These will be two effects of the same motivation.

Given the nature of the health care professions, every professional action is an interaction. Therefore, a nurse's excellence and success depend not only on herself but also on her patient. The power of her interaction is, to some extent, dependent on the power of her patient's response. To maximize the efficiency of her actions, she must be capable of strengthening her patient's virtues. The excellence of interaction depends on the actions of those who interact.

Her action, in strengthening her patient's virtues, at the same time enables her patient to realize his rational self-interest, which was his motive for coming into the health care system.

For her to interact optimally, her patient must be capable of responding. To perfect her professional virtues, her power to act well and successfully, she must be capable of increasing the strength of his ability and willingness to act well and successfully. This can be achieved through attention to her patient's character. It can be achieved most efficiently through attention to his individual virtues—through attention to the bioethical standards. As she is analyzing him through his virtues, she is, at the same time, nurturing and strengthening his virtues and her own.

## A DIFFERENT DOOR

*Myself when young did eagerly frequent*
*Doctor and Saint, and heard great argument*
*About it and about, but evermore,*
*Came out by the same door wherein I went.*

—Rubáiyát of Omar Khayyám

The experience that Khayyám describes is quite common for students of ethics. They never get across the room. They "[come] out by the same door wherein [they] went." They hear "great argument" concerning the nobility of this or the glory of that, and when the first joy of learning has past, they realize that they have learned nothing related to their lives or intentions. If they do not become aware of this, they are worse off.

Sometimes, there is an ethical dilemma of which one may be unaware. If you have ever been a patient, you can understand this because as a patient you know that the health care professional is not aware of all the things with which you are dealing. As the nurse gains an understanding of her patient and then acts from this understanding, she may resolve a dilemma without even being aware of the fact that a dilemma existed. This is much better than not being aware of it, not acting on it, and failing to do for him what he would have done for himself, or failing to do for him what you would have done for yourself.

Whether you are aware of a dilemma or not, it is desirable that you understand as much as you can about the patient under your care. We cannot know the mind of another person directly, but the bioethical standards provide a way to get the best knowledge of another person as possible. They act as lenses to clarify the psychology of your patient. Using the bioethical standards as lenses enables you to see and understand other people. They enable you to see your patient as an autonomous person.

> Using the bioethical standards as lenses enables you to see and understand other people. They enable you to see your patient as an autonomous person.

The uses of the bioethical standards are manifold. Used as lenses to clarify the character of an ethical agent, they reveal:

- Interactions between the character structures.
- Weaknesses and strengths of an agent's character.
- Reliability of an agent's actions.
- Objects of implicit awareness through which each agent is able to communicate without understanding the internal thoughts of others.
- Virtues, or that which makes possible the virtue of an ethical agent.
- The resources that make possible the enjoyment of life.
- The objectivity of one's awareness that enables one to enter an ethical relationship.
- The limitations on what can be agreed to in the agreement.

## UNDERSTANDING

Every person has a philosophy of life, whether or not the person realizes it. This philosophy affects the person's professional philosophy and guides the approaches she takes to her role as a health care professional (Gaberson, Oermann, & Shellenbarger, 2015). That philosophy is more than ethics. A person's ethic is, so to speak, surrounded by her view of the world—the nature and the possibilities offered by reality, and a notion of what is and what is not possible to know, how one comes by knowledge, and what makes knowledge reliable.

Understanding the nature of another person can be compared with understanding something like a piece of hard cherry candy. How does a child first come to understand the nature of a piece of hard cherry candy? First, he sees an opaque redness. Then he can smell the cherry aroma of the piece of candy. He can feel its firm roundness; tap it on the table and hear its hardness. He can then taste its cherry sweetness. These sensory investigations reveal the nature of a piece of hard cherry candy.

One can understand some things about a person on a sensory level, by looking at him or listening to him, but only in a limited way. There are other ways beyond sensory input where one can come to understand another by discovering the characteristics that make him what or who he is. The characteristics that make a person who he is cannot be grasped on a sensory level, but they can be grasped through the bioethical standards acting as lenses.

Your patient is a unique individual and must be understood as a unique individual. All too often, a health professional looks on her patient globally as a homogeneous and undifferentiated living organism—more or less like herself. She understands herself inadequately and only with great difficulty. Therefore, in the short time she has with her patient, she finds it nearly impossible to understand her patient completely. However, the person who is her patient can be understood as a living, thinking organism characterized by a high degree of autonomy—that is, uniqueness.

If you see your patient as an alien mass, not surprisingly you will not understand him. If you discover him as structured by the virtues characterized in the bioethical standards and you are open to the character structures that make him who he is, you will find it remarkable how efficiently you can understand your patient.

As a nurse engages in the nurturing process, she must examine the principles that structure and motivate a patient. This is an essential, defining part of a nurturing process. To do this, one who would nurture must gain an understanding of the principles involved. The most effective way to come to understand these principles is to study them in those whom one is nurturing. One nurtures these principles in one's patient. This is the art of one's profession.

The bioethical standards serve as lenses that explain and clarify your patient's motivations. They reveal the general psychology of your patient. Ethical interactions with a patient are interactions with a patient's motivations. Using the bioethical standards as lenses enables you to see and understand other people. They enable you to see your patient as an individual person.

## THE BIOETHICAL STANDARDS AS LENS

### The Standard of Freedom Acts as a Lens

> The character structure that serves as the bioethical standard of freedom is an agent's power to control his time and effort, to take self-directed, independent actions guided toward the agent's own values and by his own motivations

The character structure that serves as the bioethical standard of freedom is an agent's power to control his time and effort, to take self-directed, independent actions guided toward the agent's own values and by his own motivations. If you would know your patient, you must look at how he reacts to the things that demand his time and effort and, if possible, why he reacts in this way. Examine his desires and the purposes he has set for himself.

He is a private individual, which means, in effect, he owns the being he is. His time and effort—his living—is his own. His actions and motivations—his control of his time and effort—imply who he is. Gain an understanding of how he uses his time and to what he puts his effort, and you will know him quite well. Sometimes a patient will act against who he is. At this first stage of your ethical awareness, you will be able to recognize this.

This is the first level of knowledge one can have of another. Analysis through freedom gives the least complex understanding of a patient, but it is far better than no understanding at all. In some cases, it will be the only knowledge of a patient a nurse can gain. Without that knowledge, she might have no knowledge on which to base decisions and actions. This is the best basis upon which further understanding is built.

## The Standard of Beneficence Acts as a Lens

The character structure that serves as the bioethical standard of beneficence is an agent's power to relate himself appropriately to the sources of pleasure and pain. It is the power to act to acquire the benefits one desires and the needs one's life requires.

If you would move to a higher level of understanding, look at the way your patient relates himself to pleasure and pain. Discover how he defines benefits and how he acts to gain benefits and to avoid harm. When you have gained this level of awareness, you will have no trouble interacting with your patient without any likelihood that you might violate his rights. You will have a workable idea as to when he would and would not give "voluntary consent." When for some reason he cannot give consent, you will have a basis on which to judge where his consent would and would not be "objectively gained."

His actions suggest his attitude toward potential benefits and potential harms. When you explicitly understand what his actions suggest, you will have a bit of ethical understanding that is wonderfully helpful to fill your ethical role successfully.

## The Standard of Objectivity Acts as a Lens

The character structure that serves as the bioethical standard of objectivity is an agent's power to achieve and sustain his awareness of his thought processes and his circumstances, which is to say, his context.

If you would know your patient, look at how clearly he is aware of himself and how he engages with the reality of his situation. It is important to know him in this way because he is dependent on that reality for his life, health, and well-being. If you understand his reactions, you understand the way he relates himself to the world. If this is possible, it is the way you need to understand him.

A patient's behavior reveals much about his awareness of objective reality and, more important, his attitude toward it. You gain an objective understanding of him when you make this as explicit as the situation allows. Objectivity is a value to everyone. It is especially a value to a nurse, even more than to a patient but a nurse's objectivity is the best asset a patient has.

## The Standard of Fidelity Acts as a Lens

The character structure that serves as the bioethical standard of fidelity is the power of an agent to adhere to the terms of a decision or agreement.

The character structure that serves as the bioethical standard of fidelity is the power of an agent to adhere to the terms of a decision or agreement. It is an individual's commitment to an obligation he has accepted as part of his role.

If you would know your patient, look at the attitude he has toward himself. His attitude toward himself shapes who he is.

You ought to do what is best for your patient. This is difficult unless your patient wants to do what is best for him. To reach this level of awareness of your patient, you must understand his attitude toward himself. You must know something about what he values. You must know the way he relates himself to his choices. It helps if you know how strongly he values himself—his fidelity to himself. If his fidelity to himself is weak, you may be able to strengthen it.

To do for himself everything he can do, he must be faithful to himself. To do for him everything you can do, you must be faithful to your agreement with him. If you are faithful to your agreement with him, you are being faithful to yourself as a health care professional. At the same time, nothing you can do will better strengthen his feeling of self-worth and his desire to exercise fidelity than your obvious expectation of his fidelity to himself. Your fidelity to him achieves this better than anything you can do.

## The Standard of Autonomy Acts as a Lens

The character structure that serves as the bioethical standard of autonomy is the rational human being, the uniqueness, independence, individual identity, and ethical sovereignty over himself as an agent of an agent.

The character structure that serves as the bioethical standard of autonomy is the rational human being, the uniqueness, independence, individual identity, and ethical sovereignty over himself as an agent of an agent.

All these lead to and create the unique person who is your patient. If you are to know another person and interact effectively with him, you must understand his uniqueness—the final product of the bioethical standards. You must know how this person is different from others—how he is who he is. You begin with the knowledge that he is an individual, reasoning person. From this, you try to discover as much about him as you can through the other bioethical standards.

## DILEMMA 8.3: TO TELL OR NOT TO TELL THE FINDINGS OF SURGERY

During the performance of a laparotomy for the removal of an ovarian cancer, Dr. Richmond discovers the presence of precancerous gonads in Amelia, his 17-year-old patient. This is a condition (testicular feminization) that occurs once in every 50,000 females. Most women who have the condition are not gratified to discover it. Dr. Richmond believes he has a duty to reveal this detail of her condition to Amelia because "she has a right to know it." (Adapted from Minogue & Taraszyewski, 1988)

## LENSES IN FOCUS

Ingrid makes an ethical analysis of each of her patients. She proceeds in this way:

She attempts to determine areas of her patient's life where he will desire control of his time and effort while he is in the health care setting. She begins with her patient. She does not begin with an empty abstraction, such as the idea of freedom. She begins with evidence gleaned from her patient's actions and purposes.

She stays on the alert for areas where she can do her patient some good. She stays alert for areas where she might do him some harm or prevent some harm from coming to him.

She engages in a close analysis of the context. She does this to determine whether and where she might harm her patient by stumbling over the standard of objectivity. She seeks to discover where her patient will benefit by receiving some item of information. Her patient is the center of her ethical attention. She nurtures his life, health, and well-being. She does this by nurturing his commitment to himself.

She seeks to learn the areas of her patient's desire for freedom. She does this also by learning about her patient. She does not reflect on the concept of freedom in her mind. She engages in ethical interaction with a person. She does not engage in ethical interaction with a concept.

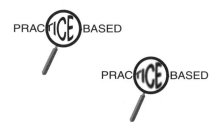

**FIGURE 8.2** Lenses in and out of focus.

All these lead her to the uniqueness of her patient. She comes to this by learning about her patient. She does not do this by examining her concept of uniqueness. She knows that her ethical interactions will be with a unique patient. It will not be with the idea of uniqueness that she carries around in her mind.

## LENSES OUT OF FOCUS

On the contrary, for Dora, a nurse who works with Ingrid, her center of attention is on her vague understanding of her guiding standards and not her patient (Figure 8.2). She regards standards as deontological rules and rules as her standard. In ethical matters, she gives her attention to these rules rather than to the well-being of her patient.

Dora's process of ethical discovery is not governed by the nature of her patient's situation. She feels a responsibility to the rules themselves. Only the rules, as she understands them, possess ethical relevance for her. Used in this way, her standards as rules make it impossible for her to stay in tune with the context.

Ingrid's use of standards assumes that the efficiency of a nurse's ethical actions is measured by the benefit the nurse's actions yield. Because she assumes this, the center of her ethical concern cannot be abstract, ethical rules. The center of her context must be the nature and the needs of her patient. The center of Dora's ethical context is a rule. Dora assumes that the benefit of a nurse's ethical actions is measured by the mechanical conformity of her mechanical actions to an externally related standard. The center of her ethical awareness is rigid, abstract, ethical rules. Ingrid does not attempt to benefit a standard. Dora does.

> *A nurse who works for a telephone-based service receives a call from a young man who reports that he is going to commit suicide and discloses his plan for the time, place, and method. The nurse determines the threat is serious and calls 911 in the caller's area. The emergency response team arrives in time to save the young man. After the caller recovers, he contacts the advice service, furious with the nurse for "infringing" on his right to commit suicide.* (Malloy, 1998)

The caller shares Dora's ethical perspective.

The bioethical standards are means to ends beyond themselves. They are not ends in themselves. There is no way, in the standards themselves, to show that the standards have any value.

Fidelity is of no value to fidelity. Freedom cannot be benefited by having its freedom respected. Obviously, these ideas are utterly senseless. However, they are ideas that, in one way or other, inspire many actions in the health care setting.

*Bob is an elderly, feeble, senile man who has entered the hospital for diagnostic studies. On her shift, Dora cares for Bob, and Ingrid cares for him on hers. Bob wants to get up and ambulate. In the context of his condition, it is foreseeable that he might fall and injure himself. Ingrid quiets him but does not allow him to ambulate. Dora, terrified by the term "paternalism," does allow Bob to ambulate. Bob falls and fractures his hip.*

Dora claims that the reason she allowed Bob to ambulate was out of respect for his right to self-determination. In Bob's context, Dora's claim does not justify her action. She placed the well-being of self-determination above the well-being of her patient. More often than not, the benefit to a patient in not being restrained outweighs the possible harm (Janelli, 2006). This is context dependent, and no abstraction, including self-determination, forms a context. It is only the circumstances and the knowledge and awareness of reasoning, desiring, and acting agents that form that context.

Ingrid claims that the reason she did not allow Bob to ambulate was through a fear that he would fall and injure himself. Unless what she did took place in a very peculiar biomedical context, Ingrid's claim justifies her action. Ingrid placed the well-being of her patient above the well-being of self-determination.

> It is only the circumstances and the knowledge and awareness of reasoning, desiring, and acting agents that form that context.

## CONFLICT

Actions that are ethically appropriate in relation to a certain patient at one time may not be ethically appropriate in relation to the same patient at a different time. Actions that are ethically appropriate to one patient at a certain time may not be appropriate in relation to a different patient at the same time or if the actions are taken in a different way. The bioethical standards signify virtues that, working together, constitute the character of a rational being—specifically,

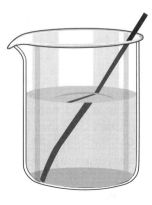

**FIGURE 8.3** Only apparently bent.

insofar as he or she is an ethical agent. It is these virtues that place the agent in a context, that make the context what it is in relation to the agent (or patient), and that shape the agent's motivations and actions.

The bioethical standards can ease a nurse into the bioethical context. They can make it easier for her to resolve ethical dilemmas. However, conflicts in the interpretation of the bioethical standards can arise. This is not a conflict in the bioethical standards themselves but only an apparent conflict (Figure 8.3). The stick looks bent in the water, but this is only apparent. The stick is not bent. When this occurs, they cannot be resolved in the context they have created. A wider context must be formed.

It is often difficult to know where and how a standard ought to be applied. Rational, ethical action on the part of a nurse without reference to the nature of her patient is impossible. On the other hand, the bioethical standards, outside of the context, do not and cannot outline the context. The context must determine the application of the bioethical standards. They are very broad abstractions, and some way must be found to bring them down into a patient's context.

---

### DILEMMA 8.4: GOING AGAINST THE PHYSICIAN'S ORDER FOR A DYING MAN

Rodney is one of Lynetta's patients in the intensive care unit. He is dying from cirrhosis of the liver. Rodney asks Lynetta for a small drink of water. The order left by the physician placed Rodney on NPO status (nothing by mouth) because of the actively bleeding ulcers in his stomach and intestine.

Despite all his medical problems, Rodney is alert and thirsty. He knows the probable consequences of a sip of water and yet continues to want it. Rodney's physician is called in the hope that he will change the order. He will not. He says that he wants to be conservative and is afraid that the water would trigger more bleeding. Despite this, Rodney still continues to plead for a drink of water. What should Lynetta do?

---

## MUSINGS

We have established that:

- Nursing as an intelligible activity relies on the nurse–patient agreement.
- The existence and nature of the nurse–patient agreement implies the appropriateness of the character structures as bioethical standards.
- The bioethical standards guide us in the most effective way of keeping the nurse–patient agreement.
- The more intelligible a nurse's practice, the more effective and rewarding.
- The bioethical standards reflect those aspects of human nature that make the nurse–patient agreement possible and desirable.

- Freedom clearly expresses the self-governance of individuals.
- Objectivity is a biological device whose purpose is the well-being of individuals.
- The freedom described in the bioethical standard of freedom is the ability to pursue one's life and guide one's actions through objective awareness. This is a freedom possessed only by individual people.
- Fidelity is a virtue that can be practiced only by individuals, one by one.

Every person is unique. So is every bullfrog and every waterfall. The weather every winter is unique. The uniqueness described in the bioethical standard of autonomy is not the uniqueness of bullfrogs, waterfalls, or winters. It is the uniqueness of individual persons.

Wherever nursing has a logical foundation, it is an activity essentially involving individual nurses and their individual patients. Every other nursing activity (e.g., education, administration, research) is an outgrowth of this.

"[T]he standards provide a means to learn more about the patient (a lens through which to see the patient) and identify aspects where the patient can be supported" (Cutilli, 2009, p. 188).

## STUDY GUIDE

1. What is necessary for a theory to be called practice based?
2. As you are aware, the purpose of a lens—for example, in eyeglasses—is to make things clearer, more accessible to one's view. Take each of the bioethical standards as a lens and apply it to your knowledge of yourself. It will be a great learning experience.
3. Now do the above with someone you know very well. What have you learned?
4. What is the meaning of the saying from the *Rubáiyát* of Omar Khayyám? Relate it to yourself.
5. What does looking at the standards as lenses add to your knowledge of your patients?
6. Use this case for class discussion; the analysis of the case only appears in the instructor's manual.

### DILEMMA: RIGHT OF A TEENAGER TO KNOW DESPITE WISHES OF HER MOTHER

Bonnie is a 17-year-old teenager who has had 2 years of extensive treatment of a particularly difficult form of leukemia. She has had a bone marrow transplant, chemotherapy, and virtually all options for treatment. Through all her treatments, improvements, and relapses,

*Continued*

Bonnie has kept in touch with two very close friends. At her last admission to a regional cancer treatment center, the family was told there were no further options and Bonnie would not live more than a few weeks or months.

She is now at home, very weak, needing almost constant care. She still shows a lively interest in what is occurring, she seems to find humor in little things, and she constantly wants to listen to her favorite music cassettes. Her mother is in charge of all treatments and has issued orders to everyone that Bonnie must not be told her prognosis. These orders are reiterated to each home care nurse. She has even gone so far as to restrict visits from Bonnie's father, from whom the mother is divorced, and Bonnie's close girlfriends, fearing they will "let it slip" that Bonnie is terminal. She refuses to leave Bonnie's room when anyone else is visiting and usually tries to direct the conversation making comments such as, "When you get better." Bonnie knows she is dying; she frequently asks Carrie, her hospice nurse, "How much time do I have left?" "Why won't anyone let me talk about my dying?" and more insistently, "I am not afraid to die, but I need to talk to my friends about this." You have spoken to her mother about Bonnie's concerns, but she refuses to listen to any discussion about telling Bonnie the truth. What should you do? (Turkoski, 2003)

## REFERENCES

Cutilli, C. (2009). Ethical considerations in patient and family education. *Orthopedic Nursing, 28*(4), 187–191.

Gaberson, K. B., Oermann, M. H., & Shellenbarger, T. (2015). *Clinical teaching strategies in nursing.* New York, NY: Springer Publishing Company.

Haddad, A. (2002). Ethics in action: Honoring a daughter's wish to donate her organs. *RNWeb, 65.* Retrieved June 18, 2004, from www.reweb.com

Husted, G. L., & Husted, J. H. (2004). Ethics and the advanced practice nurse. In L. A. Joel (Ed.), *Advanced Practice Nursing* (pp. 639–661). Philadelphia, PA: Davis.

Janelli, L. M. (2006). Physical restraint use: A nursing perspective. *Medsurg Nursing, 15,* 163–168.

Khayyám, O. (1983). *Rubáiyát of Omar Khayyam.* New York, NY: St. Martin's Press. (Original work published 11th century)

Malloy C. (1998). Managed care and ethical implications in telephone-based health services. *Advanced Practice Nursing Quarterly, 4*(2), 30–33.

Minogue, B. P., & Taraszyewski, R. (1988). The whole truth and nothing but the truth. *Hastings Center Report, 18*(5), 34–36.

Rhodes, R. (1912). Cases from Mount Sinai School of Medicine, CUNY. American Philosophical Association Newsletter on Philosophy and Medicine, *91,* 75–76.

Turkoski, B. B. (2003). A mother's orders about truth telling. *Home Healthcare Nurse, 21*(2), 81–83.

# NINE

# MORAL DISTRESS

## OBJECTIVES

- Discuss the nature and causes of moral distress.
- Examine the effect of moral distress on the person and on nursing.
- Explain what is involved in moral courage.
- Identify strategies to reduce moral distress and moral residue.
- Discuss how objectified ethical abstraction helps in dealing with moral distress.
- Determine the role of justice in relationship to futile care.
- Give examples of incivility in the health care arena.

*The world is a dangerous place, not because of those who do evil, but because of those who look on and do nothing.*

— *Albert Einstein, n.d.*

## THE NATURE OF MORAL DISTRESS

The actions that a nurse takes have an ethical aspect because they are concerned with the vital and fundamental goals of health and life. In her role as a professional, a nurse acts as an agent for her patient. The purpose of a patient (regaining or maintaining the power of his agency) determines the actions taken by the nurse. A nurse does for her patient what the patient would do for himself had he not lost his power of agency, his ability to be his own agent. She assists him in regaining the ability to take independent actions. In the interaction of a professional and a patient, they agree that, because the patient is a patient, and the nurse is a professional, the professional will act as an agent for the patient and on behalf of the patient to carry out the patient's values, goals, and purposes.

"Moral distress is the physical or emotional suffering that is experienced when constraints (internal or external) prevent one from following the course of action that one believes is right" (Pendry, 2007, p. 217). When a nurse knows the ethically right action to take as she acts as an agent for her patient but she is unable to take this action, she experiences moral distress. The nurse may feel powerless to act for any of a variety of reasons (Epstein & Delgado, 2010). For instance, organizational constraints make doing the right thing difficult or impossible. She may not be able to take the correct action because she is not able to communicate effectively with those who hold the power. To cite two examples, the action is against her organization's policy, or it is in conflict with what is viewed as the best for others. Moral distress may lead to position resignations, or even to nurses' leaving the nursing profession altogether, because it causes such emotional distress. Moral distress is a threat to the nurse's moral integrity, because she is not able to act correctly as an agent for her patient. Moral integrity, according to Hardingham (2004), involves a sense of self-worth and unity that is present when there are clearly defined values that are congruent with the nurse's actions and perceptions. A threat to a nurse's moral integrity is a threat to her identity as a nurse, because a nurse is charged with the responsibility to act as an agent for her patient when he is unable to do so himself.

## CLINICAL ISSUES THAT PROMOTE MORAL DISTRESS

In cases of moral distress, the nurse is aware of the right action, but she feels powerless and is not able to take this action.

Moral distress is an ethical matter, but it is not the result of an ethical dilemma. An ethical dilemma involves a situation in which the ethically correct action must be decided. In cases of moral distress, the nurse is aware of the right action, but she feels powerless and is not able to take this action. The American Association of Critical-Care Nurses (AACN) position statement on moral distress (2008) identifies it as a serious, and often ignored, problem in nursing. A variety of clinical issues arises in the nursing profession that can lead to moral distress: futile care disputes, disagreements between health care professionals and family members, disagreements between physician and nurse, cost issues, incivility between and among health care professionals, and triage (covered in Chapter 6) decisions.

## Futile Care

Definitions of futile care center on the idea that the treatment to be delivered will not improve the outcome for the patient

Patients' receiving futile care is one of the major causes of moral distress for nurses. Definitions of futile care center on the idea that the treatment to be delivered will not improve the outcome for the patient (Jonsen, Siegler, & Winslade, 2006; Kasman, 2004). In addition, futile care is also considered more burdensome than therapeutic (Robley, 2009), the burden including physical and emotional pain as well as loss of agency and dignity (Gallagher, Zoboli, & Ventura, 2012; Gillick, 2012). The futility of a medical treatment must be determined within the context of the individual case, because a treatment may not be successful in every circumstance (Mobley, Rady, Verheijde, Patel, & Larson, 2007; Meltzer & Huckabay, 2004; Sibbald, Downar, & Hawryluck, 2007).

The laws regulating actions related to futile care vary by state, and most are nonspecific thus allowing for negotiation. Only two states, Texas and Virginia, have laws that specify time periods during which futile treatment may be stopped by physicians with the support of the institutional ethics committee. The Texas futile care law is part of the larger Texas Advanced Directive Act enacted in 1999. This law allows a physician to refuse to begin or to continue life-sustaining treatment if the physician determines the treatment to be medically hopeless or futile. A hospital ethics committee may review the physician's decision, and if it agrees that the treatment is futile, the patient or designated decision maker has 10 days to find an institution willing to accept the patient and to continue treatment. The hospital has no obligation to continue treatment beyond 10 days. An extension of the 10-day limit may be granted if the decision maker can provide a preponderance of evidence that there is an institution that will accept the patient (Texas Health & Safety Code, 1999).

The controversy about such laws stems from the concern that physicians or ethics committees might undercut the wishes of an individual. Those opposed to such laws believe that physicians may make value judgments about the quality of life for a terminally ill person that the person might not make for himself. They believe the individual or his designated decision maker is the only one who can determine whether a life is worth living. Supporters of futile care laws counter with the idea that physicians have the appropriate knowledge about what is futile and what is beneficial (Kajnar, 2006; Ozar, 2007). They can make timely decisions that reduce periods of pain and loss of dignity and control over one's life that will be extended while family members argue and/or negotiate over which course of action they prefer.

However, negotiation itself negates the purpose of identifying care as being useful or futile.

However, negotiation itself negates the purpose of identifying care as being useful or futile. The following explanation of medical futility is based on the seminal and developmental work of Schneiderman, Jecker, and Jonsen (1990) and Schneiderman (2011), pioneers in identifying and addressing this issue. Beginning in the early 1990s, they described the concept of futility as having both quantitative and qualitative aspects. In quantitative terms, evidence published in the literature provides support for treatments being either useful or futile. We can predict which treatments will be successful and which will not. Although absolute certainty of a treatment's success or failure can never be established, we can develop guidelines based on rational thinking and on scientific verification. For example, Sasson et al. (2008) verified circumstances under which prehospital Basic Life Support (BLS) may be terminated without disadvantage to the patient. Delivering futile care from a quantitative aspect indicates the care is based on uncommon rarities or even statistical impossibility.

## DILEMMA 9.1: PATIENT'S BENEFIT VERSUS FAMILY'S DESIRES

Martha has bone cancer and is suffering excruciating pain. Treatment has been unsuccessful. She is dying. She is heavily medicated but is still in terrible pain. The question of placing her in palliative sedation is discussed with the family. They are against this because she will not be able to talk with them.

In qualitative terms, we can predict which treatments will bring about an improvement in a particular human situation and which will merely prolong the suffering and loss of agency that exists.

A medically useful treatment includes the expectation of a benefit that can be perceived by the patient as such.

Justice is also an important part of futile care decisions. Justice is concerned with the fair distribution of burden and benefit.

In qualitative terms, we can predict which treatments will bring about an improvement in a particular human situation and which will merely prolong the suffering and loss of agency that exists. The immediate individual context must provide the foundation for a decision. A medically useful treatment includes the expectation of a benefit that can be perceived by the patient as such. The goal of the nurse is to restore her patient's agency. Her actions are based on the values, goals, and purposes of her patient. Medical futility should then depend on achieving the patient's goals. Treatment should be aimed at releasing the patient from the need for treatment and then on the patient's being able to achieve life goals.

Justice is also an important part of futile care decisions. Justice is concerned with the fair distribution of burden and benefit (Schneiderman, 2006). Can we ask a patient to endure treatment with only a 1-in-100 chance that it will improve his situation? Futile treatment places this unfair burden on a patient. For example, a specific treatment such as renal dialysis may be known to have beneficial effects for particular types of patients. For a patient with stage 4 liver cancer who is slipping into a coma, however, dialysis will have very little if any chance of improving his situation. It may even cause his death.

In light of this, a symphonological examination of futile treatment is itself futile. What rational human being would choose care that fails to:

- Provide a benefit that the patient will be able to appreciate?
- Improve the patient's ability to take self-directed, independent actions guided toward his own values and motivations?

- Increase the patient's awareness of his thought processes, his circumstances, and his context?
- Adhere to the terms of his commitment to himself?
- Promote the patient as a unique, rational human being?

Why then is futile care even an issue? The answer lies in communication problems among health care providers, patients, and family members.

## Communication Among Health Care Providers, Patients, and Significant Others

Moral distress can arise from issues surrounding futile care. Between nurses and physicians differences in perceptions about futile care are based on differences in their professional roles. Factors such as competing values, hierarchical processes, and availability of resources can lead to communication difficulties (Oberle & Hughes, 2001). Physicians bear the burden of making or avoiding decisions, and nurses must carry out the orders and be witness to the consequences. Physicians report conflict over initiating or foregoing futile care based on the Western philosophy of saving or curing all patients (Boyle, Miller, & Forbes-Thompson, 2005). At the same time, nurses report distress from inability to influence decisions and having to prolong patients' suffering (Meltzer & Huckabay, 2004; Oberle & Hughes, 2001; O'Connor, Winch, Lukin, & Parker, 2011).

Communication issues for patients and significant others begin primarily with lack of reliable information (Gillick, 2012). For example, in a study of significant others regarding their primary goals for patients with end stage Alzheimer's disease, 50% chose a comfort approach, 21% said they would want a life prolonging treatment, and 18% said they would want something in between. After viewing a video about the disease process and care of the patient at end stage, 89% said they favored a comfort approach, and no one wanted life prolonging treatment (Volandes et al., 2007). It is a matter not only of lack of knowledge about disease processes but also of lack of knowledge about care processes and inappropriate expectations for medical care. Patient's loved ones misunderstand that doing "everything possible" does not ensure a good outcome and may only prolong suffering (Clabots, 2012).

### DILEMMA 9.2: THE DEMANDS OF JUSTICE

A certain patient is in a persistent vegetative state. There is no predictable chance that he will recover from his condition. He has requested that if he were in this state he be allowed to die. Do beneficence and respect

*Continued*

for his autonomy require that he be kept alive or that he be allowed to die? It can be argued that:

- He must be allowed to die. The unique individual that he once was no longer exists. The recognition of his right to autonomy includes recognition of the fact that there is no autonomous being to be kept alive.
- He must be allowed to die on the basis of beneficence. Biological survival in the sense of the preservation of electrochemical processes is in no way the equivalent of a human life. If there were any foreseeable possibility of his attaining even the lowest level of a human life, the demands of beneficence might be entirely different. There is no hope for a worthwhile and human life, and respect for his once human dignity requires that he be allowed to die.

The agent has an exclusive right to decide. His decision is authoritative. On the other hand:

- He must be kept alive. One possesses life only once and life is precious above everything else. Without life, nothing else is of any value. The patient's staying alive is a tribute he pays to himself and to his life. Beneficence demands that he be assisted in staying alive.
- He must be kept alive because no one has a right to terminate the life of an autonomous individual. What the patient was in the past is no longer relevant. His autonomy now is the unique nature of his present existence—even if it is only these electrochemical processes. Recognition of his present autonomy demands that his life be preserved.

## Incivility Between and Among Health Care Professionals

Incivility has been defined by Clark, Olender, Kenski, and Cardoni (2013) as "rude or disruptive behavior often resulting in psychological or physiological distress for the people involved and, if left unaddressed, may progress into threatening situations (or result in temporary or permanent illness or injury)" (p. 98).

Nurses have an ethical responsibility to interact respectfully with patients, colleagues, and students. This is self-evident, and yet there continues to be bullying within the health care setting and within academia. This problem is escalating. Incivility has been defined by Clark, Olender, Kenski, and Cardoni (2013) as "rude or disruptive behavior often resulting in psychological or physiological distress for the people involved and, if left unaddressed, may progress into threatening situations (or result in temporary or permanent illness or injury)" (p. 98). Incivility and bullying in nursing are complex problems and include such behaviors as denying coworkers access to resources, refusing information or help, embarrassing verbal exchanges, or spreading rumors (Matt, 2012). Emerging evidence suggest that incivility in the workplace has significant implications for nurses, patients, and health care organizations (Luparell, 2011; Matt, 2012), as well as students and faculty in nursing programs (Anthony, Yastik, MacDonald, & Marshall, 2014; Shanta & Elaison, 2013).

Beauchamp and Childress (2009) attribute incivility in health care to, among other things, a lack of discernment. They defined *discernment* as "the ability to make fitting judgments and reach decisions without being unduly influenced by extraneous considerations, fears, personal attachments, and the like" (p. 40). Using the principles of symphonology, undue influence can be avoided thus ensuring appropriate responses to incivility in the health care arena and in educational settings.

> *. . . reflection on the bioethical standards within a given context enable faculty to choose a response to incivility that ethically aligns with agreements made and supports an understanding of one's nature and needs for personal development. Thus, the application of a symphonological model for ethical interaction can be considered as a new perspective from which to frame solutions to incivility [and the moral distress that results].* (Burger, Whitfield-Harris, Kramlich, Malitas, & Page-Cutrara, 2014)

## Cost

The value of an individual life, in and of itself, is not calculable. Although cost does not play a role in determining the futility of a treatment for an individual, patients and families are concerned that decisions related to futile care may be based on economics (Gillick, 2012; Robley, 2009). Retrospective reviews of medical records have shown that the cost of care at the end of life is high. About 27% of all Medicare spending occurs in the last year of life (Lubitz & Riley, 1993), and this figure holds stable over time (Fleishman et al., 2012). A review of 6,832 medical records of elderly people in Oregon and Washington indicated that end-of-life costs were significantly higher for people who received futile care. However, further analysis revealed that large reductions in futile care would result in only small cost savings (Fleishman et al., 2012). This suggests that end-of-life costs are high, but futile care does not add significantly to them.

## THE MANIFESTATIONS OF MORAL DISTRESS ON THE PERSON

Distress indicates suffering, trouble, and disturbance. Moral distress is a dreadfully negative experience for the nurse who suffers from it. When a nurse is not able to act as an agent for her patient in the manner she knows to be ethically correct, she can suffer greatly. She may suffer emotionally with feelings of powerlessness, ineffectiveness, anxiety, and self-doubt. If not able to act in an ethically correct manner, she may struggle to act at all. As she feels a threat to her moral integrity, she may abandon herself, her patient, her position, or her profession. Gunther and Thomas (2006)

The nurse may suffer emotionally with feelings of powerlessness, ineffectiveness, anxiety, and self-doubt.

reported that some of the nurse–participants in a study they conducted indicated that even years after suffering from moral distress related to an unforgettable patient care event, the nurses were still trying to understand and justify the outcomes.

## Bioethical Standards Out of Focus

*Just as a nurse engages in the nurturing process with her patient, a nurse must also nurture herself.*

To nurture is the commitment and objective of a nurse. It is the motivation for a nurse when she made the agreement with herself that she would become a nurse. Just as a nurse engages in the nurturing process with her patient, a nurse must also nurture herself. She must examine the principles that structure and motivate her. The bioethical standards serve as lenses during her examination. They come in as principles as she examines and understands her motivations. Ethical interactions are interactions with her motivations. Using the bioethical standards as lenses enables her to see and to understand herself as an individual person. When a nurse is suffering from moral distress, the bioethical standards related to self are out of focus (see Chapter 8).

Freedom is the nurse's power to control her time and effort, to take self-directed, independent actions guided toward her own values and by her own motivations. Beneficence is the nurse's power to relate herself appropriately to the sources of pleasure and pain and to act to acquire the benefits she desires and the needs her life requires. Objectivity is the nurse's power to achieve and to sustain her awareness of her thought processes, her circumstances, and her context. Fidelity is the nurse's power to adhere to the terms of a decision or agreement. It is her commitment to an obligation she has accepted as part of her role as a nurse. Autonomy is the rational human being; it is the nurse's unique, independent individual identity, and ethical sovereignty over herself. Each of these creates each singular nurse. When a nurse is unable to take the action she knows to be ethically correct in acting as an agent for her patient, her bioethical standards are out of focus and she suffers from moral distress. She is not able to keep her agreement with herself or her patient or to take the action that the unique people, situation, and context require based on their values and motivations.

## EFFECT OF MORAL DISTRESS ON NURSES AND NURSING

*Moral distress can lead to negative patient outcomes, and has consequences for nursing and health care facilities as nurses leave their positions, and even their profession.*

Moral distress can lead to negative patient outcomes, and has consequences for nursing and health care facilities as nurses leave their positions, and even their profession. The AACN (2008) position paper on moral distress indicates that it causes dissatisfaction with the work environment and is a major contributor to nurses leaving their work environment. The AACN paper also asserts that it affects the nurse–patient relationship and can affect the quality, quantity, and cost of nursing care.

## DILEMMA 9.3: PHYSICIAN'S ORDERS VERSUS BENEFIT TO THE PATIENT—A NURSE'S DILEMMA

Blessing is a 41-year-old refugee from Africa who came to the United States with her five children a year ago under the sponsorship of a religious organization. She is a victim of torture and was pregnant with her sixth child, conceived during a rape, when she arrived. The religious organization assisted her financially and were her only contacts following her move. She speaks very limited English. The religious organization became concerned about her a few months after the birth of her child as she started acting paranoid and would not leave the apartment she had been renting, even though she was served papers indicating that she had to move. Law enforcement had to remove her from the apartment and took her to a hospital for a psychiatric assessment. She is actively psychotic, paranoid, angry, and demanding to be returned to her apartment with her children. She does not understand her circumstances. She will not eat, drink, or use the restroom until she is returned to her apartment. An intravenous (IV) line is ordered, and she voids large amounts of urine without a receptacle every few hours. Medical service places orders for a straight catheter following bladder scans every couple hours. She has to be restrained to complete these orders. The nursing staff expresses distress and concern regarding these orders given her past history of torture and rape. They are to follow the physician's orders but feel to do such would be more harmful than helpful to Blessing.

## Moral Residue

Moral residue is an accumulation of the residual damage that is left after each morally distressing situation is encountered by a nurse and she has had to act against what she knows to be the ethically correct action to take.

Moral residue is an accumulation of the residual damage that is left after each morally distressing situation is encountered by a nurse and she has had to act against what she knows to be the ethically correct action to take. Epstein and Delgado (2010) assert that "after these morally distressing situations, the moral wound of having had to act against one's values remains." They describe moral residue as long lasting and powerfully integrated into a nurse's thoughts and views of herself. Gunther and Thomas (2006) report that caregiving experiences can result in an accumulating residue of moral distress for nurses that, in turn, can affect their future experiences in their everyday work life. According to Epstein and Hamric (2009), there are three potential results from moral distress and moral residue. A nurse may become morally insensitive and no longer recognize or engage in morally sensitive situations. A nurse may conscientiously object and move forcefully to make her opinion known by such actions as documenting her disagreement in the chart or by asking for a consult. Last, the third result is viewed as the most damaging by Epstein and Hamric; the nurse may suffer from burnout.

The third result is viewed as the most damaging by Epstein and Hamric; the nurse may suffer from burnout.

## Burnout

Formation of objectified ethical abstraction (discussed in detail later in this chapter) is a process that can increase the emotional strength and staying power of a caregiver. The increase in strength and staying power that can result from utilizing the process of forming an objectified ethical abstraction can solve the problems of caregiver strain because burnout is the loss of emotional strength and staying power

Under ideal circumstances, a nurse will want to give care. A professional will want to see her patient's pain and suffering decreased through her efforts for a very personal reason. Pain and the loss of autonomy are both forms of suffering. Ideally, a nurse hates suffering in general and specifically hates it as it affects each patient. A nurse gains a deep sense of personal satisfaction simply by taking part in decreasing the pain, loss, and suffering of another person for whom she cares. "Compassionate fatigue," thought to be a form of burnout, is brought on by health care professionals coming in almost constant contact with suffering (Gentry, Baranowsky, & Dunning, 2002). Formation of objectified ethical abstraction is a corrective remedy for "compassionate fatigue" and a preventive measure against burnout.

## MORAL COURAGE

*Stand up for what is right even if you stand alone.*

*— Anonymous*

Moral courage is the ability to do what is right or moral despite elements that would influence a person to act in another way (Lachman, 2011). Moral courage is the ability of a nurse to engage in strategies to decrease her moral distress and put the bioethical standards related to herself back in focus. Gallagher (2010) reaffirms that courage is a virtue and suggests that a nurse with sufficient moral courage is able to speak up and to challenge unacceptable practices and policies. *However, this is not without risks.*

> Moral courage is the ability of a nurse to engage in strategies to decrease her moral distress and put the bioethical standards related to herself back in focus.

> Moral courage is the ability to do what is right or moral despite elements that would influence a person to act in another way.

"Healthcare professionals often face complex ethical dilemmas in the workplace. Some professionals confront the ethical issues directly while others turn away. Moral courage helps healthcare professionals who often face complex ethical dilemmas in the workplace" (Murray, 2010). Moral courage is the ability to do what is right or moral despite elements

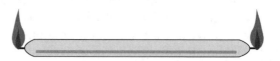

**FIGURE 9.1** Burnout.

that would influence a person to act in another way (Lachman, 2011). Lachman, Murray, Iseminger, and Ganske (2012) have suggested an Acronym: CODE—C for moral courage; O for obligation and adherence to the American Nurses Association (ANA) Code of Ethics for Nurses; D for danger management; and E for the expression and action component.

A nurse with moral courage is able to assert her belief in the ethically correct action to take, to communicate this effectively with others, and to engage in strategies to work toward a resolution. When a nurse has a practice-based bioethical decision-making model that she is able to utilize, it enables her to communicate with others when situations of moral distress arise. She is prepared better to interact in situations with moral courage. "The relationship between moral courage and moral distress is not straightforward. It is tempting to say that if nurses have sufficient moral courage they need not experience moral distress. However, given that organizations are not always supportive and do not always react appropriately, but rather may act defensively to concerns about standards of care raised by conscientious practitioner, even the most morally courageous staff may fear to speak up" (Gallagher, 2010, para. 15).

Professional obligations are spelled out in the ANA Code of Ethics for Nurses. Armed with an understanding of their obligations, nurses must assess the risks in speaking out when acting in ethically charged situations. Sometimes, the risk may be too great and further analysis of the problem is warranted. Danger management is an important aspect of moral courage and ways need to be found to decrease risk to self and others and, at the same time, "stand-up" for what is right.

> When a nurse has a practice-based bioethical decision-making model that she is able to utilize, it enables her to communicate with others when situations of moral distress arise.

> Sometimes, the risk may be too great and further analysis of the problem is warranted. Danger management is an important aspect of moral courage and ways need to be found to decrease risk to self and others and, at the same time, "stand-up" for what is right.

## Using Moral Distress Reduction Strategies

A nurse can engage in moral distress reduction strategies to decrease her suffering from moral distress and to reduce moral residue. Epstein and Delgado (2010) offer a variety of strategies for nurses to use to reduce moral distress. They suggest nurses speak up about the problem and voice their concerns, be deliberate and accountable with their voice and action, build support networks of multidisciplinary colleagues, and be more productive by focusing on needed changes in the work environment. They also suggest that nurses participate in moral distress education, target common root causes of moral distress in the work environment, work on developing policies, and work on designing a workshop to address moral distress. The AACN (2008) also suggests that nurses recognize and name moral distress, affirm the professional obligation to act and commit to addressing it, be knowledgeable about using professional resources to address it, and actively participate in professional activities to expand knowledge about it. They also suggest developing skills through mentoring and using resources to decrease moral distress, as well as implementing strategies to accomplish desired changes in the work environment. This can help preserve the personal integrity and authenticity of nurses. The AACN also encourages employers to take action and to have an open, respectful work environment with interdisciplinary forums to recognize and to address moral distress.

## Objectified Ethical Abstraction

A nurse who is able to communicate effectively, as well as to utilize resources such as mentors, interdisciplinary colleagues, and professional organizations, will likely decrease her experience of suffering from moral distress. Even when utilizing these reduction strategies, situations will arise when a nurse is unable to act in the manner she knows to be the ethically correct manner and she may still suffer from moral distress.

Utilizing the strategy of objectified ethical abstractions (OEA) can assist the nurse in managing her distress and suffering. Formation of objectified ethical abstraction is a process that can increase the emotional strength and staying power of a nurse. The increase in strength and staying power that can result from using the process of forming an objectified ethical abstraction can help resolve the problem of moral distress and burnout because they are both the loss of emotional strength and staying power.

## Forming the Objectified Ethical Abstraction

A nurse hates suffering in general. A nurse gains a deep sense of personal satisfaction simply by taking part in decreasing suffering. Caring does not require a nurse to lose sight of herself in the suffering she observes and/or experiences while acting as a professional nurse. Formation of the objectified ethical abstraction is a corrective remedy and a preventive measure against moral distress and burnout. She can use the technique of orienting herself emotionally onto an objectified ethical abstraction to decrease her suffering.

To form the objectified ethical abstraction, a nurse begins by observing her patient's suffering. Then, through an act of abstraction, she turns her awareness to many instances of suffering, including her own suffering and the suffering of all of her patients. She looks on this abstraction, *suffering,* as if it were a concrete thing in itself. From here she broadens her abstraction to include all suffering. Finally, she looks upon this abstraction of suffering as if it were an independently concrete existing object. By regarding this abstraction of suffering as concrete, she takes actions that are motivated toward an almost visible entity.

A nurse takes suffering to represent a concrete reality in order to generate the emotional attitude that enables her to have strength to work toward stopping it. Suffering is an abstraction because it is taken (abstracted) into the mind from every individual instance of suffering and exists as an individual reality only in the mind. Suffering is objectified because it is treated as a concrete object existing apart from the mind. Suffering, as an abstraction, is an ethical abstraction. Suffering is the one supreme human adversary the health care system was created to combat.

## Use of Objectified Ethical Abstractions

Caring and a dedication to beneficence do not require a nurse to lose sight of herself or the facts of her life to share her patient's suffering. Ideal circumstances in the health care setting will increase a nurse's self-awareness and strengthen her attachment to her life. She can create ideal circumstances through the technique of orienting herself emotionally onto an objectified ethical abstraction.

Her hatred of suffering and her consequent desire for the well-being of her patient are given a new strength and endurance as suffering becomes a target to take action against. It enables a nurse to relate to her patient without alienation on the one hand or codependence on the other.

## Interacting With the Objectified Ethical Abstraction

By interacting with the objectified abstraction, as well as by interacting with her patient, a nurse is focused on more than the concrete present moment. The objectified abstraction gives the present moment a new and wider meaning. It enables the nurse to relate to her patient without alienation on the one hand or codependence on the other. Her hatred of suffering and her consequent desire for the well-being of people are given a new strength and endurance.

It is too much to deal with every patient's suffering, as well as one's own suffering. If a nurse is not spurred on by antagonism to the existence of suffering, her actions will be hindered and weakened by her unacknowledged awareness of suffering's vicious presence. The entire purpose of the health care system is to help patients overcome suffering, recover their well-being, and/or attain a peaceful death. A nurse who is not motivated by a hatred of suffering is out of sync with her profession and to her own nature. The absence of this motivation is not appropriate to a health care professional or a human being.

A nurse's actions and purposes are made easier if she knows why she is doing what she is doing and she has a firm idea of the end result being pursued.

A nurse's actions and purposes are made easier if she knows why she is doing what she is doing and she has a firm idea of the end result being pursued. When a nurse knows what she is working toward accomplishing in general and what she can accomplish here and now with her patient, the means to accomplish it become less tedious and stressful. In one way, she is keeping her attention directed on her patient, for she is combating her patient's suffering. In another way, by keeping her thoughts on the defeat of suffering and the victory of freedom from suffering, she is keeping her attention directed toward the abstraction of suffering. This unites the nurse and her patient by giving them a common enemy and also a common goal. At the same time, it puts a psychological distance between them. This distance frees them from an unhealthy dependence on each other and does this in such a way as to bring them closer together.

Before the professional formed her ethical abstraction and objectified suffering, she regarded suffering as a concrete object and took it instance by instance. She was focused on her patient, who, in turn, was focused on his suffering. By focusing her attention on the abstraction, the nurse places both the patient and his suffering back into perspective. Then she can see the health care setting in relation to her role and purpose and her role and purpose in relation to this patient's situation. Through this, the professional and her patient are closer. At the same time, she has an emotional defense. She has distanced herself from stress and suffering without distancing herself from her patient. This distance, instead of hindering and weakening her action, gives her an abstract experience of the meaning and purpose of her action and gives her action long-term strength and endurance.

*This unites the nurse and her patient by giving them a common enemy and also a common goal.*

*Through this, the professional and her patient are closer. At the same time, she has an emotional defense*

## MUSINGS

Using a symphonological approach to building relationships with patients and significant others can help alleviate the moral distress surrounding futile care and other things that contribute to moral distress in the health care arena. Focusing on the standards will ensure the conversation is patient centered, identifying and promoting his autonomy, improving and supporting objectivity, maintaining his freedom, moving in the direction of beneficence, and remaining faithful to the values, goals, and purposes of his life.

When a nurse has a practice-based bioethical decision-making model that includes strategies that she is able to use to cope with suffering, as well as to communicate with others when situations of moral distress arise, she is better prepared to engage in sufficient moral courage and to confront the challenges of her profession. When a nurse is able to communicate intelligently the action she knows to be ethically correct, she will have a better chance of being able to follow through with this action with the approval of those in power. And even if she is not able to take the action that she knows to be the ethically correct action to take, she can be assured that she has done her best in acting as an agent for her patient and has kept her agreement with herself and her patient to the best of her ability. When she is able to communicate successfully the ethically correct action to take given the unique person, situation, and context based on the individual values and motivations, she is able to put the bioethical standards back into focus for herself and for her patient and make a difference for, at least, some of her patients and herself.

## STUDY GUIDE

1. Have you ever experienced moral distress? If so, explain why it happened and what you did about it.
2. Give some examples of cases in which futile care was being given and ask yourself why?
3. Having moral courage to speak out can be dangerous. Discuss why.
4. Apply objectified ethical analysis to something that you have experienced that gave you distress. How could it have helped?
5. How can the bioethical standards applied to a situation in which you are experiencing moral distress help you resolve the problem?
6. Use this case for class discussion; the analysis of the case only appears in the instructor's manual.

---

### DILEMMA: DISAGREEMENT AMONG HEALTH CARE PROVIDERS REGARDING LIFE-SUSTAINING INTERVENTIONS

Mr. Judd, age 64, comes into the hospital to have a tumor (later discovered to be benign) removed from his jaw. During the surgery, he suffers a cerebrovascular accident (CVA). Three weeks after the CVA, the physician asks the family about withdrawing food and fluids and allowing Mr. Judd to die naturally. Mr. Judd has no living will or durable power of attorney for health care. His wife and children turn to Amanda, Mr. Judd's primary care nurse, for advice. On assessment, Amanda finds that Mr. Judd responds occasionally to simple commands, such as, "Squeeze my hands," "Turn your head," "Blink your eyes," and so on. Based on these observations, Amanda tries to talk to the physician. The physician insists that food and fluids be withdrawn. He believes that Mr. Judd will never get any better. Are there any further steps that Amanda ought to take?

---

## REFERENCES

American Association of Critical-Care Nurses (AACN). (August 2008). Position Statement: Moral distress. Retrieved from nej.sagepub.com on September 8, 2013.

Anthony, M., Yastik, J., MacDonald, D. A., & Marshall, K. A. (2014). Development and validation of a tool to measure incivility in clinical nursing education. *Journal of Professional Nursing 30*(1), 48–55.

Beauchamp, T. L., & Childress, J. F. (2009). *Principles of biomedical ethics* (6th ed.). New York, NY: Oxford University Press.

Boyle, D. K., Miller, P. A., & Forbes-Thompson, S. A. (2005). Communication and end-of-life care in the intensive care unit. *Critical Care Nursing Quarterly, 28*(4), 302–316.

Burger, K., Whitfield-Harris, L., Kramlich D., Malitas, M., & Page-Cutrara, K. (2014). Application of the symphonological approach to faculty-to-faculty incivility in nursing education. *Journal of Nursing Education 53*(10), 563-568.

Clabots, S. (2012). Strategies to help initiate and maintain the end-of-life discussion with patients and family members. *MedSurg Nursing, 21*(4), 197–203.

Clark, C. M., Olender, L., Kenski, D., & Cardoni, C. (2013). Exploring and addressing faculty-to-faculty incivility: A national perspective and literature review. *Journal of Nursing Education, 52*(4), 211–218.

Epstein, E. G., & Delgado, S. (September 30, 2010). Understanding and addressing moral distress. *OJIN: The Online Journal of Issues in Nursing, 15*(3), Manuscript 1.

Epstein, E. G., & Hamric, A. B. (2009). Moral distress, moral residue, and the crescendo effect. *Journal of Clinical Ethics, 20*(4), 330–342.

Fleishman, R. J., Mullins, R. J., McConnell, K. J., Hedges, J. R., Ma, O. J., & Newgard, C. D. (2012). Is futile care in the injured elderly an important target for cost savings? *Journal of Trauma and Acute Care Surgery, 73*(1), 146–151.

Gallagher, A., Zoboli, E. L., Ventura, C. (2012). Dignity in care: Where next for nursing ethics scholarship and research? *Revista De Escola Enferma, 46*(Esp), 51–57.

Gallagher, A., (March 21, 2010). Moral distress and moral courage in everyday nursing
practice. *OJIN: The Online Journal of Issues in Nursing, 16*(2), Manuscript 8.

Gentry, J. E., Baranowsky, A. B., & Dunning, K. (2002). The accelerated recovery program for compassion fatigue. In C. R. Figley (Ed.), *Treating compassion fatigue* (pp. 123–137). New York, NY: Brunner-Routledge.

Gillick, M. (2012). Doing the right thing: A geriatrician's perspective on medical care for the person with advanced dementia. *Journal of Law, Medicine & Ethics, 40*(1), 51–56.

Gunther, M., & Thomas, S. P. (2006). Nurses' narratives of unforgettable patient care events. *Journal of Nursing Scholarship, 38*(4), 370–376.

Hardingham, L. B. (2004). Integrity and moral residue: nurses as participants in a moral community. *Nursing Philosophy, 5*(2), 127–134.

Jonsen, A. R., Siegler, M., & Winslade, W. J. (2006). *Clinical ethics: A practical approach to ethical decision making in clinical medicine.* New York, NY: McGraw-Hill.

Kajnar, H. (2006). Shared decision making in medicine. In F. Porzsolt & R. M. Kaplan (Eds.), *Optimizing health: Improving the value of healthcare delivery* (pp. 74–86). Boston, MA: Springer.

Kasman, D. L. (2004). When is medical treatment futile? A guide for students, residents, and physicians. *Journal of General Internal Medicine, 19*(10), 1053–1056.

Lachman, V. D. (2011). Strategies necessary for moral courage. *OJIN: The Online Journal of Issues in Nursing, 15*(3), Manuscript 3.

Lachman, V. D., Murray, J. S., Iseminger, K., and Ganske, K. M. (2012) Doing the right thing: Pathways to moral courage, *American Nurse Today, 7*(5).

Luparell, S. (2011). Incivility in nursing: The connection between academia and clinical settings. *Critical Care Nurse, 31*(2), 92–95.

Lubitz, J. D., & Riley, G. F. (1993). Trends in Medicare payments in the last year of life. *New England Journal of Medicine, 328*(15), 1092–1096.

Matt, S. B. (2012). Ethical and legal issues associated with bullying in the nursing profession. *Journal of Nursing Law, 15*(1), 9–13.

Meltzer, L. S., & Huckabay, L. M. (2004). Critical care nurses' perceptions of futile care and its effect on burnout. *American Journal of Critical Care, 13*(3), 202–208.

Mobley, M. J., Rady, M. Y., Verheijde, J. L., Patel, B., & Larson, J. S. (2007). The relationship between moral distress and perception of futile care in the critical care unit. *Intensive and Critical Care Nursing, 23*(5), 256–263.

Murray, J. S. (September 30, 2010). Moral courage in healthcare: Acting ethically even in the presence of risk. *OJIN: The Online Journal of Issues in Nursing, 15*(3), Manuscript 2.

Oberle, K., & Hughes, D. (2001). Doctors' and nurses' perceptions about ethical problems in end-of-life decisions. *Journal of Advanced Nursing, 33*(6), 707–715.

O'Connor, A. E., Winch, S., Lukin, W., & Parker, M. (2011). Emergency medicine and futile care: Taking the road less traveled. *Emergency Medicine Australia, 23*(5), 640–643.

Ozar, D. (2007). The value of an ethics consultation. In D. Steinberg (Ed.), *Biomedical ethics: A multidisciplinary approach to moral issues in medicine and biology* (pp. 186–190). Lebanon, NH: University Press of New England.

Pendry, P. (2007). Moral distress: Recognizing it to retain nurses. *Nursing Economics, 25*(4) 217–221.

Robley, L. R. (2009). Medical futility: Where do we go from here? *Nursing Critical Care, 4*(3), 47–48.

Sasson, C., Hegg, A. J., Macy, M., Park, A., Kellermann, A., & McNally, B. (2008). Prehospital termination of resuscitation in cases of refractory out-of-hospital cardiac arrest. *Journal of the American Medical Association, 300*(12), 1432–1438.

Schneiderman, L. J. (2011). Defining medical futility and improving medical care. *Journal of Bioethical Inquiry, 8*(2), 123–131.

Schneiderman, L. J. (2006) Seeking justice in health care. In F. Porzsolt & R. M. Kaplan (Eds.), *Optimizing health: Improving the value of healthcare delivery* (pp. 15–20). Boston, MA: Springer.

Schneiderman, L. J., Jecker, N. S., & Jonsen, A. R. (1990). Medical futility: Its meaning and ethical considerations. *Annals of Internal Medicine, 112*(12), 945–954.

Shanta, L. L., & Eliason, A. R. (2013). Application of an empowerment model to improve civility in nursing education. *Nursing Education in Practice, 14*(1), 82–86.

Sibbald, R., Downar, J., & Hawryluck, L. (2007). Perceptions of "futile care" among caregivers in intensive care units. *Canadian Medical Association Journal, 177*(10), 1201–1208.

Texas Health & Safety Code. (1999). Chapter 166.

Volandes, A. E., Lehman, L. S., Cook, E. F., Shaykevich, S., Abbo, E. D., & Gillick, M. R. (2007). Using video images of dementia in advanced care planning. *Archives of Internal Medicine, 167*(8), 828–833.

# TEN

# THE POWER OF ANALYSIS THROUGH EXTREMES

## OBJECTIVES

- Interpret what can be learned from the crocodile paradox.
- Give examples of how the implicit can guide decision making.
- Explain the method of analysis through extremes.
- Give personal examples of how extremes analysis can be used in practice.
- Define gentle coercion.

Ethical errors occurring in the health care setting result in harm to the patient and others. Ethical errors can be avoided by ensuring that the agent is interacting with the correct person and that the actions to be taken are ethically justifiable.

Analysis of a situation by examining the extremes establishes the nature of the case through the lenses of the bioethical standards. Awareness of this nature brings awareness of what is to be done, for whom it is to be done, and why it is to be done. Awareness of the right person for whom one ought to take an action is a precondition of awareness of what action ought to be taken and why. Analysis by the appropriate standards can then guide the awareness of how it is to be done. The right beneficiary has been found if all the following are true:

- His autonomy is such that a rational, controlled, and nonaggressive agreement can be formed.

> Ethical errors can be avoided by ensuring that the agent is interacting with the correct person and that the actions to be taken are ethically justifiable.

- His freedom guides the actions to be taken.
- The contextual demands of objective awareness are justifiably understood from his vantage point.
- Benefit and harm are well defined by him and appropriate to the context.
- His vision of fidelity (i.e., of the agreement) is appropriate.

The wrong beneficiary has been found when any of the following are truc:

- His autonomy is such that a rational, limited, and nonaggressive agreement cannot be formed.
- The way he proposes to use his freedom in the context is such that it would not be possible to justify his decisions and actions.
- He cannot exercise objective awareness in guiding his actions.
- His understanding of benefit and harm is nonobjective or aggressive.
- His vision of fidelity lacks respect for the rights of others.

## THE FOURTH HUMOROUS VIGNETTE: THE CROCODILE PARADOX

One balmy day on a South Seas island paradise, a woman was washing her laundry in the sea. Her baby was lying on the sand a few yards away. A crocodile lurked in the nearby bushes. All of a sudden, while the woman was distracted by a spot of bear fat on a lace scarf, the crocodile rushed over and snatched her baby.

The woman pleaded, "Please don't eat my baby." Crocodiles, as any crocodologist will tell you, are remarkably straightforward, reliable, and sincere. To tell the truth, their attention tends to be narrow, and their awareness is dominated by instinct and tradition. Nonetheless, they have a charming sense of humor.

The crocodile decided to amuse himself by offering the child's mother this mocking bargain: "If you can tell me what I am going to do, I will give your baby back to you. But if you cannot, I will eat your baby."

This was rather unkind because the crocodile was determined to eat the baby. If the woman said that the crocodile would not eat the baby, she would not be telling him what he was going to do and so he would eat the baby. If she replied that he was going to eat the baby, this would be what he was going to do only if, in fact, he did eat the baby.

What a dreadful impasse! Hum. We will have to think about this.

## ANALYSIS THROUGH EXTREMES

When you have eliminated all that is impossible, whatever is left, however improbable, must be the case. (Sherlock Holmes [Doyle], 1930)

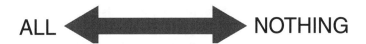

**FIGURE 10.1** Extremes.

Extremes is a method of analysis through which a nurse or any health care professional can clarify a bioethical context by identifying the relationships—the rights and responsibilities—of the people involved in that context. It involves carrying a situation to ridiculous extremes in a thought experiment in order for issues to become clear (Figure 10.1). Although some dilemmas do not lend themselves to extremes analysis, it is a very powerful instrument for analyzing those that do.

The value of analysis through extremes arises from the fact that it is usually easier to determine what is the wrong thing to do than it is to determine what is the right thing to do. Determining the wrong thing to do greatly assists one in determining the right thing to do.

The discovery of that which is definitely wrong—that which is ethically "impossible"—is a powerful tool when what is definitely right is not self-evident and not easy to discover.

What is right and what is wrong may be established in relation to the standards. To ascertain that a certain approach would be the wrong application of a standard helps one to discover the right application. Even where the right application of a standard is vague and unclear, the wrong application will probably be more evident. And its wrongness—its ethical invalidity—will clarify the right approach and the right application.

With an objective and contextual awareness, under ideal circumstances, the right thing would be visible, and the wrong thing would also be visible. This clear vision can be achieved by focusing on the extremes of each standard taken as a right (e.g., the right to freedom, the right to objectivity, and so on). Through this, one can determine whether the ethical nature of the health care setting would be better expressed in giving absolute and complete support for each standard as a right to a certain beneficiary, or whether it would be best that this beneficiary enjoy no right to the exercise of the virtue given that the way in which he would exercise it would involve unethical actions and would establish unethical conditions. This will establish the nature of the case overall and the most appropriate action to be taken.

The questions to be asked are, "Which extreme—absolute support for a beneficiary or no support for a beneficiary—will most perfectly maintain the rationality and objectivity of the agreement?" "Which extreme will most perfectly satisfy appropriate commitments and expectations?" and "Which extreme will most perfectly avoid the violation of a right?"

Extremes analysis proceeds by determining what the final results would be of the patient having absolute control over the exercise of each standard. This is in contrast to that person's having no control over the exercise of a standard. Through this analysis, it can be seen which alternative is more just and desirable. When this is determined, the ethical status of an individual patient and the actions that are and are not appropriate to the context will become evident.

## CASE STUDY ANALYSIS THROUGH EXTREMES

In analyzing these cases, we will focus on the context by determining whether the beneficiary's (normally the patient's, but not always) complete control of the standard or the absolute control of that standard by another would be relatively more rational, more objectively desirable, and more justifiable. The following is an absurd dilemma in every way but one: It perfectly illustrates the nature of an agreement that a rational nurse would not make and how such a dilemma ought to be resolved. This is the same type of analysis one would make in preventing suicide for a patient with a mental health diagnosis.

### CASE STUDY 1

Maggie, a nurse in the cardiac step down unit enters the room of 23-year-old Peter, just as Peter's girlfriend is storming out. Peter's girlfriend is obviously angry. When Maggie approaches Peter's bedside, she sees that Peter's sutures have torn and he is hemorrhaging. Maggie explains the situation to Peter and tells him that she is going to take the steps necessary to stop his hemorrhaging. He tells her that he does not want her to stop his hemorrhaging. He has broken up with his sweetheart, and he has nothing left to live for. He wants to die.

This puts Maggie in a dilemma. She has an agreement with Peter that she will act as his agent—to take those actions that he cannot. On the other hand, Peter has made a very unusual request of her. Should she take whatever steps are necessary to save Peter's life or, as the agent of her patient, should she simply accede to his wishes?

In other words, is Maggie (and, by extension, every other nurse) only "the agent of a patient, doing for a patient what he would do for himself if he were able"? If this were the case, much of a nurse's education would be wasted. A nurse is a person—a rational human being. She has an active sense of balance and proportion. She is more than her definition. A person capable of being nothing more than the agent of a patient,

A person capable of being nothing more than the agent of a patient, regardless of the context, would not be capable of being a nurse.

regardless of the context, would not be capable of being a nurse. A nurse should substitute her judgment for her patient's only in the most extreme cases. This is a most extreme case.

As this case is analyzed, this is what is revealed.

Should absolute consideration for Peter's autonomy be the guiding standard of interaction, or should no consideration be given to Peter's autonomy? Peter is a unique, rational human being. His uniqueness is formed from his rationality. The course of action Peter proposes turns an emotional upset, which he feels very intensely, against his rationality. This course of action turns Peter against his own nature. If his uniqueness is such that the emotions engendered by a romantic disappointment would inspire him to turn against his life, this is contrary to the essential nature of rationality. It is irrational. He ought not to be supported in this, because no professional agreement could possibly demand irrationality on the part of the professional. No one, including the nurse herself, ought to assume that her professional agreement should replace her human understanding with duties. A nurse must expect to encounter and accept unusual religious practices or personal outlooks to which people have dedicated themselves, but never an impulsive choice like Peter's.

In this case, is it more appropriate that Peter should exercise absolute freedom or no freedom whatsoever? The decision he has made would negate his freedom—an unhindered future—through his death. Because Peter has abandoned his freedom, it is appropriate that the health care professional give no consideration to his plans to destroy himself. This is the best possible and most logical course of action the health care professional can take.

Should Peter's perspective be regarded as absolutely objective and definitive and be given all consideration, or should it be regarded as entirely nonobjective and be given no consideration? When objectivity is reduced to the level of emotional stimulus and response, objectivity is abandoned. Peter, himself, has abandoned his objective awareness.

*When objectivity is reduced to the level of emotional stimulus and response, objectivity is abandoned.*

Should perfect consideration be given to the benefits Peter plans to pursue, or should no consideration be given to them? Peter sees his greatest benefit in abandoning all the benefits of his future life. In the context of his life, the harm he has suffered is nearly insignificant. He already has abandoned beneficence toward himself.

Should Peter's present state of fidelity to himself determine his nurse's action or have no influence on her course of action? Fidelity to an event (his suicide) has displaced fidelity to himself—the self that could live a long and satisfying life.

It may be that Peter's future life would be so marred by the loss of his sweetheart that his life would, objectively, not be worth living. However, for the health care professionals attending him, it is impossible to see that this would be so. In Peter's present emotional state, it is impossible for him to see that this would be so. Therefore, although it might be a mistake to interfere with him, it is far more probable that the benefits the health care setting provides are better brought about by ignoring his wishes and restraining him—even forcibly if necessary—in order to get the hemorrhaging stopped.

Maggie has a responsibility to do for Peter what Peter would do for himself if he were able. In his present emotional upset he is unable to do anything for himself. She has a professional agreement with Peter. However, no rational person would make an agreement with another to care for his life and health and, at the same time, let him die as a result of what can only be understood as an emotional impulse. Health care professionals are expected to be rational beings—the more rational the better. A person who is rational, whether health care professional or patient, cannot logically be expected to make an irrational agreement or keep an agreement by taking an irrational action.

In many circumstances, when a patient wishes to die, his wish is rational, condoned, and ought to be condoned. Peter's case does not fall into this category.

Now that Peter is in a better emotional place and well on the road to recovery, we can return to our sojourn on the island paradise.

> *However, no rational person would make an agreement with another to care for his life and health and, at the same time, let him die as a result of what can only be understood as an emotional impulse*

## RESOLUTION OF THE CROCODILE PARADOX

When the crocodile made his good-natured but horrifying offer, this is what happened:

The mother replied, "When you offered me this agreement, the implication was that you would listen to my reply. You said, 'If you can tell me what I am going to do, I will give your baby back to you.' I cannot tell you anything unless you listen to what I say. You will not hear what I say unless you listen to what I say. **So, what you are going to do is listen to what I say and then you will give me back my baby, because I told you what you are going to do.**" Immediately the crocodile lost his air of urbane gentility, and with a surly lack of grace, he returned the woman's child. He had failed to consider the implications of what he said.

Nothing can establish the validity of a proper resolution nearly so well as drawing out the absurd implications of its contrary. The implication to be drawn from Peter's dilemma is quite obvious. Implications seldom are obvious, but quite often extremes analysis allows one to confidently draw out the relevant implication. For instance, the implication of Maggie's letting Peter die would be that bioethical interaction, in its most serious moments, can be determined by an emotional turmoil.

> *That which is implied by the context is often the most important part of the context. Thus, the power of the implicit is vital to ethical decision making.*

That which is implied by the context is often the most important part of the context. Thus, the power of the implicit is vital to ethical decision making.

## CASE STUDY 2

Elizabeth is from a large and well-to-do family. She is 24 years old and living on the streets. Her family has paid to have her admitted to several, private, psychiatric facilities for treatment of her schizophrenia. Elizabeth always signs herself out. Because she is judged not to be dangerous, she cannot be held against her will.

Elizabeth's symptoms can be well controlled with psychotropic medication. However, she does not take the drugs and says she does not like the way she feels when she is taking her medication. She writes beautiful poetry and says she finds "my own reality" much more interesting than the boring and tedious life she experiences when on the medication. She prefers the friends she makes on the street to the dullness of "so-called normal people."

Her sister arranges to have her poetry published and sends the meager proceeds to her. She is occasionally picked up for vagrancy and brought in for treatment. Her parents are always contacted. Elizabeth does not maintain contact with them otherwise. Eloise, a social worker, has been assigned to her case. What should be done? (Davis, Aroskar, Liaschenko, & Drought, 1997)

In this case, should absolute consideration for Elizabeth's autonomy be the guiding standard of interaction, or should no consideration be given to Elizabeth's autonomy? Elizabeth is a rational human being, but her ability to use conventional reason is impaired with misperceptions and perceptual disturbances. She is living in "a world of her own." Nonetheless, the way she is living violates no one's rights. As far as we know, she is asking no one to make a commitment to her and she has no expectations of anyone's doing so.

A series of interdependent questions suggests itself in this case: How can the greatest potential harm be avoided and how can the greatest potential good be produced? Is it more desirable for Elizabeth to be happy in her world than to be unhappy in ours? Should Elizabeth sacrifice her happiness for the sake of reason or demand that reason serves her happiness?

> Is it more desirable for Elizabeth to be happy in her world than to be unhappy in ours? Should Elizabeth sacrifice her happiness for the sake of reason or demand that reason serves her happiness?

Elizabeth can avoid the greatest potential harm—the loss of her happiness—by continuing her present lifestyle. Happiness is, and unhappiness is not, desirable. If it is necessary at present for Elizabeth to be happy to remain in her world, then this is her best decision, even in a strange way, her most rational decision.

In this case, is it more appropriate that Elizabeth should exercise absolute freedom or no freedom whatsoever? The ultimate goal of psychiatric care should be to bring Elizabeth to a place where she is able to control and preserve her existence and to flourish. (In this, the goal of psychiatry is no different from the goal of medical science.) At present, her activities do not threaten her survival. They allow her the only form of flourishing she can enjoy. The arena of Elizabeth's life and her agency is maximized in her present lifestyle and the friends she makes on the street. Elizabeth's life is more purposeful and much more interesting than the boring and tedious life that she experiences when on medication.

It is a great temptation to try to control the lives of others or, somewhat more beneficently, to try too hard to help others control their own lives. Sometimes the best thing to do is to do nothing. In Elizabeth's case, she has a right to absolute freedom.

Should Elizabeth's perspective be regarded as absolutely objective and definitive and be given all consideration or as entirely nonobjective and be given no consideration? In this case, there is, at least, an apparent, conflict between objectivity and reason. In several cases cited in this book, the resolution suggests that the power to reason ought not to be sacrificed for the sake of objective awareness.

This is particularly true when the revelation of a new objective fact would be so emotionally devastating that it would be impossible for the hearer to exercise reason. When awareness of an objective fact, in the immediate moment, makes it impossible to reason about one's course of action in the future, objectivity loses all value. **The alternative here for Elizabeth is not a subjective awareness unrelated to objective reality but objective awareness tied to a smaller context—a context with which a patient is psychologically and cognitively able to deal.**

As ethical tools, objectivity and reason do not refer to a person's ability to do crossword puzzles or balance a checkbook. Reason and, therefore, objectivity are tools to the achievement of flourishing and happiness. In Elizabeth's case, happiness would not be achieved by adopting a more conventional lifestyle. So, in a very real sense, it would be irrational for her to change her lifestyle. If any way could be found to enable her to be happy in a different reality, then this might be acted upon. At present, however, there is no such way.

Should perfect consideration be given to Elizabeth's plans to pursue her own sense of beneficence or should no consideration be given to this? Elizabeth's desire is to continue the lifestyle she is living now. Furthermore, no way can be discovered that would enable her to experience her life in this way under different circumstances (e.g., living at home on medication).

Should Elizabeth's present idea of fidelity to herself determine her course of action or have no influence on her course of action? Elizabeth, in her own reality, is experiencing life in an emotional way that many people might envy. Considering that Elizabeth's family is well to do, they might exercise fidelity to her by adding something onto the meager proceeds that Elizabeth's poetry brings to her.

A nurse should not overlook the use of gentle coercion with Elizabeth. **Gentle coercion is when the nurse engages a patient in a conversation with the intent to persuade him by increasing his understanding and encouraging him to take self-ownership. It is an appeal to a patient's reasoning power.** **It never gives way to actual coercion.** Gentle coercion to induce Elizabeth to adopt a more self-controlled lifestyle, of course, is justified. Placing Elizabeth in a state of slavery to appearances is not. (This is what a nurse does every time she educates a patient about changing his lifestyle; she encourages and persuades in a caring manner.) A new term is being used for this in many mental health facilities: *motivational interviewing*, which is often used for groups.

The implication of compelling Elizabeth to conform would be that a humdrum and conventional lifestyle is an ethical standard, a standard so important that, in enforcing it, every individual standard can be violated.

## CASE STUDY 3

Jerry is an AIDS patient. He has a rare lymphoma with several large tumors in his abdomen. Jerry is responding to treatment and will probably be able to return to his home. He has asked his physician and his nurse to keep his confidence. He does not want his wife or his homosexual partner to know that he has AIDS. The physician encourages him to tell his wife and lover, but Jerry refuses. He says that he is very careful about using a condom, and he does not want to upset his present lifestyle with his wife and lover. (This case will be discussed from the aspect of the purely ethical aspects, rather than the legal aspects. Of course, the nurse has the responsibility to be aware of the legal aspects of her practice and act accordingly. Ethics and the law do not always complement one another, however. This is one of many of the causes of moral distress).

Should absolute consideration or no consideration be given to Jerry's unique desires?

Jerry's disease has robbed him of many potential benefits he would have enjoyed without it. He is now imperiled at every turn. Whatever happens may strip him of one of the few benefits he has left. If Jerry were to lose the relationship he has with his wife and/or his lover, the quality of his life would be greatly diminished. In addition to everything he now faces, either loss would be a type of "little death." Suffering the little death of a destroyed relationship is insignificant in comparison to the real death that Jerry's wife and/or lover would suffer if he were to infect them.

Jerry's physician has no right to allow these two people to be placed in jeopardy based on Jerry's promise to practice safe sex. Jerry's nurse also has an ethical obligation to speak out if this is necessary.

Should absolute consideration or no consideration be given to Jerry's freedom? The uniqueness of a person's position does not give him the freedom to threaten another person's right to life. The range in which one has a right to freedom has ethical boundaries. It stops far short of any action that would endanger the life of another person. The fact that one might be careful while exercising this action is not relevant.

*Suffering the little death of a destroyed relationship is insignificant in comparison to the real death that Jerry's wife and/or lover would suffer if he were to infect them.*

Even more so, it does not give a biomedical professional a right to cooperate with him in this by maintaining a life-threatening confidentiality.

Should absolute consideration or no consideration be given to Jerry's outlook on the situation? One cannot develop as an ethical agent and one cannot flourish as a human being without taking certain actions and developing certain attitudes. One does not maintain an ethically developed attitude toward one's own life if one does not inform another person that his or her life is about to be placed in danger. By informing Jerry's wife and lover, the physician would honor his own life and, at the same time, fulfill his human and professional obligation to them.

Should absolute consideration or no consideration be given to Jerry's benefit seeking? Jerry's physician has an opportunity to extend a significant degree of beneficence toward Jerry. This opportunity is very much outweighed by the harm Jerry's physician has the opportunity to do to the others. It is the function not only of epidemiologists but of all health care professionals to prevent or to stop the spread of disease. There is no obvious reason why AIDS is an exception.

Is absolute consideration or no consideration due the health care professional agreement? What consideration ought to be given to the rights agreement? The biomedical professional–patient agreement is not an agreement that can include a clause allowing them to conspire together to violate the rights of others.

If Jerry can exercise absolute freedom, he need not even take precautions. If he has no freedom, then although he will be inconvenienced, no one's life will be placed in jeopardy. No one whose life is endangered can really be thought of as being free. Life must be given precedence over sexual passion. His view of the situation cannot be regarded as objective. Sexual passion is not noted for producing objective judgments. Only by breaking a confidence with Jerry can his wife and lover be enlightened with an objective awareness to which they have a right. The benefit to Jerry is relatively trivial. The detriment to his wife and lover could be fatal. A health care professional has no right to exercise fidelity to a patient when this would violate the rights of a third party. Out of respect for his own life, the physician should exercise a greater fidelity to potential victims.

The implication of maintaining Jerry's confidence is that a health care professional ought to keep his professional agreement, even if this means violating the rights' agreement. If violating the rights' agreement is justifiable, then there is no ethical reason to keep the professional agreement. The rights' agreement is the foundation of the health care professional–patient agreement. It is a fact that legally, Jerry would be liable if he knowingly infected his partner. Use of a condom is not an excuse for not informing one's partner. Here, the law and ethics are in harmony (Epstein, Thomas, & Ritecki, 2003).

> A health care professional has no right to exercise fidelity to a patient when this would violate the rights of a third party. Out of respect for his own life, the physician should exercise a greater fidelity to potential victims.

## CASE STUDY 4

Alfred came into the hospital 4 days ago for a coronary bypass. The surgery went well, and Alfred seems on the way to recovery. A few hours ago, his family was in to visit him. The room was filled with quiet conversation, and the family seemed to share a sense of intimacy.

After his family has gone Lois, his nurse, brings his heparin injection to the room. For no apparent reason, Alfred refuses the medication. Lois knows that Alfred's failure to take the medicine puts his life in jeopardy. She explains to him the reason for the drug and stresses its importance. On one hand, Lois's reasoning tells her that Alfred should take the heparin. There is every reason why he should take it, and no apparent reason for him not to take it. On the other hand, Alfred is adamant. He absolutely refuses to receive the injection of heparin. He also refuses to discuss the reasons why he will not let Lois give him the injection. There is no apparent reason why Alfred's freedom does not give him the right to make this decision. There seems to be an irresolvable conflict between Lois's reason and Alfred's freedom.

If you think about the ethical dilemmas that Alfred's case involves, three things are obvious:

1. Justifiable ethical decisions depend not on the facts of the ethical context but on those facts that are known. Justifiable ethical decisions cannot depend on facts that are not known. No decision of any sort can be made on the basis of facts that are not known or on the basis of a person's refusal to recognize or reveal them.
2. An ethical agent may often feel guilt over the results of a decision that was made on inadequate knowledge. The guilt the agent assumes may very well be worse than the unfortunate result of the decision. If the agent made the decision on an objective reading of all the knowledge that was available, the decision would be perfectly justifiable regardless of its results. Alfred ought to be fully informed concerning the foreseeable consequences of his decision.
3. An ethical agent's reasoned beliefs are sufficient to justify ethical actions. There is nothing whatsoever that an ethical agent can act upon except his reasoned beliefs.

The health care professional might invite Alfred to come along on an analysis through extremes. Lois might dialogue with Alfred as follows:

> You have every right to decide what is going to happen to you, but if you refuse the heparin, you may suffer a stroke or a heart attack. You may die or become paralyzed.

Do you want to make these decisions entirely alone without any expert input (autonomy)? If you give your attention to yourself and to the circumstances here in this room, you will probably enjoy a long life (freedom).

Do you want knowledgeable guidance? Do you want to look through the eyes of people who can see the consequences of different decisions? Do you want to control everything that goes on in this room, or do you want to make it an informed cooperation? If you keep your thinking narrowed down to your present mood, you may change your mind when it is too late (objectivity).

Do you want to make your decision without any knowledge of its consequences or what these consequences would mean to you (freedom)? You will never again react to family or friends. You will never decide on where you want to visit or where you want to go on vacation. You will never again drink a cool beer on a warm day or spend an evening reminiscing with your wife in a quiet restaurant (beneficence). (The best thing a health care professional can find out about a patient is those things in life he most enjoys. These are always useful as incentives.)

> The best thing a health care professional can find out about a patient is those things in life he most enjoys. These are always useful as incentives.

There are a lot of decisions you do not have to make right now. You do not have to decide where you want to go in the next several weeks or what you want to do. But I think you are going to want to be around to make those decisions.

Alfred, you will be dead a long time. How about taking a few years to complete a good life (fidelity)? Okay? (The offer of an agreement.) Let's get at it. (The assumption of an acceptance. This is an example of gentle coercion.)

If he still does not want to take his heparin, he may, in self-defense, reveal the reasons why not. Then you will have much more to work on with him. But hopefully, in this way you can show him—without telling him—the unique person he is; the way he is reacting to his present condition makes him the wrong person— making the wrong decision for himself.

To act otherwise would imply that force is a valid form of ethical interaction or that his experience of comfort and control in the present moment is more important than his experience of comfort and control throughout the rest of his life.

## DISCOVERY VERSUS CHOICE

> That which will be discovered will be the lesser of two harms, or the existence of a harm opposed to a benefit.

The outlines of a context can be discovered by analysis through the standards. Analysis of potential benefits and harms—the most fulfilling exercise of the standards as virtues is revealed through their foreseeable consequences. That which will be discovered will be the lesser of two harms, or the existence of a harm opposed to a benefit.

The ethically appropriate beneficiary can be discovered in the structure of the context by analysis through extremes. Not only this, but there is always the possibility that another dilemma, perhaps more important than the first, may be discovered through extremes analysis. Extremes analysis will reveal who is certainly the wrong person, thing, time, way, extent, and reason.

*Extremes analysis will reveal who is certainly the wrong person, thing, time, way, extent, and reason.*

When it is perfect, an agreement will be with the right person. When agreement is not with the right person, it is radically imperfect. That which would ordinarily be the right thing to do will be the wrong thing to do, and every category will be failed.

## THE PERFECT BIOETHICAL AGREEMENT

*One who is the right person when no right is violated becomes the wrong person when a right is violated.*

One who is the right person when no right is violated becomes the wrong person when a right is violated. The right person, when interactions are in sync with the nature of the health care setting and the nurse's role, becomes the wrong person when interaction is out of sync. The right person under the terms of a rational agreement, when the agreement becomes irrational, becomes the wrong person.

When there is no possibility of an innocent person's rights being violated, when the agreement between a patient and the health care system is consistent with the nature and purpose of the health care system, and when the agreement is free of irrational terms, the bioethical agreement is perfect. The fact that extremes analysis has revealed one person to be the right beneficiary of ethical interaction does not imply that he is to be the exclusive beneficiary of ethical actions. Others must be considered, albeit in an indirect way and to a lesser extent.

*The fact that extremes analysis has revealed one person to be the right beneficiary of ethical interaction does not imply that he is to be the exclusive beneficiary of ethical actions.*

If one went from extremes analysis to an exclusive concern for the rights of one beneficiary, one would have discovered the context, only to abandon it. The purpose of extremes analysis is to establish the right beneficiary and what is right for that beneficiary. It does not and cannot give one a license to ignore balance and proportion in relation to everyone else involved in the situation.

*The purpose of extremes analysis is to establish the right beneficiary and what is right for that beneficiary. It does not and cannot give one a license to ignore balance and proportion in relation to everyone else involved in the situation.*

For instance, your patient wants to talk to you about the condition of his wife, but you see that the patient in the next bed, who is not your patient but is unattended, is in intense pain. You check and discover that he has not been given his pain medication. You arrange for him to get his pain medication. Then you go to your patient to discuss his distressful situation. A health care professional's agreement with a patient does not include the provison that she will not assist someone who is in severe pain before consoling the patient with whom she has an agreement. This is an example of giving up a smaller good to gain a greater good.

You are about to give your patient his aspirin as ordered. He believes that this will help him to sleep. A visitor in the patient's room has a heart attack. You give the aspirin to the visitor. You would do this even if it meant that your patient would have to toss and turn all night. Then, after the person who had the heart attack has been treated, you would, of course, obtain aspirin for your patient. This is an example of giving up a smaller good to prevent a greater harm.

You go into a drugstore to buy medicine for your husband who will die without it. The pharmacist informs you that he will sell the drug to you, but only at a wildly inflated price—a price that you cannot pay. A dilemma arises: Under these circumstances, would you be justified in stealing the medicine from the druggist? Should the druggist or your husband be the beneficiary of your ethical action?

It would be understandable if you were to place a greater value on the life of your husband than on the property rights of the druggist. Many people would be inclined to forgive you if you were to steal the medicine. Then, later on, you could reimburse the druggist the normal cost of the medicine. The druggist has an implicit agreement with his customers that he will charge a standard price for his medicine. He proposes to break this agreement. You hold him to it. This is an example of doing a smaller harm to prevent a greater harm.

You have promised your kids that you will take them to an amusement park. Your neighbor is rushed to the hospital. She must have a delicate operation and she wants you to go with her to help her understand what is happening during the process. Obviously, it would be more rational of you to make your neighbor the beneficiary of your action. However, because of this, you would certainly not conclude that you should never again take your children to an amusement park. This is an example of doing a smaller harm to attain a greater good.

## GUIDELINES

Freedom and objectivity for various reasons are the most powerful standards for extremes analysis.

Freedom and objectivity for various reasons are the most powerful standards for extremes analysis. Most instances of analysis through freedom will reveal how freedom is to be exercised and if its exercise will produce irrational consequences or involve a violation of rights. Most instances of objectivity will reveal what justifiable decisions and choices will be achieved and whether they would presuppose an irrational agreement.

It is very rare that it happens when one analyzes through the extremes of two or three standards that the others are going to show something different. After two or three, the others will follow suit unless the first, second, or third, or one of the next three, were analyzed inappropriately.

Most instances of analysis through fidelity will reveal what fidelity requires—whether, for instance, it might require a violation of rights. Most instances of analysis through beneficence will reveal how the idea of beneficence squares with the nature of the health care system or whether it presupposes an irrational agreement—an agreement inappropriate to the health care system.

The greatest value of autonomy is in confirming analysis through the other standards. There is a venerable philosophical axiom—*Operatio sequitur esse*—that describes the fact that the characteristic actions of an existent arise from the nature of the existent. So it is with the nature—the autonomy—of a person. The knowledge of who he is follows on and requires the awareness of what he does and why.

Another effective way to discover the autonomy—the individual nature—of a person is through his passions. The patient's emotional reaction to circumstances may be the most reliable indicator of the condition of his autonomy. Therefore, a flawed autonomy will be demonstrated by emotional reactions toward the wrong thing, or the wrong person, for the wrong reason, at the wrong time, in the wrong way, and to the wrong extent. This will reveal a lack of justifiable cause and effect actions and reactions (Aristotle as cited in McKeon, 1941).

Autonomy is the interwoven character structure that produces a person's actions and that he experiences as himself. The fact that he is likeable and attractive or upsetting and unattractive is in the eyes of the beholder. It forms no part—nothing—of his autonomy.

Only an autonomy that produces irrational or coercive decisions and actions is a flawed autonomy.

## STUDY GUIDE

1. What can be learned from the crocodile and the importance of the implicit to ethical decision making?
2. What are the main purposes of analysis through extremes? How is it used?
3. Extremes analysis is a useful tool. It is *not* meant to be used as definitive, only as a guide, a very helpful guide. Could you use this in your personal life? How?
4. Give an example of where extremes analysis might be most useful in your practice.
5. Use this case for class discussion; the analysis of the case only appears in the instructor's manual.

### DOES DAN HAVE THE EXCLUSIVE RIGHT TO THE INFORMATION ABOUT HIS GENETICALLY TRANSMITTED ILLNESS?

Dan is in a nursing home suffering from Huntington's chorea. He will remain there until his death, because he is no longer able to care for himself. He and his ex-wife have been divorced for the past 4 years. She comes in occasionally to visit him with their two children, Lauren

*Continued*

(age 6) and Brian (age 9). Dan has made it quite clear to the physician and nurses that he does not want his ex-wife or children to be told his diagnosis. However, if the children do not know of his condition, they will not be able to make an informed decision about having children of their own. Does Dan have a right to have his request honored?

## REFERENCES

Davis, A. J., Aroskar, M. A., Liaschenko, J., & Drought, T. S. (1997). *Ethical dilemmas & nursing practice* (4th ed.). Stamford, CT: Appleton & Lange.

Doyle, A. C. (1930). *The complete works of Sherlock Holmes, Vol. I: The sign of fours.* New York, NY: Doubleday.

Epstein, R., Thomas, J. C., & Ritecki, G. W. (2003). Please don't say anything: Partner notification and the patient-physician relationship. *Virtual Mentor, 5*(11). Retrieved April 2014 from http://www.ama-assn.org/ama/pub/category/print/11504.html

McKeon, R. (Ed.). (1941). *The basic works of Aristotle.* New York, NY: Random House.

# ELEVEN

# ELEMENTS OF HUMAN AUTONOMY

**OBJECTIVES**

- Examine the nature of each of the elements of autonomy.

- Illustrate how each element adds to the knowledge of the patient.

- Demonstrate the relationship between reason and desire in ethical decision making.

- Examine the relationships among agency, rights, and ethical interaction.

- Give examples of the specific role of purpose related to the elements of autonomy.

Ickarow is a free-spirited bird that lives freely in a backyard. One day Ickarow noticed that when he flies from tree to tree, the air presses against his body and slows him down. Ickarow, oblivious to the need for analysis, has decided to fly up above the air so that he will be able to fly faster, more easily, and more efficiently. Ickarow was misguided and made a poor decision. A professional nurse who hopes to arrive at an objectively justifiable ethical decision without a prior exercise of observation and full analysis of the situation is as misguided as Ickarow was when he thought he could fly better in a vacuum. She has lost her context as fully as Ickarow. She will never understand the ethics of her profession, no more than Ickarow understands the mechanics of flying.

## ANALYZING AUTONOMY

Ethical decision making must be preceded by ethical judgment. It cannot be any better than the judgment on which it is based. Before an ethical agent can know what action to take, she must understand the independent uniqueness of the persons involved, the nature of the circumstances in which the action is being done, and why the action is being taken. This knowledge is gained only through objective judgment. A perfected judgment is developed by understanding the elements of autonomy and the uniqueness of each individual involved. The validity and value of every later judgment must be formed in the light of the first judgment, including the assessment of autonomy.

The autonomy of an individual is the unique nature of that individual. The elements of autonomy are the elements of human nature. They are the principles that give every individual person a human nature. They are properties or characteristics possessed by a human person simply because he or she is a human person. They form the nature of the person.

The elements of autonomy will serve the following aims for a nurse:

> If a professional nurse's objectives are to be met successfully, the road to success is the understanding of the patient's unique character.

- They can further facilitate her acquaintance with the nature of her patient. If necessary, they will enable her to make a rigorous analysis of her patient's nature and see into his values and motivations. If a professional nurse's objectives are to be met successfully, the road to success is the understanding of the patient's unique character. The measure of her ethical competence is how well her actions reflect that understanding. The best way to achieve that understanding is to understand what he has created out of his human nature (his virtues). At the same time, the nurse must never forget the human nature out of which he created these virtues.
- They enable a nurse to clarify the precise nature of the dilemma she faces. The ethical aspects of the patient's situation develop immensely from the way it affects him, the way he evaluates it, and in his reaction to it. Many ethical dilemmas will arise when these evaluations and reactions are inappropriate to the situation. These evaluations and reactions arise from the way the elements of autonomy are lived and experienced by this patient. How a patient lives the elements of autonomy within the limits of what they make possible is very revealing of who the patient is.
- There are certain circumstances in which, for various reasons, the elements of autonomy serve better to resolve dilemmas than do the bioethical standards. Generally, these will be when a nurse must do more than simply interact with a patient and must essentially act for a patient. The elements of autonomy are especially effective in the analysis of two types of dilemma:

1. When a nurse cannot speak to her patient but must speak for her patient (e.g., when she speaks for an embryo or an infant; when her

patient speaks a foreign language or comes from a significantly different culture; when her patient is comatose or otherwise incapable of communicating).

2. When a nurse is acquainted with her patient's unique and individual nature well enough that she can actively engage the elements of his autonomy (his objectivity just as his way of reasoning, his idiosyncratic ways of dealing with topics in which he cannot or will not deal objectively, his benefit-seeking as revealed through his motivating desires) into her analysis. This is very rare.

One becomes autonomous when he takes his inborn distinctive characteristic elements and develops them as virtues or vices. No one can be human and be completely unfamiliar with that which makes him autonomous. Everyone is familiar with the elements of human autonomy, at least on an implicit level. It is quite advantageous for a nurse to become familiar with them clearly, openly, and explicitly.

### DILEMMA 11.1: PLAYING THE ODDS OR BETTING ON A SURE THING

Vladimir, a concert pianist, has sustained an injury that may affect his ability to play the piano. Two operations could be performed. One operation has a 90% chance of restoring gross movements of the hand and eliminating pain. Another experimental operation has about a 10% success rate in restoring fine motor coordination. However, if this operation were to fail, Vladimir would lose much of the gross movement of his hand. Vladimir must make a decision. The decision regards the possibility of either achieving a value or the loss of a value. The value of being able to play the piano must be considered in the context of other activities that Vladimir values. The decision that Vladimir must make is an ethical decision. The action he will take, based on this decision, is an ethical action.

Vladimir must take into consideration these two essential facts: The success rate for one operation is 90%; for the other, it is 10%. When making his decision, Vladimir must consider the value he places on his ability to play the piano. He must also consider the disadvantages of losing gross motor coordination. The situation can guide Vladimir's action through the desires that enable him to understand himself and his life. By means of these desires, Vladimir can reason to the comparative desirability of both operations. A professional nurse can assist him in this process. To interact effectively with Vladimir, a professional nurse would need to join him in this process. The nurse would need to have an understanding of his ethical context and the context of his central and vital purposes.

## DESIRE AND THE ETHICAL CONTEXT

Imagine a world in which desire is not a part of human nature. This world is a tropical island floating among the clouds. On this island, all the necessities of survival—including fruit trees, cool water, and all survival essentials—are readily at hand. There is no motivation for seeking alternatives or change due to discontent with the current situation and, there is no awareness that human life can be more than the basic necessities. The sense of human desire is either gone or was never present. In this world, there are no specific human realities. There are no human purposes, no human choices, and no human actions. In this world, every action is conducted on an animal level. Therefore, nothing is either good or evil. Nothing is either right or wrong.

In such a world, ethics, as a study, would not only be nonexistent, but it would also be inconceivable. In this world where there is no human desire, there would be no important, vital, or fundamental goals. If there are no essential goals, there is no need for a system of standards to motivate, determine, or justify these goals. If desire was not an element of human nature, there would be no ethical realities of any sort. Ethical realities exist in the world only because desire is an element of human nature.

> Ethical realities exist in the world only because desire is an element of human nature.

## DESIRE AS "THE ESSENCE OF MAN"

The great ethicist, Benedict Spinoza (1632–1688), said that desire is the essence of man. Although Spinoza was concerned with the universe and not the context of the health care arena, his ideas regarding desire are still useful. Desire is all of the physiological and psychological processes that constitute the life of an individual person. *Desire* is defined as "that, which being given, [the person] itself is necessarily [given], and, being taken away, [the person] is necessarily taken [away]; or, in other words, that without which [the person] can neither be nor be conceived, and which in its turn cannot be nor be conceived without [the person]" (Spinoza, 1685/1949, p. 89).

The term *desire* as an element of individual autonomy has a specific meaning. It does not refer to any single desire for any single value. It does not even refer to the whole collection of a person's desires. It refers to the defining fact of human existence. It is the nature or "essence" of every individual person (Husted, 1988). This makes desire much more than simply a psychological reality. It makes every process sustaining the life of a person an aspect of desire. From this perspective, every fact about an individual human being, and in fact about all human beings, can be explained in terms of desire.

> This makes desire much more than simply a psychological reality.

This definition perfectly defines desire in a professional context. Conceptualizing desire this way is important and valuable to a nurse in understanding her profession. In simpler terms and in more detail:

- There is a minor difference in the chemical composition of males and females, but basically every person has the same chemical composition.
- Everyone's physiology is basically the same.
- Everyone has the same world to think about.
- Everyone's life depends on the same basic conditions.
- All people are limited, in the same ways, in the actions that they can take.
- Everyone has the same rights to life and action.

Despite all this, each and every person is different, unique, and autonomous in a vitally important way. There is one human attribute in which every individual person is different from every other. This attribute is human desire as a psychological reality.

*Desire* can be appropriately defined as "all of the physiological and psychological processes that constitute the life of an individual person." This gives the concept of desire an organic grounding. Without this organic grounding, human desire would be arbitrary, whimsical, transient, and unimportant as it would be determined from influences outside of the agent. This would make it of no greater ethical value than any other externally determined activity. Desire is an expression of the essential being of a human agent. Desire, given an organic and purely psychological grounding, includes those conditions and actions of the organism of which a human is conscious and the conscious ideas that motivate her to take purposeful action. All these constitute the desire of the ethical agent.

## DESIRE AND THE NURSE'S ORIENTATION TO NURSING

A professional ethic should be suitable and appropriate for the profession whose members it is set to guide. Every profession arises out of human purposes and desires. Nursing and the biomedical sciences arose out of the desire to regain health and well-being, as well as to alleviate pain. Therefore, a nursing ethic ought to be suitable and appropriate to this desire. Also, the fact that human desire is important validates the need for nurses.

A nursing ethic needs a logical basis for empathy with the desire to regain health and well-being. Without this basis, a nursing ethic becomes pointless. There will be no necessary and permanent connection between dilemmas and ethical analysis. Dilemmas will be subject to being resolved by customs and convenience.

An explicit empathy with human desire is the only logical basis for empathy with an individual's desire. If a nurse does not have empathy with human desire, she will not have empathy with a patient's desire for health and well-being. A nursing ethic that approves of the desire for health and well-being would also approve of the desire for autonomy, freedom, and happiness. No health professional who lacks empathy with desire as a human reality has a stable empathy for any individual patient or any individual person. Caring is empathy for another person's desires; without empathy, caring is quite cold and impersonal. No bioethical standard is desired by a patient for its own sake because a bioethical standard exists for the purposes to which agents direct it.

> If a nurse does not have empathy with human desire, she will not have empathy with a patient's desire for health and well-being.

Wen is in the hospital. His nurse, Evelyn, is quite aware of Wen's uniqueness. Evelyn's recognition of Wen's uniqueness, however, is utterly valueless to Wen. In itself, uniqueness is without any ethical importance. Uniqueness becomes autonomy—an ethical standard and concern—insofar as a person expresses this uniqueness by acting on his personal desires. If Evelyn recognizes that Wen is an accountant, a wood-carver, a husband, and the father of two children and that he lives beside a river, her recognition of Wen and his circumstances is of no great ethical advantage. A census taker who talks to Wen in his workshop recognizes this much.

Another nurse, Jennifer, begins with the awareness that Wen is motivated by desire. She recognizes that Wen desires to earn a living, perfect his skill at carving horses, retain the love of his wife, happiness for his children, and to return to his home beside the river. Jennifer empathizes with Wen's desires. This fosters understanding between Jennifer and Wen. It provides the basis for an ethical interaction between them. A nurse will seldom encounter an ethical dilemma that she can easily resolve with complete accuracy. Ethical dilemmas involving unique and inconvenient desires make it even more difficult to reach a clear-cut resolution.

## DILEMMA 11.2: TRAUMA VERSUS TREATMENT

Nine-year-old Wally was badly burned in a fire at his home. Iris, his nurse, comes to take him for debriding. Wally begins to cry and tells Iris he does not want to go. His face trembles, and he screams, "I'll go when my Mommy comes." Wally's mother was killed in the fire. Without any further discussion, Iris agrees not to take him.

The short-term benefit that Wally received by not undergoing the pain of debriding might not, all things being equal, compensate for the long-term detriment. Iris must consider the possible effect on Wally if he is told under these circumstances that his mother is dead. Iris has, in a sense, done Wally some good. She may have done him greater harm. It is not possible to calculate the amount of good or harm that Iris has done Wally. The harm Iris did was permanent. Perhaps the good was also permanent.

Everyone desires to give and receive that which is good. Everyone desires to avoid that which is harmful, but in every concrete situation, it is not always easy to recognize what is good and what is harmful. This is often one of the last skills that a nurse masters.

## DESIRE AND ETHICAL DECISION MAKING

In a solitary context without the presence of others, what a person ought to do is determined by what he wants to do and what he can do. The action he wants to take depends on his purpose and why he is acting. There are other principles of ethical action to be considered, but ethical decision making begins in desire and is shaped appropriately by concern for every element of autonomy.

In an interpersonal and interactive context, there would never be any reason for ethical decision making if it were not for desire. Agents form an agreement and begin to interact. They need a way to define the purposes of their interaction. They need a way to keep their desires in harmony. The desire that originally motivated them provides that way.

## SELF-PRESERVATION OF DESIRE

It is desire, the desire to be a nurse, that brings a nurse into the nurse–patient agreement. The patient's desires, however, are forced on him. It is these desires that determine the decision a professional nurse ought to make and the actions she ought to take. The desires that illness or injury force on a patient make nursing what it is. Whatever a person does and whatever a person is are determined first by desire. Spinoza asserted that, "Desire is the essence of a man, that is to say, [desire is] the effort by which a man strives to persevere in his being" (1685/1949, p. 201).

At one end of our existence, this desire motivates us to fill our basic needs. On the other end, it inspires the highest creations of the human mind. Desire can be thought of as more than this. It can be thought of as the energy of life. All the processes that preserve and enhance the life of the organism arise from desire. Life desires itself. From metabolism to reason, two forms of the energy of life, these processes serve to preserve and/or to enhance the life of the organism. Reason does this fully as much as any other vital process. Reason, itself, can be thought of as a form of desire. It is a process that produces understanding. The achievement of understanding satisfies the desire for understanding. Understanding serves human agency and human life.

A person lost in a forest might feel a desire to create shelter for himself. He might examine all the resources around him and figure out a way to build a shelter. If he cuts his arm, the laceration will likely heal itself. In several ways, the processes of feeling, examining, building, and healing are very different. However, they are alike in one very significant way: They each are a way nature has programmed the living organism to preserve its existence as a living organism. In a widened sense and comprehensive view of *desire*, each process can be thought of as a form of desire.

In the case of a patient, there is the closest and most intimate connection between these different forms of desire. A patient's rational decision to enter the health care setting is motivated by his desire to regain his health and decrease his suffering. His desire to end the pain he suffers and to regain his health arises from and is an extension of his unconscious bodily processes. These physiological processes are those that the body sets in motion in the healing process. We can view the whole healing processes by which the body regenerates itself, the conscious feeling of desire, and the reasoning process that produces the decision, as three expressions or steps of one natural drive. In one way or another, this whole process can be seen as the working of desire.

Biomedicine thinks of the patient as a unitary being who is to be understood holistically. The patient is not a mind bringing a body into the health care setting. Nor is a patient a body bringing a mind into the health care setting. If we look at humans holistically, we see their lives, as they live them, as conscious and embodied desire. In humans, reason is the instrument by which this desire preserves itself. Desire begins the process. Reason is the way that desire keeps going. The biomedical arts are ways in which people preserve their lives. Medicine is the product of desire and reason.

> In humans, reason is the instrument by which this desire preserves itself. Desire begins the process. Reason is the way that desire keeps going.

## REASON AS THE BASIS OF THE BIOETHICAL STANDARDS

Every patient choice, value, and action begins in desire. A nurse ought to understand this easily. All of her choices, values, and actions begin in desire. Those choices and actions that do not begin in her autonomous desire are not really hers and she experiences them as something outside of herself and as alien. The patient's experience of his desire is precisely the same. A patient, being in a state of enforced passivity, experiences most of his choices and actions as alien and not his own. He experiences them as being forced on him. A nurse has a significant advantage in understanding her patient if she understands this part of his experience. Her task, for his benefit and for her benefit, is to make them the product of his virtues.

> Every patient choice, value, and action begins in desire. A nurse ought to understand this easily. All of her choices, values, and actions begin in desire.

Everyone's choices, values, and actions begin in desire. They should not, however, be allowed to continue in desire alone. A professional's ethical thinking begins with a focus on desire. It should be turned over to reason, however, soon afterward. This is true because of the nature of ethics, the structure of the world we live in, the nature of desire, and the irreplaceable necessity of reason. Ethical action is action toward vital and fundamental goals. Any action taken toward vital and fundamental goals must be sustained by reason. Otherwise, there would be no way for a nurse and her patient to be aware that they are vital and fundamental goals and ought to be pursued as vital and fundamental goals.

> They should not, however, be allowed to continue in desire alone.

## DILEMMA 11.3: RIGHTS OF CHILDREN

Little Sandy is in the hospital to have his tonsils removed. Sandy is screaming and crying. He does not want to have the operation. The surgeon brings in the consent form for Sandy's mother to sign. Sometime later, Sandy's nurse gives him the preoperative medications.

Sandy's dilemma appears to be a simple case with an easy solution. It seems this way only because we take so much for granted. Sandy's tonsils are infected. It would be reasonable for them to be taken out. On the other hand, Sandy is already an autonomous individual. Autonomous individuals have rights. Although at first glance this situation seems to present no particular problems as Sandy must be operated on, it does yield some interesting ethical questions:

1. Does Sandy's mother have an ethical right to sign the consent form?
2. Does Sandy's nurse have an ethical right to give him the preoperative medications?
3. Does the surgeon have an ethical right to operate on Sandy?

Also, assuming that Sandy has no rights protecting him against this procedure (and, in every culture, it is taken for granted that he has not), other ethical questions arise:

4. When and how will Sandy acquire the rights that would protect him against this procedure?
5. Do Sandy's mother, the surgeon, and the nurse have rights that would protect them against undergoing this procedure involuntarily?
6. If so, when and how did Sandy's mother, the surgeon, and the nurse acquire these rights?
7. When and how will Sandy acquire the rights that his mother, the surgeon, and the nurse possess?
8. Will Sandy ever acquire the right to decide for his child? If so, when, why, and how?

Sometime in his life, Sandy will acquire the right to decide for his child. If he does not, then neither did his mother ever acquire the right to decide for him. It seems as though reason is on the side of Sandy's tormenters. In reason, Sandy ought to have the operation. In reason, there is no reason for Sandy not to have the operation. There is no reason except Sandy's desire not to have it. At the same time, it is a fact that Sandy is an autonomous ethical agent. If Sandy's autonomy will not protect him, nothing ever will. The most rational course of action to be taken is for Sandy to have his tonsils removed. Sandy's lack of rights in this circumstance is because reason is against him. Sandy's case shows the fragile interweaving of reason, autonomy, and individual rights.

A conflict between reason and autonomy is built into the nature of rights. On one hand, people possess rights by virtue of their rationality. On the other hand, they can interact with others only if others give their voluntary consent to the interaction. This voluntary consent, in addition, must be objectively gained. People possess rights by virtue of their capacity to reason, but they can interact with others only according to the autonomy of those others.

Conflicts can arise, even among benevolent people, over the question of rights. Most of these conflicts involve:

- One person's belief that reason demands or justifies an action.
- Another person's belief that this action would violate his autonomy and his right to be what and who he is.

Everyone has a right not to be aggressed against, coerced, or defrauded. This is the implicit agreement. It is the basis of ethical interaction. In addition to the universal rights agreement, a special implicit agreement is formed between nurse and patient. Special conflicts can arise here. Conflicts sometimes arise as to what constitutes aggression, coercion, or fraud. Although one person's reason tells him the other's rights have not been violated, the other's reason will tell him they have. Here autonomy must prevail. Some middle ground must be found between the reasoning of one person and the autonomy of another.

## DILEMMA 11.4: THE RIGHT TO BE ONE'S OWN AGENT

Roger is an elderly man who was brought into the hospital because of dehydration as a result of the flu. While Roger is in the hospital, his physician realizes that Roger's pacemaker needs to be replaced. The physician and nurse go in to talk to Roger about the scheduling of the operation. After the physician leaves, Roger tells his nurse that he has no intention of having the operation. The last time he had a pacemaker put in, he suffered a stroke that left him confined to a wheelchair.

Even at his advanced age, Roger has autonomous purposes for his life. When he analyzes the benefit of having the pacemaker replaced (another year of life) against the drawbacks (the possibility of having another stroke and becoming completely dependent on others, or the possibility of not surviving the operation), he decides that his most reasonable course of action is not to have his pacemaker replaced.

On the other hand, when his pacemaker runs down, Roger may die immediately. This certainly seems to place reason on the side of Roger's physician. The physician feels, not without probable justification that reason is on her side. The operation to replace the pacemaker would probably be a success and would give Roger another year of independent living. Whatever rights Roger has in this situation, he does not have by virtue of any reasoning he has done. What Roger has to gain is objectively much greater than what he has to lose. It is almost beyond doubt that the course of action suggested by the physician is the course of action Roger should take. The physician believes that Roger is old and senile. She has Roger declared incompetent, and the operation is performed.

This situation places the rights that Roger has by virtue of his autonomy into conflict with the rights the physician has by virtue of her reasoning. This dilemma yields another set of interesting ethical questions:

1. Was the physician justified in the course of action she took?
2. Does a health care professional's education, training, and experience give her extraordinary rights?
3. What is the ethical role of a nurse in this situation?
4. The judge who declared Roger incompetent may have been legally justified. Was he ethically justified?
5. Is there any significant difference between Roger's situation and Sandy's?

If reason is allowed to override one's exercise of his autonomy in conflicts among rights, this will solve a large number of problems, although it will also create an infinite number of problems. If reason is allowed to override autonomy, then when anyone feels that his or her reason justifies a course of action, he or she will have a right to violate the autonomy of another. Under these circumstances, no one would have any rights at all. If one is to have any rights, then reason cannot be allowed to override autonomy. Suppose that the reasoning behind one person's argument is superior to the reasoning behind another person's argument. Ignoring the fact that, in most cases, it would be difficult or impossible to prove this, there would always be a third person whose reasoning is superior to the second. Then, there would be a fourth whose reasoning was superior to the third. This could go on forever, and no ethical decision could ever be made.

Spinoza addressed the question of what is good and what is evil on its most basic level. He describes good and evil in the following way: "We call a thing good which contributes to the preservation of our being, and we call a thing evil if it is an obstacle to the preservation of our being, that is to say, a thing is called by us good or evil as it increases or diminishes, helps or restrains, our power of action" (1685/1949, p. 196). Reason and beneficence counsel a nurse to look at the issue of good and evil from her patient's point of view. Unless she does this, it is impossible for her to form and keep an agreement with her patient according to the purposes that brought him into the health care setting. This point of view and these purposes are the reasons why there is such a thing as the health care professions. A professional nurse cannot ethically dispense with reason and beneficence in her ethical decision making.

*Reason and beneficence counsel a nurse to look at the issue of good and evil from her patient's point of view.*

As defined previously, *desire* includes much more than the well-known psychological position. A nurse understands her patient best if, by desire, she understands all the processes that contribute to her patient's survival and to the enhancement of his life. The psychological reality of desire is the best known process of this type, but every process that contributes to the survival of the organism belongs to the same family. By including every such process under the concept of desire, a nurse can have a well-balanced understanding of her patient. The patient's psychological desire is only a small part of the context. Only this understanding of his desire enables the professional to interact with her patient in his entire context. This understanding of desire, as an element of autonomy, is the understanding of a person. For a nurse to know her patient as a living reality is far more important than it is for her to know any isolated psychological factor.

## REASON AND DESIRE

*Desire is, like fire, a useful servant but a fearful master.*

— *(Author unknown)*

Every person is inspired by a desire to pursue the good as he sees it. The good is the object of desire. The good is a form of the true. The true is the object of reason. That which can be good, however, is only good if it is true and if it actually exists or can be brought into existence. The pursuit of the good ought to be guided by the knowledge that it does exist, either actually or potentially. It also ought to be known that whatever is being pursued is truly good. This must be discovered by reason.

That which can be good, however, is only good if it is true and if it actually exists or can be brought into existence.

Ethical action is the pursuit of vital and fundamental goals. The goals of the health care professions are vital and fundamental values. For the health care professions, as is the case for all ethical action, it is reason that makes the pursuit of these values possible. When there is good or the possibility of good in the world, when happiness is possible, when belief needs to be refined, and when survival is a problem that must be faced, there is an ethical universe. This universe calls for practical reason and ethical action.

*Socrates said of reason that it is man's means to pursue the good. Aristotle said of reason that it is man's means to happiness. For the American logician and philosopher of science Charles Sanders Peirce, reason is important because it is man's means of refining his beliefs. For novelist–philosopher Ayn Rand, reason has ethical importance because it is man's means of survival.*

In an ethical universe, desire is a human's source of action. Reasoning power allows a person to discover understandable relationships and associations in his or her experience of the world. Reason allows the individual to adapt his or her actions in the pursuit of that which he or she experiences as good. Reason is the companion of all ethical action and the designer—the choreographer—of understandable, intelligible connecting causal sequences.

A human is, in the classic definition, a rational animal. A person's relationship with reason is so intimate that one cannot easily imagine what it would be like to be deprived of reason. Without the use of reason, one would have no more autonomy or freedom than an earthworm. Animals, when they are not driven by basic needs, do little more than sleep.

It is through reason that nurses are able to consider the rationale for their actions, the scope and extent of their participation in decision making, and the manner in which decisions are to be made and to be implemented (Milstead, 2015). A nurse who totally lacked reason would not be able to understand or to act on the bioethical standards. She would, in fact, not be able to act on or to understand anything at all. A nurse who lacks reason or who is unable to exercise it is unable to act or to understand. Even minor lapses of reason that can occur when under stress may make it temporarily impossible for her to be guided by the bioethical standards. Each of the bioethical standards arises as a form of desire and is activated in response to desire or is based on some form of desire. In an ethical sense, each is also a virtue, a form of reason or knowledge. Each virtue is reasoning desire.

## THE DIFFERENT ASPECTS OF LIFE

To gain understanding of the role of ethics in a patient's life, life must be defined in the same way desire is defined. As a bioethical element, life includes the entire context of a living person as any narrower definition would not be adequate for an effective bioethics. Under life, one must understand every process and action, including reason and desire, by which an organism maintains its survival and enhances its well-being. To understand life, it must be understood from the perspective of the subject who is living it. To do this, it is desirable to understand life from one's own perspective. For bioethics, an adequate understanding of life will include such things as:

*Under life, one must understand every process and action, including reason and desire, by which an organism maintains its survival and enhances its well-being.*

- The body's physiological processes.
- The integration of these processes.
- Basic needs common to all animals, including food, water, and air, which are directly and immediately tied to the animal's survival.
- Basic needs common to all human beings, including shelter, clothing, companionship, and freedom from pain.
- The life of consciousness, including perceptual experience, conceptual thought, and emotion.
- The higher order needs and values of human beings, including purpose, creativity, hope, and self-ownership, that are values directly and immediately tied to a human level of existence.

- The value of various activities, including walking, flying an airplane, cooking, and working, that are conditions of physical self-expression.
- The meaning of *aesthetic* values, including music, reading, painting, hobbies, and discussion, which a person examines and/or experiences in his life at its best.
- That with which a person is engaged and to which he is committed, including the meaning of the products of his acts of choice.
- Memories of the past.
- Anticipations of the future.

A nurse can define life from the perspective of an outsider. There are, however, a number of reasons why she ought to define life from the perspective of the living subject:

1. Medical science defines it from this perspective. If medical science thought of life simply as physiological survival, there would be no such things as psychiatry, physical therapy, and plastic surgery.
2. If a nurse defines her patient's life solely in terms of its basic physiological processes, she will never be able to deal with ethical questions concerning risk, euthanasia, abortion, and cloning. If she defines life in terms of its basic physiological processes, then she truly will never experience her patient.
3. If life, as an ethical concept, were defined in terms of physiological processes, then life as an ethical concept would pertain to all organic matter.

All organic matter is characterized by physiological processes. All organic matter has basic needs that must be met if it is to survive. If a nurse broadened her understanding of life as an ethical concept, to denote all physiological processes, she would have to broaden her understanding to include all living matter in her ethical concern. If she concerned herself with the freedom and autonomy of all organic matter, she, herself, could not survive. Nurses, as humans, need to consume organic matter in order to remain alive. It would not be logical if a bioethical standard demanded the self-destruction of the health care professional who recognized it.

A nurse's ethical concern is not with organic matter, it is with a patient. It must be with a patient in his entirety. The only kind of patients there are, are patients in their entirety. Her ethical commitment to her patient does not arise from the fact that he is organic matter. It arises from and is formed by the fact that his life is all the things it is. A patient's life is his autonomy. In addition to his physical needs and processes, his life involves his desire, his reason, his purposes, and his power of agency.

> The only kind of patients there are, are patients in their entirety
>
> A patient's life is his autonomy. In addition to his physical needs and processes, his life involves his desire, his reason, his purposes, and his power of agency.

4. It is not possible for a nurse to deal with her patient's life entirely on an abstract level. If a nurse defines her patient's life entirely in abstract terms, she will never be able to deal with her patient on an ethical level. People involved in ethical interaction are individual and

concrete. Only an understanding of life as one element of an individual patient's autonomy will serve to guide ethical action. People are too different and life is too many things for the individual to be understood in entirely abstract terms. Only if a nurse defines the life of her patient as she defines her own life will she look at her patient as an ethical agent looks at another person in an effective ethical interaction.

> Only if a nurse defines the life of her patient as she defines her own life will she look at her patient as an ethical agent looks at another person in an effective ethical interaction.

In every case, the benefits that enhance the patient will benefit the professional nurse. Their interaction ought to enhance both of their lives. This is the place for a concern for life to begin. A nurse's agreement is not with organic matter. Nor is the life that is at the center of her agreement a disconnected abstraction. Her agreement is with the virtues of an individual human being.

## LIFE AS THE BASIS OF THE BIOETHICAL STANDARDS

A health care ethic that is not suitable and appropriate for patients and health professionals is riddled with problems. The chief problem is that it is not a clear and comprehensible field of study. Not every ethical system is automatically understandable and clear. Ethics is, or ought to be, derived from a study of individual people as living, rational beings. There is no logical ethic of redheads, diabetics, poets, or long-distance runners. A logical and intelligent ethic relevant only to males or only to females is impossible. Such an ethic would be a mistake or a prejudice masquerading as an ethical system. A rational, solitary ethic is one whose motivations can be justified by the benefit it brings to the person who follows it. A rational, interpersonal ethic is one whose motivations can be justified by the benefits and harmony it brings to the interaction of the people who are guided by it. Human survival, on every level, is contingent upon rational belief. Rules and conventions are not substitutes for rational belief. They weaken the conditions of human survival.

> Ethics is, or ought to be, derived from a study of individual people as living, rational beings.

## LIFE AS THE PRECONDITION OF ALL ACTION AND VALUES

Nothing can be sought after or desired by anyone unless the person is alive. Life is the precondition of all values. As Spinoza (1685/1949) described it: "No one can desire to be happy, to act well, and to live well, who does not at the same time, desire to be, to act, and to live, that is to say, actually to exist" (p. 206). In the field of ethics, one faces two options:

> As Spinoza described it: "No one can desire to be happy, to act well, and to live well, who does not at the same time, desire to be, to act, and to live, that is to say, actually to exist"

- One can choose a ritualistic ethic. This is an ethic based on and arising out of rules, customs, and conventions.

This action is not interaction. It is not constant. It is episodic. When the occasion for ethical action arises, nurse–patient interaction ends. A nurse interacts instead with a duty, an emotion, a number, or a social pretense.

- One can choose an agreement-based ethic. For a professional nurse, an agreement-based ethic is an ethic based on her patient's purposes, and the nature of her professional practice as identified in the nurse–patient agreement.

Nursing is far more logical and understandable under an agreement-based ethic. If a nurse follows rules and conventions, her ethical actions are objectively purposeless and are imposed from the outside. The final value of her ethical system is what a professional is supposed to do. This is not the same thing as the life, health, and well-being of her patient. To pursue the well-being of a patient is to act purposefully. This is the highest potential of the profession. It is the highest potential of a nursing ethic. A nursing ethic ought to be all about what nursing practice and human life are all about.

## LIFE AS THE FINAL VALUE

Life is the entirety of a living being.

Before one can value anything else, one must value one's self.

Life is the entirety of a living being. As an element of human autonomy, it is the completeness of the person that one experiences as one's self in one's world. The fact that something is valued by one person provides no motive to any other person to value it, unless the second person values the first person. Before one can value anything else, one must value one's self. Things are valued by a person because the person is valued by herself and her valuing is respected by herself. In the health care setting, if judgment and choice are to be determined by the rights and values of a patient, then identifying the patient's life as the central term of the nurse–patient agreement is effortless.

It is important for a nurse to recognize that:

- Life is the requirement and precondition of all of a patient's other values.
- Life is the prerequisite and precondition of a patient's rights. To respect a patient's right to autonomy and freedom and not to be concerned for his life and well-being is not logical. At the same time, to be concerned with a patient's life and well-being and not respect his right to autonomy and freedom is to have lost one's ethical direction.
- Life is the purpose of a patient when entering the health care environment. A patient's concern for his life, in all those aspects of his life that are of a nurse's professional concern, must be shared by his nurse, or there is no easily understood reason for her being his nurse. Life is the central term of the agreement that a nurse makes with her patient.
- A patient's motivation in entering the health care environment is the fact that his capacities and potentialities are radically restricted and reduced from his previous functioning. When a patient regains his capacities and potentialities, his life is very much expanded.

- A patient, *except in the most extreme circumstances,* can have no rational desire before his desire to live. However, in extreme circumstances, a desire for death is not an irrational desire. It arises from recognition of the nature of life.

## THE ROLE OF PURPOSE

It is possible to make ethical decisions with an individual person, either oneself or one's beneficiary, serving as the reference point of ethical analysis. A person does this when he or she makes human purposes the center of his or her ethical system. There are few consistent followers of either a ritualistic or a purpose driven ethical system. Most people haphazardly form the ethical system they adopt from a combination of what they have been taught by relatives and their observations of what they perceive as effective, ethical actions occurring in their real life. Ethics, as a formal study, arose from the necessity of making decisions in the face of adversity. A person can observe what succeeds and what fails early in life from such things as the experiences of family living, negotiating with playmates, and the demands of school work. A person can observe and learn from this, but not everyone does.

Amy, a nurse on a cardiac step-down unit, is an example of a person who haphazardly formed her ethical system. Her system is more largely influenced by the ethical instruction programed into her by others than it is by her experience of both successful and failing human interactions. Her actions are much more ritualistic than purposeful. Her actions have more in common with singing a song or reciting a poem than with cooking a meal or mowing the lawn. The goal of singing a song or reciting a poem is simply the activity itself and nothing beyond it. The goal of cooking a meal is the finished meal. The goal of mowing a lawn is having an attractive lawn. Amy's ethical actions have no purpose beyond the actions themselves. Her ethical actions, like singing and reciting, are their own reason for being. In the context of a person's everyday life, there is certainly nothing wrong with singing a song or reciting a poem. These can be enjoyable activities. However, purposeless activity is not at all appropriate in a bioethical context.

Purposeless activity is not at all appropriate in a bioethical context.

## THE ANATOMY OF PURPOSE

When circumstances, resources, knowledge, and ability make one's purpose possible to achieve, then purpose and action are justifiable and reasonable. When it is not possible to achieve one's purpose, then the purpose and action are not justifiable or reasonable. To pursue a purpose that includes a number of other valuable purposes is even more justifiable. If the one purpose excludes a number of other valuable purposes, it is less justifiable than it would have been, if not completely unjustifiable and unreasonable.

Desires are formulated into purposes. There are three types of purpose that determine the ethical aspects of a situation:

- **A purpose set by an individual agent's desire and decision.** Desire motivates an agent's action toward every goal. Desire is the dynamic principle that is the basis of every human purpose.
- **A purpose set by the recognition of rights.** By recognizing the rights of others, one sets uncoerced cooperation as the principle of purposive interaction.
- **A purpose planned and acted on by individuals through explicit agreements and promises.** This purpose must always be motivated by desire and, ethically, must recognize the rights of everyone involved. For a decision and action to be justified:
  □ Its goal must be a predetermined purpose.
  □ There must be a reason to believe that it will accomplish this purpose.
  □ It must not be prohibited by the nature of the nurse's professional role.
  □ It must not violate the rights of the patient.
  □ It must not interfere with the understanding that brings them together.

## PURPOSE AS THE BASIS OF THE BIOETHICAL STANDARDS

Purpose is the goal-obtaining approach taken by a desiring being. Purpose describes action directed toward vital and essential concerns, needs, and values.

Purpose is the goal-obtaining approach taken by a desiring being. Purpose describes action directed toward vital and essential concerns, needs, and values. Finally, purpose signifies the needs and values toward which an agent's actions are directed. Purpose is the central element of a practice-based ethic. In any action that a person takes, success or failure depends on whether the person accomplishes his or her purpose. In an ethical context, whether an aspect of the context is good or evil depends on whether it assists or hinders the purposeful actions that are called for in the context. The intentional quality of the action is determined by the purpose. An ethical action is defined in terms of its purpose.

The practical quality of an action is determined by its appropriateness to the achievement of its purpose. Purpose intends some envisioned progress. Progress is achieved through a conscious process. This process follows the context in which progress is most complete or most probable. For nursing, this conscious process consists in the standards of the profession. These standards lead a nurse to exercise intelligent cognitive discrimination and insight into the contextual relationships that make progress possible.

A person's actions always include the intention that inspires the action. Intentions always include the goal for which the action is intended. If a person's purpose is to gain happiness, then those actions that will bring about conditions that produce happiness are right and good. Those actions that bring about conditions that undermine happiness are wrong and harmful. For purposes of returning a patient to a level of agency at which he can speak and do things for himself, those actions that bring about the physical and psychological conditions of agency in a patient are right and good. Those actions that weaken the physical or psychological conditions of his agency are wrong and harmful.

*A person's actions always include the intention that inspires the action. Intentions always include the goal for which the action is intended.*

Steven is in the hospital with peripheral vascular disease. His nurse, Joy, is educating him about how he must care for himself when he leaves the hospital. To do this, Joy:

- Tries to find out all she can about Steven so she can advise him according to his specific situation.
- Gives him all the information he needs so that he can enjoy the maximum freedom of action.
- Tells him whatever he needs to know in order to enable him to gain and to retain his power of agency. She tells him nothing that he does not need to know or that might hinder his gaining and retaining his power of purposeful action.
- Allows Stephen the space he needs in order to make autonomous decisions.
- Does whatever she can in order to promote Stephen's welfare. She does nothing that might hinder Stephen's welfare, nothing that might hinder his power to take autonomous actions.

## THE FACETS OF PURPOSE

*The standard of any action, including ethical actions, is the purpose that the agent means to accomplish by the action.*

The standard of any action, including ethical actions, is the purpose that the agent means to accomplish by the action. The long-established answer to the question of why the chicken crossed the road is a good example of this. The chicken wanted to get to the other side. If a chicken, or a person, wants to walk across the road, then getting to the other side is the standard of success. If a person wants to learn to use a computer, then his or her standard of success is the ability to use a computer. If a student wants to learn to fly, then the standard of success is being able to take off, stay up, and come down. If a nurse wants to recognize the freedom of her patient, then that patient acting on his freedom is the standard of the nurse's success.

Every event that fulfills an agent's purpose is an event that demonstrates the success of an ethical agent. The reason for an ethical decision-making model is to guide the action of an ethical agent in accomplishing the purpose. The world presents various alternatives that an agent chooses from according to his or her desires. When an agent chooses from alternatives, this act of choice forms a purposeful frame of mind. A purpose is the object of a desire that a person brings to the forefront and retains in his or her attention. A choice is an objective relationship between a feeling of desire and a possibility of achievement that a person perceives in the world. A choice is a mental action that closes off alternative mental actions of choice. All action is purposeful behavior.

Any purposeful ethic involves choice. An ethical system not based on purpose and choice is ritualistic and formalistic. A ritualistic or formalistic ethic cannot motivate actions appropriate to nursing, nor can it guide a nurse's actions appropriately. It cannot enable her to justify objectively the actions she takes. A nurse armed with a formalistic ethic would not know what questions to ask in a context, nor would she know what would constitute the answer to a contextual ethical question. A process of ethical justification has to do with these questions and answers. Such a process is simply an explanation of the questions a person has asked and the answers on which she has acted. Purpose as an element of autonomy, in and of itself, is of primary importance in resolving an ethical dilemma. Each of the other elements of autonomy is important only as it relates to purpose.

> A purpose is the object of a desire that a person brings to the forefront and retains in his or her attention.

> Purpose as an element of autonomy, in and of itself, is of primary importance in resolving an ethical dilemma. Each of the other elements of autonomy is important only as it relates to purpose.

## DILEMMA 11.5: REFUSING TREATMENT IN THE CONTEXT OF LOSS OF HOPE

Jody Smith, a retired nurse with three adult children and numerous adult grandchildren, lives in a small rural area on a limited income. Two months ago, she fell and broke her left hip. After surgery for an artificial hip replacement, she was transferred to a rehabilitation center where she had a left-side cerebrovascular accident (CVA). Upon her readmittance to the acute care facilities, she received aggressive therapy for the CVA. Completely paralyzed on her left side, Mrs. Smith has decided that she no longer desires aggressive therapy and frequently asks the staff why she cannot die in peace. "The rehabilitation is so painful and I'll never walk again. What's the use?" Both the physicians and her family are much more optimistic. The orthopedic surgeon is convinced that Mrs. Smith will walk again, and the neurologist believes that Mrs. Smith will make a full recovery from the CVA and be able to return home and care for herself. Both physicians have excluded Mrs. Smith from their conversations, assuring her children that she will be "as good as new." They ignore Mrs. Smith's request to discontinue anticoagulants and rehabilitative therapy. She refuses to cooperate with the physical and occupational therapists. She will not take her medications, and refuses to perform simple tasks, relying instead on staff members to meet her activities of daily living. What should be done? (Guido, 2013)

## AGENCY AS THE BASIS OF THE BIOETHICAL STANDARDS

A person's agency is the power to act on autonomous desires that spring from his or her own reasoning. Agency makes a human life what it can be and will be. Agency requires autonomous desire.

A person's agency is the power to act on autonomous desires that spring from his or her own reasoning. Agency makes a human life what it can be and will be. Agency requires autonomous desire. Without autonomous desire, behavior is involuntary. Involuntary behavior does not arise from agency. For instance, if a person is jostled in the street and bumps into a wall, that behavior does not arise from agency. His behavior arises from a force outside of his agency. Agency requires reason or autonomous thought. Behaviors that arise entirely from emotions and reflex behaviors are not actions. Actions express the specific nature of the agent who acts. Only rational beings possess agency. Only reason in action expresses the specific nature of a rational being.

The health care setting is designed to promote the regaining of agency in the service of a patient's individual purposes. If ethical action does not properly begin with attention to agency, with actions that arise in a patient's autonomous desire and reason, then all of bioethics is misdirected. For these reasons, every bioethical standard has the same purpose:

- The standard of autonomy protects those actions of a patient that express his unique character structure.
- The standard of freedom protects actions arising from the individual agency of a patient.
- The standard of objectivity supports the actions that arise from the individual agency of a patient. It does this by allowing him to act on his own knowledge and awareness.
- The standard of beneficence protects the actions of an agent and his power of agency.
- The standard of fidelity protects his objective attention to his self-interest and to the values he pursues, as well as a person's self-awareness of the interactions of several agents as they act toward interwoven purposes.

## THE BIOLOGICAL FUNCTION OF AGENCY

Agency is an agent's power. It is the instrument of reason and desire.

Agency is an agent's power. It is the instrument of reason and desire. The function of purpose is to move an agent from a lesser to a greater level of autonomy, freedom, objective connection to reality, power to pursue values, and fidelity to his life. The function of agency is to move an agent from a less refined reason and a less complete knowledge to a more refined reason and a more complete knowledge. It guides reason through rational desires and in actions leading to the fulfillment of desire. It enables an agent to attain a more desirable condition of being. Finally, agency serves to increase its own competency and strength. In taking physical actions, a person increases the strength of her body. In taking the actions necessary to increase understanding, a person increases the strength of her mind.

In taking the actions necessary to increase understanding, a person increases the strength of her mind.

## AGENCY AND RIGHTS

In the life of every (noncriminal) individual and in the history of humanity, it becomes evident that the range and effectiveness of people's activities are greatly enhanced if they do not have to devote time and effort to guarding themselves against aggression, coercion, and fraud. So, as a sort of evolutionary instrument, an implicit agreement arises among rational beings, an agreement not to aggress against, not to coerce, and not to defraud one another. It is also the essential basis of the existence of laws. Laws arise because there is a need for them. In fact, the need existed long before the laws were in place. This implicit agreement arose before the laws were possible. It arose with the human ability to make agreements.

Before any laws were ever made, the necessary relations of justice existed. "To say that nothing is just or unjust except that which is commanded or forbidden by positive law is as absurd as saying that before a circle is actually drawn its radii are not equal" (De Montesquieu, 1848/1949, p. 108). To the extent that a society is free, the laws that it recognizes as most fundamental are reflections of individual rights. These laws are an explicit statement of the implicit agreement on nonaggression. When laws have no rational justification, no evident need, and no moral basis, they are resented and notoriously difficult to enforce. This is not true of laws based on the implicit agreement. Most criminals do not even resent such laws!

This preexisting agreement against aggression arises from the human condition. Without it, there would be no basis for honoring any inconvenient explicit agreements. No legal system could possibly be effective. There would be no basis for agreement on a legal system. The only check on people's criminality would be the limits of their imagination and the range of their daring.

Making an agreement is not at all synonymous with having reason to believe that an agreement will be kept. When there is no positive reason to believe that an agreement will be kept, there is no practical reason to make an agreement. Dependable explicit agreements are made possible by this implicit agreement of rights as the product of an implicit agreement among rational beings, made and held by virtue of their rationality, not to obtain actions, nor the products or circumstances of action from one another, except through voluntary consent, objectively gained.

> This implicit agreement gives structure to explicit agreements and to laws. It gives moral force to every explicit agreement and every other implicit agreement.

This implicit agreement gives structure to explicit agreements and to laws. It gives moral force to every explicit agreement and every other implicit agreement. This holds true of the unspoken agreement between nurse and patient. The nurse–patient agreement is, in effect, guaranteed by the implicit agreement that constitutes rights. It is an agreement that nurse and patient have a right to expect that each will fulfill his or her role according to the purposes that motivate their interaction. It is an agreement that there will be fidelity and benevolence on each side.

The English philosopher John Stuart Mill (1806–1883) said that one person cannot advance the interests of another by compulsion. One person cannot rightly compel another person to do something because it is better for that other person to do it, because it will make the other person happier, or because, in the opinion of the first person, it would be wise for the second person to do it (1819/1988). Rights determine the actions an agent can take. Everyone has the right to be free from the coercion of others. Everyone constantly relies on the agreement that people will not deal with each other coercively. A person can act freely in any social context as long as he or she does not coerce another. In coercing another, a person gives up the right to exercise freedom. It is well said that: [The right to] self-determination is an individual's exercise of the capacity to form, revise, and pursue personal plans for life . . . free from outside control. . . . In the context of health care, self-determination overrides practitioner determination (President's Commission for the Study of Ethical Problems and Medicine and Biomedical and Behavioral Research, 1982, p. 32).

A nurse, because she is the agent of her patient and through the implicit agreement she has with him, has agreed to protect the rights of her patient. She has an ethical obligation to protect her patient from anyone who would violate his rights. Above all, she cannot, herself, break the rights agreement.

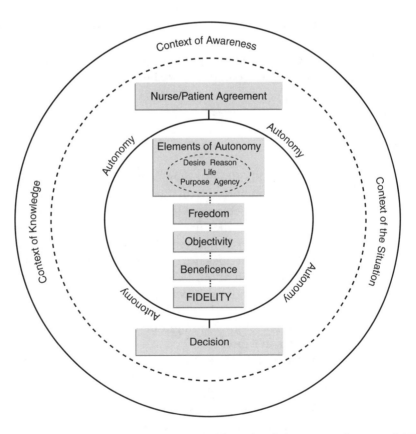

**FIGURE 11.1** Husted's symphonological bioethical decision-making model II.

## MUSINGS

No one can be human and be completely unfamiliar with that which makes him or her autonomous. Everyone is familiar with the elements of human autonomy, at least, on an implicit level. It is quite advantageous for a professional to become familiar with the elements explicitly.

To interact on a human level is to interact on a highly intimate level. People interact with each other on an intimate level when they understand each other's desires. Desire is the basis of meaning and purpose in every human life. Intimacy rests on meaning and purpose.

The interweaving of their desires is the ethical basis for the nurse–patient agreement. This agreement is seldom, and probably never, verbalized. It is an implicit agreement arising immediately between them. The ultimate basis of this agreement, therefore, is not anything the nurse or the patient says. It is who they are that determines what they ought to do.

A professional's exercise of reason is her greatest source of ethical confidence and strength. As the agent of her patient, confidence and strength are values that she offers him and herself. She owes it to herself to exercise reason in developing the virtues that her profession requires.

There is one activity more central to human life than any other. This is the discovery and pursuit of autonomous purposes. It is the activity that relates an individual's abstract aspirations and the biological functions necessary to the organism's continued survival. There is no reason why both cannot come into the health care system.

## STUDY GUIDE

1. Think about your own desires and how you did or did not use reason to follow through on them. What were the consequences for you? Were there consequences to others? Could the consequences be mitigated?
2. "Desire is, like fire, a useful servant but a fearful master" (Author unknown). What would this mean for the nurse or for the patient?
3. If a person does not desire to do good but does something good, what can be said about this person? What might be the consequences for a patient under this person's care?
4. If a person desires to do good but fails to use his or her rational nature (or reason), what might be the consequences for the patient under this person's care?
5. Does the element of life prohibit the withdrawal of food and fluids from a dying person? Would there be a context in which it would or a context in which it would not?
6. The fun parable about the chicken crossing the road highlights a number of important points regarding the role of purposes. What are some? How do they relate to your practice?

7. What does it mean to return the patient to a circumstance in which he or she can be his or her own agent? Why is this important? What if it is not possible?
8. Use this case for class discussion; the analysis of the case only appears in the instructor's manual.

---

### AGGRESSIVE TREATMENT OF A DISABLED PREMATURE INFANT

Donna is a nurse in the neonatal intensive care unit. Maureen, her patient, has given birth to a very premature infant. The infant does not quite weigh 2 pounds and cannot breathe spontaneously on his own. The amniocentesis reveals that the infant has Down syndrome. A sonogram shows that the baby suffers from a severe heart defect. Maureen asks Donna for information and advice. Her baby has only about a 5% chance of living. If the baby does live, he will have severe mental and physical handicaps. The neonatologist wants to treat the baby aggressively. Maureen asks Donna if she should allow this treatment.

---

## REFERENCES

Bioethics Case Study. (2000). Transplant. Retrieved October 25, 2006, from http://www.mhhe. com/biosci/genbio/olc_linkedcontent/bioethics cases/g-bioe-04.htm

De Montesquieu, S. (1949). *Spirit of the laws* (T. Nuggent, Trans.). New York, NY: Random House. (Original work published 1848)

Guido, G. W. (2013). *Legal issues in nursing* (6th ed.). Stamford, CT: Appleton & Lange.

Husted, J. H. (1988). Spinoza's conception of the attributes of substance. *The metaphysics of substance: The Proceedings of the American Catholic Philosophical Association, 61,* 81–131.

Mill, J. S. (1988). *On liberty.* New York, NY: Penguin. (Original work published 1819)

Milstead, J. (2015). *Health policy and politics: A nurses' guide.* Sudbury, MA: Jones and Bartlett.

President's Commission for the Study of Ethical Problems and Medicine and Biomedical and Behavioral Research. (1982). *Making health care decisions: The ethical and legal implication of informed consent in the patient-practitioner relationship.* Vol. 1. Washington, DC: U.S. Government Printing Office.

Spinoza, B. (1949). *Ethics* (J. Gutmann, Ed.). New York, NY: Hafner. (Original work published 1675)

# TWELVE

# VIRTUES AS RESOURCES

## OBJECTIVES

- Discuss the two meanings of virtue.
- Explain how the bioethical standards are virtues of an agent.
- Relate the agreement to each of the standards.
- Interpret the meaning of the swan principle.
- Demonstrate how the four ways of caring can benefit or harm the patient and self.

The term *virtue* in its original sense meant that a thing was capable of some excellent activity or function. For instance, the virtue of a boat is its tendency to stay afloat. The virtues of a horse are its swiftness and endurance. The virtue of a physician is his or her ability to heal. The virtues of a wrestler are strength and skill. The virtue of a painter is the ability to portray. In its classic sense, the virtues of a person came to mean all those excellences that arise from exercising control of one's decisions and actions through reason. This is the sense in which the term virtue is used throughout this book (see Chapter 1 for the beginning discussion of virtue).

In its classic sense, the virtues of a person came to mean all those excellences that arise from exercising control of one's decisions and actions through reason. This is the sense in which the term virtue is used throughout this book.

Physicians and advanced practice providers directly serve and promote a patient's life, health, and well-being through medical interventions. This is the direct and immediate goal of physicians and providers. The virtue of a physician or provider is to do this excellently. For other health professionals, including nurses, this is a mediate goal because it is dependent on and acted on following the direction of the physicians and providers. In matters concerning a patient's medical well-being, a physician mediates between other professionals and the patient. A physician decides what to do to cure a patient.

Ideally, a nurse would have an immediate relationship with her patient. There is a small advance in her role that a nurse can assume that can make this possible. This advance makes it possible for a nurse to be truly more a professional, to provide greater benefits for her patient, and to derive the full benefits of her profession. A nurse can make it her immediate goal to promote and serve the life, health, and well-being of her patient by serving and promoting the virtues of her patient. This the nurse does by nurturing and sustaining her patient's power to act according to his nature. The nurse does this by encouraging and supporting the patient's ability to fulfill his rational desires to serve and to promote his life and well-being and to further his pursuit of his rational self-interest. Many nurses, of course, already do this.

The virtues of a patient are identical to the virtues of a professional, and in fact they are identical to the virtues of any human being. The virtue or excellence of a human being is a form of well-being or power to sustain his life as the kind of living being he is. Virtue, then, is a form of health (Aristotle, as cited in McKeon, 1941). "Virtue gives the human being morale and morality. Virtue internalizes good values and its essence is to realize the nature of the good, which is shown and manifested in good deeds. . . . Virtue is action orientated" (Nasman, Nystrom, & Eriksson, 2012, p. 52).

The ethicist Benedict Spinoza (1675/1949) described virtue thusly: "reason demands . . . that every person . . . should desire everything that really leads man to a greater perfection, and absolutely that everyone should endeavor, as far as in him lies, to preserve his own being" (p. 202). This is precisely what the health care setting is all about. Professional nurses can directly promote and support a patient's virtue to preserve his own being. A nurse, given the fact that she is with the patient over an extended period, can do this as no other biomedical professional can. She can be the custodian of his power to sustain his life as a human being. An effective nurse is a companion who interacts with, safeguards, and nurtures and supports her patient's virtues.

In addition to everything else they are, the bioethical standards are the virtues of an ethical agent. They are characteristics of people that enable them to sustain their existence as the people they are. They are qualities of character that enable a person to develop. They enable a person to act to fulfill rational desires. The bioethical standards, as virtues, are:

1. Autonomy: The ability to sustain one's unique qualities of character that enables a person to be the person he or she desires to be. This ability makes one an excellent human being and a person who is able to sustain life as the person he or she is.

2. Freedom: The ability of people to maintain purposeful courses of action is an ability that makes them able to sustain their lives and identities and is a form of health and a virtue.

3. Objectivity: The virtue that enables one to perceive one's path to a greater perfection and to take the actions that are necessary for one to preserve one's life and health. The ability to grasp and interact with the facts of reality that are relevant to sustaining one's life and well-being is an ability that is a form of health and an invaluable virtue.

4. Beneficence: The ability to envision and take actions in pursuing one's benefit or in acting to avoid harm is a power that makes one able to sustain one's life as the kind of being he or she is and is a virtue.

5. Fidelity: The ability to maintain one's self-awareness and one's determination to continue on courses of action that serve his or her life and well-being is a form of ethical health and is a virtue.

A nurse ought to recognize these abilities as the virtues of her patient and of herself. Her justifiable interaction with her patient depends on her motivating and supporting his virtues. This is the meaning of "doing for her patient what he would do for himself if he were able." When she acts as a nurse, her actions are justified. They are also invaluable to her as a person. If the professional nurse establishes a nurse–patient agreement, she is, incidentally, most likely to avoid legal actions. Patients are not generally well versed on the law. Few patients ever say, "Looking back, I see where my nurse violated the law. I am going to take her to court." Patients take health care professionals to court when patients perceive a violation of ethical professional responsibilities and believe that professionals have made them worse off than they should have been. If she is sympathetic to, and honors, her patient's virtues, the possibility of her being a defendant in a lawsuit is remote.

For a patient to sustain his life as the kind of being he is, two things are necessary. First, he must sustain his life. It is the immediate responsibility of a physician or advanced practice provider to assist him in this. Second, he must sustain his awareness of the person he is. The natural and immediate opportunity of a nurse is to assist him in this. The ideal health care setting will enable a patient to sustain his life as the person he is. This is the ethical environment of medicine and of nursing. To achieve this environment, both a provider and a nurse are necessary. Neither alone is sufficient.

## DILEMMA 12.1: IS IT EVER RIGHT TO SELL ONE'S ORGANS?

After her gallbladder surgery, Ruth Sparrow had a serious problem, but not with her health. The surgery was successful, and she was doing well. The problem was money. Her bill was close to $20,000,

*Continued*

and she had no savings to fall back on to pay for it. She said to the hospital: "I will give you a kidney, if you will mark my bill paid in full." They turned her down. Then she ran an ad in the paper: "Kidney, runs good, for sale—$30,000 or best offer." Although she received many crank calls, some were serious and asked for her blood type. The paper pulled the ad because it is against federal and state laws to buy or sell a human organ or tissue. What do you think? (Bioethic Case Study, 2000)

## THE BIOETHICAL AGREEMENT AND ITS STANDARDS

In one way or another, every ethical decision that a professional nurse makes, every professionally justified action she takes in relation to her patient, involves the terms of the implicit (professional) agreement that establishes her dynamic relationship with her patient. This agreement structures her practice. The practice-based ethic of this relationship is derived from this agreement. It is based on the bioethical standards. As noted earlier, the bioethical standards are the assumptions and inferences of the nurse–patient agreement (and any agreement).

1. **The standard of autonomy.** To grasp the terms of a specific nurse–patient agreement, a professional nurse needs to be aware of her patient's unique nature (autonomy). Every patient is a unique personality. To interact with a patient is to interact with a unique personality.

   When a nurse acts as a researcher, an educator, or an administrator, she will not be aware of the unique characteristics of any individual patient. She must, however, always be aware of the unique characteristics of patients as patients. If any professional action, however indirect, is to be justifiable, it must be an action oriented toward the welfare of unique patients.

   A great actress, to be able to perform effectively in a play every night, must rehearse her role. Only by rehearsing her role can she perfect her performance. Every night she performs the same actions with the same people, and perfection requires rehearsal. The actress's role weakens and stagnates without rehearsal.

   The situation of a professional nurse is completely the opposite of this. Every day she faces different ethical demands; she must take different actions, with different people, in very different circumstances. A professional nurse can perfect her role only if she does not rehearse it. To perfect her role as a professional, she must meet the differing demands of every patient's situation. She cannot do this before she is in the situation. The delivery of ethical nurturing and development, in relation to each individual patient, is a role that she cannot rehearse.

   If an actress does not rehearse her role, she will never perform it other than the way it is "in general." She will never discover the possibilities, the nuances possible to the situation, and the psychological aspect of her role. An actress can discover why she does what she does and why she ought to do it before she does it, *but a nurse cannot.* An actress only appears sincere, but a nurse is sincere. A talented actress can take the role of a nurse, but a talented nurse cannot take the role of an actress. These methods of portraying feeling "in general" exist in every one of us. Also, we use them without any relation to the why, wherefore, or circumstances in which a person has experienced them. True art and performing "in general" are incompatible. The one destroys the other. Art does not tolerate "anyhow," "in general," [or] "approximately" (Stanislavski, 1963, p. 108).

If a professional nurse prejudges and rehearses her ethical actions, she will make decisions and take actions toward a specific, unique patient only somewhat appropriately at best. The life a playwright creates is entirely predictable. The playwright gives it in the play. Life in the real world is unpredictable. The two professions require, for their perfection, two completely opposed approaches. The delivery of ethical nurturing and care in relation to each individual patient is a role that nurses cannot rehearse.

> The delivery of ethical nurturing and care in relation to each individual patient is a role that nurses cannot rehearse.

2. **The standard of freedom.** To interact with a patient, a professional nurse must interact with the patient's freedom. Every action that a patient takes arises from his freedom. The precondition of a nurse's interacting with the freedom of a patient is that she recognizes and respects his freedom. A nurse who fails to respect her patient's freedom is not interacting with her patient. She, therefore, fails to honor the agreement she has made with him.

3. **The standard of objectivity.** For people to interact within an agreement, they must understand the terms of the agreement. This understanding cannot exist unless the relationship between the parties is based on a rational trust, and rational trust cannot exist unless the relationship is based on objective understanding. Except in rare circumstances, a nurse who does not communicate and interact with her patient based on objective awareness violates the agreement she has made with him.

4. **The standard of beneficence.** Every agreement has a purpose. This purpose is a goal to achieve through interaction. An agreement without a final goal would not be logical. It would be an agreement to do nothing; therefore, no agreement exists at all. The achievement of this final goal is the purpose of beneficent action—action that achieves a benefit. Every agreement, by its nature, calls for beneficent action. A nurse who fails to act beneficently toward her patient fails to fulfill the agreement she has with him. This is a profoundly unfortunate failure. In this failure, a professional fails herself.

5. **The standard of fidelity.** Wherever there is an agreement, there must be fidelity and commitment to the agreement. An agreement that parties will not honor is a contradiction in terms. No professional can ever justify an ethical decision or action that violates the implicit agreement she has with her patient.

All these considerations form the ethical context of the interaction between professional nurse and patient. The ethical effectiveness of this interaction depends on the nurse's attainment of optimal awareness, which is the widest possible context of ethical knowledge, and on her bringing about, as nearly as possible, ideal conditions for what she and her patient intend. An increase in a nurse's ethical awareness facilitates all of this is. "I urge you to be proactive in the best interest of your patients . . . and stretch beyond your comfort zone" (Meyers, 2000, p. 9). It takes pride to stretch beyond one's comfort zone. Comfort and pride cannot live together. Pride is a most desirable virtue in a professional. Comfort (i.e., stagnation) is the only alternative to pride, and it is not a virtue.

> It takes pride to stretch beyond one's comfort zone. Comfort and pride cannot live together. Pride is a most desirable virtue in a professional. Comfort (i.e., stagnation) is the only alternative to pride, and it is not a virtue.

## THE SWAN PRINCIPLE

Two people sitting on a park bench feeding the seagulls and swans discussed the parallels between their current setting and the health care setting. Some patients, like seagulls, are aggressive and demanding, whereas others are timid and lack direction. Some patients, like seagulls, can be annoying, whereas others are charming. Some patients, like seagulls, can be resourceful, whereas others are helpless. It is easy for a nurse's emotional responses to different types of patients lead her away from the efficient practice of her profession. It is a temptation to avoid the demands of demanding patients and to take advantage of timid patients. On a very basic level, seagulls and patients are very much alike, although, of course, patients are infinitely more complex and valuable than are seagulls.

The seagull feeders turned their attention to the calm dignity of the swans floating in the pond and discussed how splendid it would be if nurses in their proper setting could achieve the self-assurance and serenity of the swans. The swans appeared perfectly placid and self-contented. They were aware of their circumstances and serene within them. Fanaticism, passion, and extremism of one sort or another, until they unravel, can produce an ethical assurance and certainty, but they are not virtues. Only ethical competence can produce a reliable attitude of confidence and resilience. Without ethical awareness, professionals can be caught by surprise, and then their serenity and confidence are gone. Ethical serenity and confidence can arise only from a nurse's awareness of herself and of her professional role. This awareness must produce a constant attitude, arising from, in Aristotle's words, a firm and stable character.

A great nurse is one who is not a mere instrument. A great nurse is one who (given the context of her knowledge and the situation she faces) interacts in a way that accomplishes all that she can accomplish. A great nurse is a vital and active agent engrossed in her profession. She is part of a team but not a mere functionary (Fedorka & Husted, 2004, p. 52).

It is imperative to a nurse's role that her attention and attitude focus on her patient. As a professional, her role is that of the agent of her patient through the exercise of his virtues.

Every nurse needs a framework to guide her professional practice. The clearer her state of professional consciousness, the more effective and competent she will be in her role. A framework will clarify her consciousness. This framework is the ethical aspects of her role as a professional. The framework of her role will ideally be explicit as an ever-present thought she can clearly express to herself. It ought to provide her with a constant, driving, motivating strength. Her explicit awareness of her role will take and keep her out of her comfort zone. At the same time, it will bring her to a calm, swanlike, and reality-based dignity.

It will proceed somewhat as follows: "My patient's virtues (autonomy) are such that he is moving toward this goal (freedom) in these circumstances (objectivity) for this reason (beneficence). My virtues (autonomy) are such that I must act with him to assist him (his freedom) within the possibilities (of beneficence) in his circumstances to achieve every possible benefit that can be discovered (by objective awareness)."

Awareness of this framework unites and integrates a nurse's thoughts and actions and makes her actions an extension of her thinking. It is important to recognize as well that throughout her life, every professional nurse is the agent of a very special patient whom she motivates and inspires to a point of recognizing and using her own agency and guiding her ethical actions. That patient, of course, is the professional nurse herself.

> Every nurse needs a framework to guide her professional practice. It will proceed somewhat as follows: "My patient's virtues (autonomy) are such that he is moving toward this goal (freedom) in these circumstances (objectivity) for this reason (beneficence). My virtues (autonomy) are such that I must act with him to assist him (his freedom) within the possibilities (of beneficence) in his circumstances to achieve every possible benefit that can be discovered (by objective awareness)."

## DILEMMA 12.2: THE RIGHTS OF A CONFUSED PATIENT

Marilu is caring for an 82-year-old woman, Lillian. Lillian has been quite active in charitable affairs. One day while delivering food for Meals on Wheels, she slipped on a patch of ice. Lillian fractured her clavicle in the fall. She was taken to surgery, and the fracture was repaired. Her postoperative orders included 10 mg of valium and oxycodone/acetaminophen (5/325 mg). Lillian became very confused and within 2 days did not know her name. Her physician diagnosed her as senile. He began making plans for her to be transferred to a nursing home. He contacted her daughter, who lived in a different state, to get her permission. Her daughter gave her consent and decided to wait to visit until her mother was transferred to the nursing home. Marilu is convinced that Lillian is not senile, but the physician refused to consider the reasoning that she is very elderly and is overmedicated. Marilu believes that if Lillian is taken to a nursing home, she will never return to her normal life. She has every reason to believe that Lillian would not want to go to the nursing home until all other avenues were tried. What should be done?

## PROFESSIONALS, PATIENTS, AND CARING

Helen Keller, the famous lecturer and author, remarked that "Life is a great adventure or it is nothing." Every nurse comes into her profession expecting that it will be a great adventure, but sometimes, under the pressure of caregiver strain, health care professionals, especially nurses, become burned out. When this happens, their profession stops being a great adventure and becomes meaningless. A professional who suffers from burnout has lost her enthusiasm, her strength, and her endurance. She has stopped caring. Perhaps from the beginning, her caring was flawed (Nelson, 1992). She may never have defined *caring*.

"Caring is the essential fuel of a nurse's interaction with her patient. It is an essential means of understanding the needs and purposes of her patient. Without this, nothing can produce a successful chain of cause-and-effect interactions between them" (Husted & Husted, 1997, p. 17). Caring is the moral integrity of a nurse's (or any professional's) practice (Hartman, 1998).

> "Caring is the essential fuel of a nurse's interaction with her patient. It is an essential means of understanding the needs and purposes of her patient. Without this, nothing can produce a successful chain of cause-and-effect interactions between them" (Husted & Husted, 1997, p. 17).

Caring can open the way to understanding the needs of a patient, although it does not produce understanding of the ways to meet these needs effectively. Exclusive attention to caring assumes that there are only simple bioethical dilemmas and that professionals can deal with these dilemmas instinctively. It further assumes that ethical dilemmas are only in the mind or in the emotions of the professional and not in the world of the patient. To experience caring is a virtue, to concentrate on caring only is a flaw; in the same way, to concentrate on any standard rather than on a patient is an error and a mistake.

A caring perspective can interfere with, or replace, an interactive relationship. Caring, in and of itself, does not provide guidance. An intellectual understanding and an emotional understanding of the patient in his circumstances must produce guidance. Logical consistency must guide this understanding. There is no reason why logical stability and consistency cannot coexist with compassionate caring. In fact, each perfects the other. Caring without logical stability and consistency is caring for the wrong reason, in the wrong way, or to an illogical extent and will produce injustice. Injustice to the patient, to the nurse, or to both is unjustifiable. Likewise, logical stability and consistency without caring will distort the whole reason for being a health care system and will also produce injustice.

Caring can mean different, and even opposed, things, including:

1. Sharing the values and motivations of another because they are values and motivations for this other. For instance, sharing a patient's struggles to regain his lost well-being through empathy for the patient.
2. Being concerned with and attending to something or someone. For instance, sharing a patient's struggles to regain his lost well-being simply because he is one's patient.
3. Undergoing mental suffering or grief. For instance, feeling overburdened from sharing a patient's struggle and struggling with a patient as a burden.

4. Being under the power of one emotion and devoting oneself to strengthening an opposed emotion. For instance, feeling overburdened from sharing a patient's struggle and struggling to feel a concern that one does not feel for a patient.

---

### DILEMMA 12.3: RIGHTS OF A PATIENT WITH A PSYCHIATRIC DIAGNOSIS

Jason is a patient in a psychiatric hospital. He was admitted on a legal hold against his will. He has been diagnosed as a paranoid schizophrenic. His physician has prescribed 5 mg Haldol and 2 mg Cogentin. Jason refuses to take the medication. He tells his nurse, Jessica, that the physician is trying to poison him. Aside from what he tells her, Jessica has no reason to believe that Jason's physician is trying to poison him. Would she be justified in giving Jason an injection of the medication against his will so that he would get the benefit of it? Would doing so violate Jason's rights?

---

## WAYS OF CARING

"Caring is a concept central to the nursing profession. Although references to caring in the literature are abundant, there is little clarity about the definition and process of caring" (Scotto, 2003, p. 289). *Caring*, therefore, is in need of clarification.

There are several ways of caring: *Theatrical caring* is the way that one feels for a character in a movie or on a TV program. It is not a caring for a person. It is a type of playacting. One rejoices at the success of a character, or one is distressed at his or her failure. But it is not the character (patient) as a person for whom one cares. At best, theatrical caring is an exaggeration of common courtesy. At its worst, it is an unpleasant, exaggerated, pompous display of self-importance.

Another way of caring might be called *reaction formation caring*. This is when a nurse tries to produce caring when she does not care and because she does not care. She is unwilling to admit to herself that she does not care, and so this kind of caring becomes a disguise to cover her indifference. She cannot face the fact that she is indifferent to her patient, so she sees the façade of a caring person as herself. Reaction formation caring does little to support and nourish a patient, and, for a nurse, it is a process of self-deception and self-destruction.

A third way of caring is *codependent caring*. This consists of a nurse's trying to find her sense of ethical worth by working to make herself and her patient mutually codependent (Armstrong & Norris, 1992; Summers, 1992). It begins with self-sacrifice on the part of a professional nurse. She escapes the need to think and understand by neglecting herself and by focusing exclusive attention on her patient. When she finds her patient's response insufficient to fill her needs, she begins to feel victimized, resentful, and still dependent. Then, according to Summers (1992), "compassion may disappear and a hardened facade may cover the nurse's . . . feelings of powerlessness, fear or shame" (pp. 70–71). Through this way of caring, a nurse may attempt to find herself by actually abandoning herself and discarding her own needs. She attempts to fulfill herself through a course of action that destroys her (Morris & Trigoboff, 1996).

> Another way of caring might be called affinity caring. It is that which a nurse feels when she shares the desires and purposes of the person for whom she cares.

Another way of caring might be called affinity caring. It is that which a nurse feels when she shares the desires and purposes of the person for whom she cares. Care providers must be able to change their perspective to that of another to provide effective ethical care (Vanlaere, Timmermann, Stevens, & Gastmans, 2012). A nurse cares for a person because he is a person and because he is this person. She cares for him because she values what he values and because she shares an adventure with him. This is a nurse's great adventure. Affinity caring is genuine caring. It supports and nourishes a nurse and her patient. It is caring for a person. This is the way of caring that nurses can and ought to be noted for. "Nursing is about interacting with people . . . in a meaningful way that can make a real difference in their lives" (Trossman, 2000, p. 8).

## WHAT GOES AROUND . . .

Most occupations or professions offer benefits specific to themselves. For instance, an architect can design his or her own home. Plumbers can avoid the (allegedly) exorbitant prices plumbers charge. Surveyors are able to get out into the outdoors. Accountants are able to stay in, out of the outdoors. Teachers have a wonderful opportunity to learn. Clowns are able to enjoy the enjoyment of children. One occupation said to have a notable side benefit is that of the horse groom. There is an ancient saying to the effect that "The outside of a horse is good for the inside of a man." This saying arose, supposedly, because horse grooms, those who care for the well-being of racehorses, must give painstaking care to the horses in their charge. In addition to this, they have much time for themselves. Yet they are unable to travel far from the stables on any given day. This puts them in the habit of taking care of themselves. Notoriously, they tend to live a long life in good health.

There is also a notable benefit found in nursing. There is an approach to the profession that makes nursing one of the most rewarding of all occupations. This approach offers a benefit that is as great as any benefit any other occupation on Earth offers. A nurse must give counsel to her patient. She must also, as everyone must, give counsel to herself. As a nurse, she must inspire action in her patient. As a person and as an ethical agent, she must inspire action in herself. Throughout her entire life, a nurse is the nurse of a nurse. She is a nurse to herself. She gives counsel to and serves the virtue that is her own.

> Throughout her entire life, a nurse is the nurse of a nurse. She is a nurse to herself. She gives counsel to and serves the virtue that is her own.

## DILEMMA 12.4: WHO GETS THE DONOR HEART?

A donor heart becomes available, and there are two heart transplant candidates in the same hospital who are a match for the donor heart: Mr. X and Ms. Y. Mr. X has been on the waiting list a long time, and he is near death. He is 64 and has suffered from a heart condition for years. He has had two angioplasties and two bypass operations to correct a blockage of the heart's blood vessels. He still smokes, eats fatty foods, and is very overweight. He has been counseled about smoking, diet, and exercise each time after a procedure, but he says it is too hard to change. Ms. Y has just been put on the list and could be sustained with medication for some time until another heart became available. She does not smoke and is not overweight. She tries to watch her diet. Who should get the heart? ("Heart Transplant," 2000)

## VIRTUES AND HAPPINESS

A nurse ought to support, nurture, and safeguard the virtues of her patient. Even more so, she should act to support, nurture, and sustain her own virtues. In supporting her own virtues, a nurse will enhance her patient's life through enhancing the performance of her professional role. This in turn, of course, will enhance her own life.

Ethics has to do with action and interaction. People interact to maximize the power of their action. They interact because they can accomplish more through interaction than they can by acting alone. If people did not enhance their lives by interacting, they would not interact because they would have no reason to do so. People also act alone to enhance their lives. There is no such thing as a human action that does not make a difference. Nearly every human action either benefits or harms the one who acts. Every action is an action toward a goal. This is another reason why a nurse should support and nurture the virtues of her patient.

In recognizing and respecting the bioethical standards, a nurse safeguards the abilities of her patient's agency. To act freely, to make himself aware of the facts of his circumstances, and to pursue benefits are abilities a patient shares with every human being. In safeguarding the abilities of her patient's agency, a nurse honors her patient's rights. To be the person one is, to initiate action, and to control one's time is every person's right. In honoring her patient's rights, a nurse supports and nurtures the virtues of her patient. In nurturing the virtues of her patient, she helps him help her succeed. She achieves the virtue of professional competence and excellence as a nurse. In safeguarding, supporting, and nurturing the virtues of her patient, in acting as the protector of her patient's virtues, a nurse creates and strengthens her own character.

A nurse observes in her patient that he needs a certain ability and virtue. She does this by observing why he needs that ability. To observe that he needs it and why he needs it is the same observation. These observations are the bridge between a nurse and her patient. The ethical virtues are the bioethical standards and standards of a professional nurse's ethical action.

---

### DILEMMA 12.5: DESIRES OF A PATIENT VERSUS FAMILY'S REQUEST FOR LIFE-SUSTAINING TREATMENT

Mrs. C. is a 52-year-old woman with metastatic ovarian cancer who is hospitalized with a bowel obstruction and pain. She has undergone multiple therapies, including surgery and chemotherapy, but now her disease has progressed. She is not a candidate for surgery to relieve a bowel obstruction. She has no advance directive but has expressed a desire to be kept pain free, even if this requires her to be sedated at the end of life. She was started on intravenous morphine. This afforded her good pain relief until 3 days later, when her condition deteriorated and she lapsed into a coma. Her family requests that the morphine dosage be decreased so that she can be more alert and interactive. The family also asks that total parenteral nutrition (TPN) be started so that she does not "starve to death" (Maxwell, 2000, p. 57). What should be done?

---

## MUSINGS

The experience of attending to her patient's virtues allows a nurse to experience and to exercise her own virtues. A professional looks into herself for her awareness of the virtues she must motivate and nurture in her patient. She will find these virtues in herself because, in filling her role as a professional and in working within the framework of her profession, she will have put them there.

> A nurse will find these virtues in herself because, in filling her role as a professional and in working within the framework of her profession, she will have put them there.

This is the professional role a nurse, in particular, can make uniquely her own: to motivate, to safeguard, and to nurture the virtues of her patient. A professional can help a patient sustain his development and remain the unique being he is. She does this by maintaining her fidelity to her agreement with her patient and, through this, her fidelity to herself.

In nurturing her patient's uniqueness, she sees the value of uniqueness and accepts herself as unique. She sees the value to her of those who are different from her. She sees her value to them. She teaches herself *reciprocity*. In nurturing her patient's freedom, in practicing fidelity to her profession, she sees the value of freedom and teaches herself *courage*—the courage to accept and encourage her patient's freedom. In nurturing her patient's objectivity, she sees the value of objectivity and embraces it as her own standard. She achieves *wisdom*. She teaches herself to rely on all the knowledge she has gained through experience and to accept the fact that her knowledge is limited. This is the virtue of *wisdom*. In approving her patient's striving for his benefit, she deals with him based on beneficence. She sees the value of beneficence to him and to herself, and prompted by reason, she teaches herself *justice*. In seeing the value to her patient of his fidelity to himself, she learns the value of fidelity and teaches *pride* in herself and in her profession. Pride in herself produces fidelity to herself.

*Pride in herself produces fidelity to herself.*

She becomes aware of the value of the virtues to her patient. She sees his struggle to regain them. From her patient's struggles, she learns the importance of destiny. From being a nurse she learns the matchless value of life. When she comes to understand the value of life, she comes to understand the importance of destiny. When she comes to understand the importance of destiny, she comes to understand the value of character. By coming to understand the value of character, she gains an understanding of the virtues. No occupations on Earth can facilitate this understanding and the acquisition of these abilities more perfectly than the profession of nursing.

Virtue is the ability to be a human being. More than this, it is the ability to be a human being successfully. By learning the value of the virtues, she learns the value of character. For a person's virtues are that person's character.

*By learning the value of the virtues, she learns the value of character. For a person's virtues are that person's character.*

The French novelist Honoré de Balzac warned us that an unfilled vocation draws the color from one's entire existence. Those who look for the glory of nursing in the right places will find it; those who do not, have looked for it where it is not to be found.

## STUDY GUIDE

1. Give some thought to your own virtues—your excellence as a professional. Describe yourself to yourself; it is a great exercise in self-understanding.
2. Not all nurses or health care professionals are excellent: some by virtue of not knowing but some by not caring. How can you mentor others, of course, in a caring way, that would help them?
3. What is the point of the swan principle?
4. Think about the four ways of caring and benefit or harm that comes to the patient from each.
5. Concentrate on using only affinity caring, and note how patients and colleagues respond. Give your colleagues some positive feedback—what goes around comes around.
6. Think about how affinity caring can stop the cycle of incivility.
7. Use this case for class discussion; the analysis of the case only appears in the instructor's manual.

### SAVING A CHILD BY HAVING ANOTHER

Mary and Abe Ayala have a teenage daughter, Anissa, who has been diagnosed with acute leukemia. Their physician recommends a bone marrow transplant. Neither Anissa's parents nor her brother are acceptable donors. For 2 years the family searches for an acceptable

*Continued*

donor. Their daughter's time is running out. Finally, they face their last hope. They decide to try to have another baby in the hope that this infant will be an acceptable donor. Are the parents justified in having a baby driven by these motivations? (Associated Press, 1990)

## REFERENCES

Armstrong, J., & Norris, C. (1992). Co-dependence: A nursing issue. *Focus on Critical Care, 19,* 105–115.

Associated Press. (1990, February 17). Baby is conceived to save daughter. *The New York Times.* Retrieved from http://www.nytimes.com/1990/02/17/us/baby-is-conceived-to-save-daughter.html

Bioethics Case Study. (2000). Transplant. Retrieved October 25, 2006, from http://www.mhhe.com/biosci/genbio/olc linkedcontent/bioethics cases/g-bioe-04.htm

Fedorka, P., & Husted, G. L. (2004). Ethical decision making in clinical emergencies. *Topics in Emergency Medicine, 26,* 52–60.

Hartman, R. L. (1998). Revisiting the call to care: An ethical perspective. *Advanced Practice Nursing Quarterly, 4*(2), 14–18.

Heart transplant. (2000). *General and human biology: Bioethics case studies.* Retrieved from McGraw-Hill: http://www.mhhe.com/biosci/genbio/olc_linkedcontent/bioethics_cases/g-bioe-04.htm

Husted, G. L., & Husted, J. H. (1997). Is a return to a caring perspective desirable? *Advanced Practice Nursing Quarterly, 3*(1), 14–17.

Maxwell, T. (2000). Ethical decision making at the end of life: A series of case studies. *Patient Care for the Nurse Practitioner, 3*(11), 57–61.

McKeon, R. (Ed.). (1941). *The basic works of Aristotle.* New York, NY: Random House.

Meyers, T. A. (2000). Why couldn't I have seen him? *American Journal of Nursing, 100*(2), 9.

Morris, M., & Trigoboff, E. (1996). Co-dependence. In H. S. Wilson & C. R. Kneis (Eds.), *Psychiatric nursing* (5th ed., pp. 776–815). Redwood, CA: Addison-Wesley.

Nasman, Y., Nystrom, L., & Eriksson, K. (2012). From values to virtue: The basis for quality of care. *International Journal for Human Caring, 16*(2), 50–56.

Nelson, L. N. (1992). Against caring. *The Journal of Clinical Ethics, 3*(1), 8–15.

Scotto, C. (2003). A new view of caring. *Journal of Nursing Education, 42,* 289–294.

Spinoza, B. (1949). *Ethics.* (J. Gutman, Ed.). New York, NY: Hafner Publishing. (Original work published 1675)

Stanislavski, C. (1963). *An actor's handbook.* New York, NY: Theatre Arts Books.

Summers, C. L. (1992). Co-dependence: A nursing dilemma. Revolution. *The Journal of Nurse Empowerment, 136,* 68–79.

Trossman, S. (2000). Health for all: RN fights to level the playing field. *American Nurse, 200,* 8–9.

Vanlaere, L., Timmermann, M., Stevens, M., & Gastmans, C. (2012). An explorative study of experiences of healthcare providers posing as simulated care receivers in a 'care-ethical' lab. *Nursing Ethics, 19*(1), 68–79.

# ANALYSES OF DILEMMAS

## A NOTE TO THE READER

In reviewing these dilemmas, the reader should recall that they are abstract case studies. In abstract case studies, of course, it sounds as though the nature of the case is very clear and the responsibility of any health care professional is equally clear and rigid. In the context of a real-life situation, however, a health care professional seldom enjoys this clarity.

It is possible that for one or more dilemmas, a reader may come to a different resolution than the resolution given. This is not surprising. There is no real-world context to which to refer and no way to gain more information. Everyone approaches a dilemma from the perspective of recent experiences, ideas, and attitudes. A nurse may unconsciously rewrite the dilemma from her perspective, or it is possible to add something to the context that the dilemma does not give. A different perspective or context may, very logically, result in a different resolution to this new and different dilemma. The authors ask the reader to perform a thought experiment: Without changing anything of the dilemma as it is given, form a different perspective of the dilemma in your mind—one that suggests the given resolution. This will significantly sharpen your understanding of bioethical decision making.

There is a very large difference between a real-life context and a case study. Nothing that follows should instill a feeling of ethical incompetence in the reader. Many of the following dilemmas are highly context dependent. In addition, some are quite difficult. Several are dilemmas nurses or other health care personnel meet in their interactions with physicians. Most of the dilemmas in some way involve nurses; not all of them do. Some involve other professionals, such as physicians, and so forth.

The final resolutions of some of these dilemmas can be discovered only in the actual context in which they arise. All that can be done in a case study analysis is to make the nature of the dilemmas clear. In some cases, we will offer only broad suggestions as to the direction the resolutions might take. The purpose of these analyses is to make the reader stronger and more knowledgeable. Many ethical agents do not allow themselves to know when their response to an ethical situation has been inadequate. Without knowledge, there is no growth. Without growth, there is no possibility of consistently appropriate ethical decision making. It is a nurse's responsibility to know. The purpose of these resolutions is to enable the reader to orient her or his thinking about bioethical matters and to develop competence and confidence at bioethical decision making.

## ANALYSES

### DILEMMA 3.1, PAGE 34

#### Patient's Conflict About Her Own Care

When people face two unpleasant alternatives, they often complain bitterly about the one they find the least undesirable. In effect, Mrs. B changes the alternatives from what they are to stopping the dialysis or not having the condition to contend with at all.

Here the problem is to determine what Mrs. B wants. There is evidence that she wants to stop the dialysis. She has told everyone within hearing that she hates it and does not want to live this way. On the other hand, when the physician describes the risks of not having it, she continues to board the van that takes her to dialysis. The evidence that she wants to stop the dialysis is much less compelling than the evidence she wants to continue it.

When she has to choose between the actual alternatives she faces, she chooses to continue the dialysis. The old platitude "Actions speak louder than words" is true. Her actions are sufficient to resolve the dilemma.

### DILEMMA 3.2, PAGE 47

#### The Demands of an Agreement

Jeffrey, a young child, is your patient. You have an agreement with him to stay until his parents arrive. If you break this agreement, why would you have any reason to keep any agreements? There is a serious implication behind a decision to break your agreement with Jeffrey. That is an assertion that you are not a professional nurse. If there is ever a reason to break an agreement, there must be a cutoff point where one side, which is breaking the agreement, is acceptable and the other side where it is not. For instance, you get a call that your own child has been in a terrible automobile accident and is on his way to the emergency room. Your agreement with your own child in this situation is prior to your agreement with Jeffrey. The cutoff point would be where keeping an agreement would necessitate breaking a prior and more basic agreement. The concert is well over on the other side of the cutoff point.

## DILEMMA 4.1, PAGE 56

## Compulsory Obligation to Others

The fact that Mabel is lying to herself has great ethical relevance in this context.

**Autonomy:** By lying to herself, Mabel has closed off her autonomy. In refusing to consider one or more relevant factors, Mabel takes herself out of any objective context. She has broken the connection between the context of knowledge and the context of her situation. Sharen needs to help her understand the context. Mabel has not considered the fact that the two outcomes open to her are opposed to each other. In the opinion of the physician, she cannot have the child and fight her cancer. Mabel can establish an objective context only by considering all the alternative possibilities and choosing one. It is her right to make this choice. The responsibility of the nurse and the physician is to give her relevant information on each alternative.

The fact that Mabel is unwilling to consider every possibility makes it difficult or impossible for Sharen to communicate with her.

But Sharen, in approaching the problem directly, is making it difficult for Mabel to communicate. Indirection might be a better direction to take. If Sharen asked Mabel as a hypothetical or rhetorical question, "Mabel, if you had to make a choice between saving the life of this baby or your own life, what do you think you would choose?" Or, "Mabel, if a woman had to make a choice between saving the life of her baby or her own life, what do you think she would choose? What do you think she *should* choose?" Or, "Mabel, when a woman gets pregnant, she makes certain agreements with the baby. Do you think she makes an agreement to, for instance, keep the baby safe?" Then in discussing this relatively nonthreatening question about her thoughts, Mabel might finalize a choice, begin to discuss it, and come to a decision.

**Freedom:** Mabel is unwilling to make an objective judgment based on every alternative open to her. Under these circumstances, she cannot engage in free action. She wants it both ways, and she is scared. Neither Sharen nor the physician can directly try to influence her freedom. Mabel is being pushed to give up her freedom of choice, but if she is not free to decide, she might be free to analyze it as a hypothetical question. Instead of a momentous decision, she will deal with an interesting discussion.

**Objectivity:** Sharen owes Mabel the truth. A patient also has some responsibility to give truthful communications to the health care professionals providing care. Is Mabel violating this standard on her own behalf?

**Beneficence:** Mabel is walled off from the influence of Sharen and other health care professionals. She is being pushed from all directions. For Sharen to benefit Mabel, Mabel will have to analyze her situation and apply some level of reason to the course of action she decides to take. Sharen needs to help her do this through compassionate understanding and truthful facts. Mabel may be willing to reconsider, if she does not, for the moment, have to face it head-on.

**Fidelity:** Sharen has to engage in open communication with Mabel and help her understand the consequences of each decision. The way in which she does, along with the physician, will have a lot to do with Mabel's understanding and her final decision. The bottom line is it is Mabel's decision to make; it is her body and hers alone. The health care professionals have a responsibility to help her gently know the objective facts and then leave her alone with her husband to make the decision. In this case, although the husband has a very vested interest, it is still not his body. Even so, he needs to be included in the discussions.

## DILEMMA 4.2, PAGE 57

### Family's Desire or Patient's Wishes?

**Autonomy:** If the desires of Edgar's family are given priority, his autonomy is obviously violated because his desires and theirs contradict each other.

**Freedom:** Not to honor Edgar's wishes is obviously a violation of his freedom. This is more so because there is no possibility of his achieving freedom in the future.

**Objectivity:** The family's optimism is a subjective feeling in conflict with the facts. Subjective feelings, except those of a patient, have no weight in a practice-based ethic. Assertion of one's values for another is neither an example of ethical analysis nor a valid application of the standard of objectivity. We can assume, because there is no evidence to the contrary, that love for Edgar motivates the family's desires for him. In health care this happens often; the family does not want to see a loved one die (this is especially true with children), but the responsibility of the health care team is to help the family make judgments based on facts and on what Edgar wants.

**Beneficence:** It is not beneficent to take over a patient's right to decide in order to indulge a misguided benevolent desire. It is not beneficent to take over a patient's right to decide in order to indulge the wishes of the family.

**Fidelity:** The physician's agreement with Edgar does not depend on the attitude of Edgar's family.

## DILEMMA 4.3, PAGE 59

### The Demands of Promise Keeping

This is not a dilemma that a nurse is very apt to find. However, the dilemma presented in this extreme case points to the principles involved in any dilemma of this kind.

**Autonomy:** The patient is unique. This uniqueness determines the nature of his desire. No one can know how his uniqueness in the situation shapes his desire. The nurse must go on the knowledge she has, but the dilemma assumes that she has very little knowledge.

**Freedom:** If she reveals what her patient has told her, she will, at least apparently, be taking action against him. If she informs the physician, she will also be taking an action for him. She will be helping him continue acting on the purpose he had in entering the hospital. This purpose inspired his original agreement. If his nurse keeps her later agreement, she will have broken her earlier and more basic agreement. This would imply that agreements are to be broken. In fact, it is implicit in the original agreement—that the hospital would function as a hospital—that no contrary agreements would have any status. This alone, in and of itself, would free the nurse from any responsibility to keep her promise.

**Objectivity:** To meet the demands of the standard of objectivity, beneficence must guide a nurse. Does objectivity call for her to keep her promise to the patient, or does it call for her to inform the physician so that he or she can take the best possible action? To discover the demands of beneficence, she has to know the probable outcomes of different courses of action given her patient's ultimate purposes.

There is no way the nurse can know what direction beneficence takes. However, all of this takes place in a health care setting, and when there is any doubt, the nature of the health care setting must determine action. There is no way to interpret the patient's revelation to his nurse as anything more than a joke. If it were a matter of any seriousness, she is entitled to believe he would not have revealed it.

**Beneficence:** Contextually, it seems as if beneficence calls for telling, but the harm of telling is not known. Action is behavior arising from knowledge. An agent should always prefer to act on what she does know rather than on what she does not know. The harm of not telling is known. If this harm is at all serious, then that which the agent knows must override that which she does not know. Beneficence, guided by reason, suggests that the nurse break her promise of secrecy.

**Fidelity:** Fidelity requires the nurse to make a choice. She must exercise fidelity either toward her promise or toward her patient. Her promise, of course, was a promise to her patient. All the same, she owes fidelity not to one aspect of her relationship to her patient but to the entire relationship and to the destiny of her patient. In the context of a purposive ethic, she owes fidelity to her patient and to what she knows.

A ritualistic ethic would demand that a nurse keep her promise, but very few nurses would. A purposive ethic would demand that a nurse keep her attention on the purpose that brought her patient into the hospital.

When a patient tells a secret to a nurse, he should not forget that the first purpose of the health care system is his health and well-being. Secrecy for the sake of secrecy must give way to health and well-being. The nurse does not take over the ownership of her patient unless she does something for him that he would not do for himself. If she does something for him that he would do, then she is simply acting as his agent.

## DILEMMA 4.4, PAGE 62

### Deception or Truth

**Autonomy:** Whatever the nature of their autonomy, it is inconceivable that Robin's parents would take a calm and disinterested view of her death.

**Freedom:** Obviously, the power of Robin's parents to move into the future would be truncated if the nurse told the entire truth. She would place an image in the parent's minds that would stay there forever.

**Objectivity:** If Robin's parents heard the gory details of their daughter's death, this could do them no good and could not fail to do them harm. It would do nothing to help them assimilate this event into their lives and begin to move on.

**Beneficence:** Robin's nurse harmed the parents emotionally and forever. Hearing the entire truth did nothing to increase their ability to reason. Robin's nurse acted dutifully, but she failed to act beneficently. Granted, the mantra to tell the truth drove her motives, but she did not consider the context.

**Fidelity:** Obviously, this action served no rational purpose. The nurse cannot justify her action by appealing to fidelity.

## DILEMMA 5.1, PAGE 73

### Right to Choose an Unhealthy Lifestyle

Martin is a biomedical professional. As such, he has a professional role. He has a responsibility to care for Frank as long as Frank needs him. Does Martin have the same responsibility? Here is a contextual kink. There is an ambiguity in the word *needs*. Frank's health is such that he needs Martin to help him change his self-destructive habits. However, insofar as Martin has no influence on Frank, insofar as Frank will not change his self-destructive habits, Frank has no need for Martin.

Suppose Frank had the services of a home health nurse who encouraged his heavy smoking and his dietary habits. From what we know of Frank, he would be no better or no worse off with or without visits from this home health nurse. These visits would change absolutely nothing. Martin's visits have precisely the same influence. Likewise, Frank would be no worse off without visits from Martin, and he is not better off with Martin's visits. Another patient might be considerably better off.

Martin has tried for 9 months to help Frank, and nothing has changed. Several options are open to Martin: He could ask that he be replaced in the hopes that another could be more persuasive (this might be a good alternative), he could ask that the physician discontinue home visits (it is not doing any objective good, and it is costly), or he could continue as things are with the belief that Frank is, at least, being monitored. We do not compel people to adhere to what is best for them. On the other hand, should Martin continue providing home services in the hope that something will give way and that Frank will begin to, at least, do better with following a regimen? A behavior modification workshop would be a great idea, but there is no reason to believe that Frank would go or that it would help. What other suggestions do you have?

## DILEMMA 5.2, PAGE 74

### Making a Decision Against Facility Policy

Nearly always when one distorts and misreads a context, it is because it has been widened beyond its relevant contours. The situation can also appear problematic if the context is narrowed too stringently. On one hand, the patient needs attention that she cannot be given in Ron's location. On the other hand, hospital policy and practice requires that an attending physician sign a transfer order. Looking at the dilemma from the narrow perspective, then, is no way to resolve it.

However, purposes that are to be accomplished in the health care setting form the context of the situation, and accomplishing those purposes is not possible here. A wider context must be sought in the context of knowledge.

The primary elements of the context of knowledge are formed by the nature and definition of the roles of those engaged in seeking to achieve the purpose. In this case, the primary elements are the definitions of a physician, a nurse, and a patient.

However one defines a physician, the purposes of the physician that do not involve the welfare of patients is far less important than the purposes that do. The latter are the defining purposes of the physician and the entire health care system.

The ethical course for Ron to follow is to transfer Mrs. Allison to the other hospital and then depend on the calm, modest, rational objectivity of the physician. This attitude of the physician is the only ethical attitude possible to her. The ethical responsibilities of any professional are set out in the definition of his or her profession. This situation is a case where the policy is bad. At the very least, someone other than the attending physician should be able to sign the transfer order. The patient should not suffer or even die because of the policy.

The nurse, for the benefit of the patient, could risk transferring the patient. Better to explain breaking protocol than why the nurse let the patient die.

## DILEMMA 5.3, PAGE 76

### Embryo Ownership

Peggy wants to be a mother. There was an agreement between Peggy and her husband that this donation would be for procreation. John donated his sperm—an almost inexhaustible resource. Peggy donated her eggs—a very limited resource. This gave John a way to punish Peggy that she could not use against him. To evaluate John's concern for the fate of his sperm, one must have recourse to one's sense of humor.

Peggy owns the eggs. Also, unless John's sperm can be extracted without harm to the eggs, they are hers. This, of course, does not involve the legal analysis. It is possible that something was signed between the two of them. On a purely ethical level, the eggs belong to the person who donated them. The authors realize that this may not be a popular decision.

## DILEMMA 5.4, PAGE 82

### Suspected Child Abuse

The elements best illuminate this dilemma. However, think about how the bioethical standards will also arrive at the same decision.

**Desire:** Shawn's desire for help is rational. Doris's desire for secrecy is not justifiable.

**Reason:** Shawn needs Alice to help him achieve the benefit of reason. Doris is not acting on reason if Alice is right in her suspicion.

**Life:** Shawn has a right to a better life if he is being abused.

**Purpose:** Shawn's purpose is justifiable. Doris's is not.

**Agency:** Alice is Shawn's agent. (If Shawn is a battered child, a great deal of good can be done. If he is not, no great harm will be done if the investigation is done in an ethical manner.)

## DILEMMA 5.5, PAGE 83

### Right to Refuse Disfiguring Interventions

**Autonomy:** Mrs. L. is, as all people are, unique; this means that she acts on her own values and ideas for her future. She has the absolute right to do this. Her husband and the surgeon acted on an implicit belief that they have the same rights over the woman as she has. This is an assumption that their right over her is more authoritative than her own rights. If assumption is a standard, then everybody has this right.

**Freedom:** The action of her husband and the surgeon entirely took away her freedom. Without freedom, she cannot take ethical action or interactions. The action they took was not an ethical action open to analysis and debate but rather an act of aggression.

**Objectivity:** So long as she is capable of evaluating the facts of the situation and knows the possible consequences of her actions, she is exercising her objective awareness. This is not even a case in which her husband and the surgeon are not sure what she wanted, such as in cases involving incompetent patients. They cannot even say that she was in extreme pain, and there is no evidence that her fear has made her unable to meet situations in a rational way. She had no opportunity to act on her objective awareness in this circumstance.

They had an intuition from right up front, face-to-face with the dilemma. She also had an intuition and a little more than an intuition. After a period of analysis she made a decision—an objective and reasoned decision. If their intuition is on par with her decision, then there is no point to consult with a patient. Her self-governance is being taken away; she has been put under an anesthetic, and all decision power is taken away.

**Beneficence:** Nonobjective beneficence is not beneficence. In her case it is coercive. Coercive beneficence is not beneficent even though they acted in her best interest from their perspective.

A young man's father sent him to college on a football scholarship so that his son could follow in his father's footsteps. This was very beneficent, save for the fact that his son wanted to be a ballet dancer. In this case, beneficence is nonobjective.

**Fidelity:** If you have an agreement with someone, for it to be an objective and ethical agreement, it has to respect the rights of those involved to decide on their own course of action. If one is not faithful to this, then the agreement is violated.

One's emotions may tell someone to violate an agreement because the evidence for a good outcome is overwhelming and, oh well, the other party will be glad afterward. One might be powerfully pulled to follow the course the husband and surgeon took—especially if the patient were one's own wife or husband whom he or she loved. However, the woman made an implicit agreement with the surgeon that he would not take the action he did. He did take this action. The implication is that the surgeon had an agreement to do to anything he wanted to do. This would mean that the woman relinquished all her rights, but no one can assume this, except through a criminal action.

There is no reason why the husband, surgeon, nurse, and others should not use gentle coercion. It is persuasion with a view to her own rational nature. This should be tried, but if that does not change her mind, the only recourse is to let her have her own desires.

## DILEMMA 5.6, PAGE 85

### Rights of a Homosexual Partner

> **Autonomy:** Cal and Art have been living together for 10 years. The meaning of this is quite clear. There is no reason to doubt that Cal would want Art to make his health care decisions. To make a valid decision, it would be necessary that someone have knowledge of Cal's situation. Art has this, and the family does not; they want everything done to keep him alive.
>
> Cal's dying process cannot be reversed. This is a sufficient reason to go against the family.
>
> **Freedom:** Cal is dying. He has no ability to exercise freedom, but health care professionals can exercise it for him. The family's only reasonable course is to accept this.
>
> **Objectivity:** It may be that the family deeply loves Cal and cannot bear to lose him. There is not sufficient evidence on which to base this. Another supposition, equally tenable, is that the family wants to keep Cal alive to punish him. The health care system cannot cooperate in this.
>
> **Beneficence:** Beneficence could not be expressed without the dismissal of hysterical resentment. The health care system, hopefully, has tried to establish beneficence into Cal's last days and will not stop that effort now. Art being with Cal would make for a beneficent ambience. Spite and beneficence do not fit well together.
>
> **Fidelity:** Cal spent a great deal of time with Art. Art was a very important part of Cal's life. Fidelity to Cal must definitely include the recognition of what Cal would want.
>
> This is a case in which the ethical and the legal are at odds. Everything should be done to work with the family for the benefit of Art. This may involve gentle coercion to use with the family.

## DILEMMA 6.1, PAGE 95

### Duty or Saving a Life?

> This dilemma is certainly extreme, but it reveals the seriocomic nature of deontology in the sick room.
>
> Picture this: A platoon of soldiers in basic training is in formation and being trained to march. Sergeant Austin is drilling them. They are beginning to look sharp. As they are marching, Lieutenant Brown steps over and says to one of the soldiers in the marching line, "Private Jones, I have a duty for you to perform. Report to Sergeant Smith for kitchen police duty." Note carefully that the lieutenant did not tell the private he was giving him a duty to continue marching. That would not have made any sense. Private Jones was already marching. To do his duty, Private Jones had to leave the column of marchers, go somewhere else, and do something else.

When a nurse goes into a patient's room, it is not possible to know what she is going to find. However, whatever she finds, if a duty were placed on her, she would have to leave the room and go to where it would be possible to perform that duty. Even in the unlikely scenario where she did not have to leave the room and abandon her patient spatially, she would have to abandon him spiritually. Does this make for efficient nursing? Does this make for any kind of nursing?

The duty that is placed on a nurse especially violates a patient's freedom, and it violates the nurse's fidelity.

## DILEMMA 6.2, PAGE 99

### Implied Consent or Violation of One's Rights?

The right of a person to make decisions for himself or herself, dispose of personal property, and so on, is firmly established in law. The facts that John Doe was deceased and could not express his wishes, that there was no family or friend to express what he would want, and that he was an excellent candidate for organ donation are all entirely irrelevant. What can be gained from minor violations of rights justified by rationalizations is very far outweighed by the consequent threat to rights. Rights is the product of an agreement among rational beings. Whoever breaks this agreement on whatever pretext proves himself or herself not to be among the class of rational beings. John Doe changed. He moved from life to death. The hospital personnel choose unilaterally to benefit from this change in John Doe's condition. There was no voluntary consent on his part. This violated John Doe's rights.

**Autonomy:** A human person does not have rights because he is alive. He has rights because he is a human person. Even the law recognizes the prenatal right to inherit and the postmortem right to bequeath. The rights of the living continue even when they are no longer living. This includes the right to dispose of or not to dispose of that which was theirs as they wished.

**Freedom:** It is not the case that what one did not explicitly forbid, he tacitly consented to. On the contrary, that which he did not consent to in the disposition of his values, unless there are compelling arguments from his perspective that can be made, one must assume he tacitly forbade.

**Objectivity:** To violate any implication of the rights agreement is to violate the rights agreement. Properly analyzing this dilemma is not possible without understanding. Also, understanding it is not possible without seeing its comic dimensions. The only principle on which the hospital personnel can justify their action is some version of "If you believe that it is so, then it is so." This reveals much more about them than about the dilemma. A safer conclusion than that their actions were justified would be the conclusion that "If they believe that it is so, then it very probably is not so," because their only reason for belief is the fact that they want it to be so.

**Beneficence:** To assume that a drowning person would want to be saved is justified. To assume that a person would want to be an organ donor without any immediate evidence is not justified. Therefore, donation is not an exercise of beneficence.

**Fidelity:** The only way to exercise fidelity would be to recognize the absence of an agreement.

## DILEMMA 6.3, PAGE 100

### Telishment

How would you explain to the young benefactor's family that they should feel no sorrow but pride and gratification at the contribution their son made to the happiness and prosperity of the village? The drawback to this practice is that to save potential victims it makes actual victims.

**Autonomy:** If the family believes that a relatively small benefit for a very large number of people is better than a large benefit for an individual, they will understand. If they understand this, they can understand anything, however absurd.

**Freedom:** You can explain to them that their son lost his freedom, but the villagers as a whole gained a far greater measure of freedom; when they see the joy on the faces of the villagers, they will be glad at what their son was able to accomplish.

**Objectivity:** Objectively the entire village is a greater number than their son.

**Beneficence:** It is well known throughout the village that they are people of goodwill with a desire to do what is best for others. Most people never have this opportunity, but through their good fortune, they have had it.

**Fidelity:** You can explain that you know they had a great affection for their son, but now they can glory in the knowledge that they were able to express the affection they had for the sum total of the villagers through the sacrifice of their son; you know how gratified they must be.

All of this may sound perfectly ridiculous, but some research experiments followed this logic, the most infamous of which was the Tuskegee syphilis experiment (1932–1972), where treatment was withheld from some subjects, even though it was known that penicillin would have cured them, so that the researchers could observe the course of the illness. This was, in effect, another form of telishment.

## DILEMMA 6.4, PAGE 104

### Right to One's Own Body

If rational self-interest is wrong, then Fauzuja Kassindja was wrong, and she should not have been given asylum.

Assuming that there is nothing in the nature of women from her country that makes them natural playthings, the fate Fauzuja Kassindja faced in her native country violated all the bioethical standards. This would set a precedent permitting anyone to do anything that whimsy urged him or her to do. Under this standard, what she did could not have been wrong.

On the other hand, if there is something in the nature of female rational animals such that they are excluded from the rights agreement, this has never been shown. In addition, this practice of female circumcision would nullify individual rights or, at least, place the recognition of rights on an arbitrary basis.

## DILEMMA 6.5, PAGE 106

### Nurse's Conflicted Emotions

When people turn away from the contemporary ethical systems, they go into emotivism, which leaves them entirely disoriented. They are unable either to pursue or to serve their rational self-interest. This is another version of the same thing. They never knew how to face the dilemma life presented them. Often, they were advised to do something obviously against their best interest; blindly following their emotions became another way of slapping their own face.

Their faces represent their reasoning capacity. It is a way of expressing one's anger at oneself. One has achieved nothing but to discover another source of frustration. Unfortunately, this is a common occurrence. Devastation follows emotions, and frustration follows devastation. A mistaken decision is not the same as a flaw in one's character.

Evelyn's mistaken decision was that an emotion was a judgment. An emotion is not a judgment. Before she declares war on her character, she ought to declare war on her badly flawed decision. It is not her capacity to make decisions but her method of making decisions that is at fault.

## DILEMMA 6.6, PAGE 107

### Benevolence or Paternalism?

**Autonomy:** Harold is unique. His motivations for refusing the amputation of his gangrenous leg must certainly be unique—but they are his motivations; it is his leg and his life. The physician, apparently, did not ask Harold why he was refusing the operation, or, if she did, Harold's answer did not satisfy her.

Harold's motivations and values are unique. So are the motivations and values of the physician. For Harold's answer to satisfy the physician, their motivations and values would have to be harmonious. If Harold's answer must satisfy his physician, then Harold's physician has the same rights in relation to Harold's life as Harold has. In fact, this would give the physician not only the same rights but also greater rights than Harold.

As one human to another, the physician has a right as a health care professional to exert gentle coercion. However, because Harold is an autonomous individual, by right he has no ethical responsibility to satisfy his physician on a decision concerning an operation that he does not want.

**Freedom:** The physician's action is an attack on Harold's freedom of choice in the matter of his own life. If this freedom is taken away, Harold has no freedom left. Without freedom, there is no possibility of Harold acting ethically. There is no possibility of Harold acting at all. Because Harold cannot engage in ethical actions, he cannot engage in ethical interactions. Therefore, Harold's physician cannot engage in an ethical interaction with him.

The ethical choice that the physician is forcing on Harold is not a choice. Harold cannot choose because he cannot think and decide for himself. It is not possible for any person to think, decide, or choose when someone forces a course of action upon him or her.

Harold's physician believes that her course of action is best for him despite his disagreement. The course of her ethical development was arrested too soon. A higher level of ethical development would produce the belief that no one can justify an interaction unless that interaction is chosen by free ethical agents with an equal ethical status and, in her case, based on a professional agreement. A health care professional does not protect a patient's right to freedom by destroying it.

**Objectivity:** This dilemma does not involve the standard of objectivity because:

1. It does not involve Harold's physician attempting to deceive him.
2. Harold has no ethical responsibility, in this context, to give his physician any objective information. Harold's physician has no right to expect Harold to tell her any truth that would assist her in her aggression against Harold's rights.

**Beneficence:** To destroy a patient's individual sovereignty is not to act beneficently toward him. There is no such thing as acting beneficently toward people by giving them a benefit they do not want.

H. G. Wells (1904) wrote "In the Country of the Blind," the story of a mountaineer who falls down a mountainside and into a fabled valley whose inhabitants are all blind. They are all very happy not being sighted. When the mountaineer tries to tell the inhabitants of the valley about sight, their doctor decides that the mountaineer is insane and that the cure is to put out his eyes. So the village elders decide they will blind the mountaineer, out of beneficence, for his own benefit.

Coercive beneficence cannot be beneficence.

**Fidelity:** Ask yourself if you would enter into an agreement with a physician if one of the terms of that agreement allowed the physician unlimited freedom to do anything she wanted.

Analysis through the bioethical standards does not justify the physician's actions.

## DILEMMA 8.1, PAGE 133

### What Is to Be Done When Intrafamily Coercion Is Suspected?

**Autonomy:** Their relationship is unique. It is uniquely complex and troubled. It will not be a simple matter for the biomedical team to adequately evaluate their relationship and advise them. Two unique personalities interacting together produce a state of affairs much more complex than a single individual. Out-of-context moralizing should be avoided.

**Freedom:** Rick and his mother both have a right to freely arrive at a decision and act on that decision. Every effort should be made to enable her to make a decision that reflects her actual values.

**Objectivity:** The consultation between Mrs. Raymond and the biomedical professionals ought to go into exhaustive detail. Mrs. Raymond, quite probably, has a long time to live. Rick's future is very uncertain at best. Rick is trying to preserve his life. At the same time, Mrs. Raymond's reasons for donating her kidney may not be well thought out. Her questions should be elaborated on until she has related the new information given to her to the entire context of her knowledge and the situation.

**Beneficence:** No one owes Rick any specific beneficence beyond performing the operation and advising him on a health regimen. No one owes him assistance in deception. Mrs. Raymond is owed the beneficence of clarity of vision. She deserves to know what she is doing. The biomedical team can help her gain this clarity of vision. She also deserves to know why she is doing what she is doing. This knowledge she must gain for herself and from herself. Skill on the part of the biomedical team might help her in this.

**Fidelity:** Biomedical care comes in various forms and degrees of excellence. Hopefully, fidelity toward the Raymonds will possess a high degree of excellence.

## DILEMMA 8.2, PAGE 137

### Family Dispute Over Donating a Child's Organs

**Autonomy:** To many laypeople, the desires that Kim expressed would be entirely alien. To her father, they are inconceivable. The fact that Kim's ethical intent is alien or inconceivable to many is completely irrelevant. Ethics is not a matter of approval or disapproval.

**Freedom:** To donate her organs would be Kim's last action and the last, but very real, exercise of her right to freedom. There is no justification for violating this right. She had this right throughout her whole life, and if it is violated, her life is violated.

**Objectivity:** Kim's desire to donate her organs does not violate any ethical standards. There is no objective reason to come into conflict with this desire. A nonobjective reason would be no reason whatsoever. The feelings of the father, although important, are not ethically relevant. It is Kim's body, her organs, and her self-governance.

**Beneficence:** The harm that would be done to someone who would otherwise receive one of Kim's organs and to Kim herself would be far greater than the harm to Kim's father.

**Fidelity:** To help Kim act on her value motivations would be to help her serve her fidelity to herself.

Kim's nurse has a professional responsibility to help her father through this crisis. To help him gently to understand and come to terms with the fact that this was his daughter's last wish is the best thing that the nurse can do for this family.

## DILEMMA 8.3, PAGE 143

### To Tell or Not to Tell the Findings of Surgery

**Autonomy:** There is no question that informing Amelia of her condition will be an assault on her self-image and will have negative effects on her (developing) autonomy. An analysis of the effects on Amelia's autonomy of being told of the condition reveals these reasons why she should not be told. It reveals no reasons why she should be told.

**Freedom:** It is certainly the case that Amelia will enjoy less freedom by knowing of her condition. Thus, at best, the standard of freedom does not support informing her of her condition.

**Objectivity:** It is hard to see how Amelia would be better off knowing of her condition. Benevolence does not call for her to be informed. The effect that being informed will have on her autonomy is an excellent reason for her not to be informed. The standard of objectivity does not justify informing her.

**Beneficence:** There is no question that not informing her is the more beneficent course of action.

**Fidelity:** The agreement between a patient and a health care professional is an agreement that the health care professional will try to make a patient's state of well-being better and not worse.

What Dr. Richmond can do immediately will make Amelia's state of well-being better, although Dr. Richmond is not the only surgeon in the world who can do this.

On the other hand, the long-term detriment of being informed will vastly outweigh the benefit that Dr. Richmond will bestow on Amelia through his immediate action. Once Dr. Richmond does this harm to Amelia, no one can undo it.

Despite the bioethical standards, many contemporary ethicists would call for Amelia to be told of her condition. Because of the complexity of this situation, let us examine it in terms of the elements of Amelia's autonomy.

**Desire:** Most 17-year-old girls would not want to be informed. One cannot know with certainty whether Amelia would want to be informed, but one can know with contextual certainty that she probably would not.

**Reason:** Knowing of her condition will make it more difficult for Amelia to think positively of herself and her life. The element of reason calls for Amelia not to be told. Knowing would do Amelia more harm than good. There is a slight suggestion, in reason, that she not be told. If reason is to be beneficent, then there is a powerful demand that she not be told.

**Life:** Not knowing threatens no part of her life. Therefore, there is nothing at all in the element of life to suggest that she should be told.

**Purpose:** None of Amelia's purposes would be served by her being informed. At the same time, one cannot doubt that her knowing would hinder some of her purposes. The element of purpose counsels that she not be told.

**Agency:** Her knowing would hinder her agency. Her self-image would be damaged. Her approach to the world would change.

Amelia has a right to know. She also has a right not to know. She has a right not to be harmed.

Contemporary ethicists offer two arguments as to why Amelia should be told:

1. Amelia will probably find out anyway.

   This is a contextual factor that one must consider in an actual context. It is, however, a factor that one can consider only in an actual real-life context. It is a logistical factor, and, as such, it is not one of the ethical aspects of the context. If there is any way that it can be brought about that Amelia will not find out about her condition, then this way should be discovered. That Amelia will find out anyway is a rationalization. It is a health care professional's excuse for doing his duty when he knows he should not.

2. It is suggested that Dr. Richmond has a responsibility to Amelia's relatives. Amelia must be informed so that she can discuss this condition with them. It might be advantageous to them to be aware of the recessive disorder that may run in their family.

Let us examine the ethical strength of this argument. Dr. Richmond may believe that he has a duty to inform Amelia's relatives. As we have seen, duty is an entirely inappropriate bioethical standard, so he cannot justifiably act on this feeling. Perhaps, however, Dr. Richmond reasons that Amelia has a duty to inform the members of her family. There is no reason to believe that Amelia has any such duty. Claiming that Amelia has a brother (and she may have a brother) does not prove that she has a brother. Claiming that Amelia has a duty does not, logically or ethically, establish the fact that indeed she does have a duty. Every bioethical standard implies that she does not.

It is probable that Dr. Richmond's reasoning, strictly speaking, is not deontological. It is not based on a declaration that either he or Amelia has a duty. His reasoning, probably, is at least partly utilitarian. He is probably motivated by the belief that by informing Amelia, "the greatest good for the greatest number" will be served—but clearly this too involves a duty. We have also seen that utilitarianism is as inappropriate to a biomedical context as deontology is. The utilitarian standard will also fail to justify Dr. Richmond's action.

The difference in this context between a symphonological ethic and utilitarian ethic is this: According to a symphonological ethic, Amelia is at the center of the ethical context. Dr. Richmond must expect nothing of Amelia but that she pursues her own welfare and the welfare of those whom she values. A utilitarian ethic, on the other hand, allows Dr. Richmond to expect Amelia to pursue the welfare of the larger number of people simply because they are the larger number rather than because she values them. She must sacrifice her well-being to their benefit.

If Dr. Richmond were motivated by a symphonological ethic, he would choose among contextual alternatives. Then he would decide according to rights and responsibilities. He would try to make his decision intelligible in relation to cause and effect. He would try to bring about ethical proportion and balance. Such a decision would call for Amelia to take on the burden of knowing about her condition only if she chose to do this. If Amelia knew all the facts, she might, out of beneficence, wish to inform her relatives.

Let us subject Dr. Richmond's position to a rational ethical analysis. Amelia should value her relatives only if she has some rational reason to value them. For instance, if they are abusive or contemptuous of her, she lacks a rational reason to value them. If she values them in spite of this, she has no ethical reward to offer those who are not abusive or contemptuous of her.

Amelia should choose in favor of her relatives only if she has a rational and objective reason to value them. This reason would have to be sufficient to make her willing to bear the burden of knowing of her condition. She has this objective reason only if her relatives, in turn, place a high value on her.

Let us see where this leaves us. If Amelia's relatives place a high value on her, they will be concerned with the effect of knowing about her condition on her. If her relatives would be unconcerned with the effect of her knowing of her condition, then Amelia has no objective reason to value them.

If Amelia does not have an objective reason to value her relatives, then to inform her of her condition so that she can inform them is simply to sacrifice her to the greater number. To inform her, Dr. Richmond would have to assume that Amelia is or ought to be motivated by self-contempt.

If her relatives place a high value on Amelia, they would not want her to undergo the trauma of knowing of her condition. They would regard the detriment to Amelia as out of proportion to the benefit to themselves.

In the context of a symphonological ethic, Dr. Richmond would have to conclude that if Amelia has no objective reason to value her relatives, then beneficence will not be a rational motivation to inform her.

If Amelia does have objective reasons to value her relatives, then her relatives will not want Amelia to know of her condition. Their balanced and proportioned desire would not be to place Amelia's benefit above theirs. Rather, they would consider Amelia's benefit of greater benefit to them.

Amelia's relatives have reason to value her only if she respects their desires. If Amelia respects their desires, then she ought to accede to their desires for her welfare to be protected.

It is not difficult to understand that her relatives would prize her increased happiness and self-confidence throughout her life more than their increased convenience.

Suppose that one of Amelia's relatives is a nurse. Should a nurse place this high a value on her convenience? How would she relate to her patients? Could you, as a nurse, place a high value on this nurse?

In the context of a symphonological ethic, there are no ethical circumstances calling for Amelia to be informed of her condition.


## Nurse's and Physician's Dilemma

This is a dilemma that falls on a physician to resolve and not on a nurse. However, in the health care system, very often a physician resolves a dilemma, but a nurse must deal with his or her resolution. Quite often, it is a nurse who must explain the physician's resolution to the patient and, perhaps, spend the better part of a day with the patient or the patient's family answering questions. These situations can be very frustrating for nurses.

Nurses should be able to analyze even the most difficult dilemmas. Knowing how to analyze difficult ethical dilemmas makes it easier to analyze simple dilemmas. It might also enable a nurse to win the respect of her colleagues in the health care system. It might make it possible for her to negotiate with them and, one hopes, to become involved with them in the decision-making process.

The implication of Dr. Richmond's duty is that his satisfaction at feeling right, which lasts for 1 hour, is of greater overall importance than Amelia's feeling of being wrong, which lasts for 60 years. This implies that in Dr. Richmond's ethical world, he lives there all alone.

*Note:* We have come against strong opposition to our position in this real case. We ask those of you who disagree to reread our rationale.

## DILEMMA 8.4, PAGE 146

### Going Against the Physician's Order for a Dying Man

*(Note that this case is very different from Dilemma 5.2 for various reasons.)* This is several dilemmas in one:

- Whether a patient in these circumstances has the right to something he wants if it may be injurious to his health.
- Whether a physician is justified in refusing him.
- Whether a nurse has a right to disobey the physician's orders.
- Whether a nurse has an ethical agent obligation that overrides the physician's order.

Obviously, a dilemma of this complexity can be resolved only in the context. However, analysis will reveal something about it.

**Autonomy:** This desire expresses Rodney's autonomy. This desire is very short range. In fact, Rodney has no long-range desires. His desire is the expression of his autonomy in his present circumstances.

**Freedom:** If it is probable that the drink of water would not increase Rodney's suffering or if his increased suffering could be alleviated, then we must consider the following: When Rodney entered the health care system, he was better able to act for himself. As time passed, he sank into a more helpless state. To refuse Rodney's dying request while he is in this state is to violate his right to freedom. Had Rodney known that he would be subjected to this violation, it is, in principle, possible that he would not have come into the health care system. In light of the fact that Rodney cannot recover, the physician's action is an action entirely lacking ethical balance and proportion. It was a callous violation of Rodney's freedom.

If it is probable that the drink of water would increase Rodney's suffering, and if his increased suffering could not be alleviated, then the violation of Rodney's freedom is not outside of the agreement between Rodney and the professionals in the health care setting.

**Objectivity:** Lynetta owes Rodney an explanation of what might happen if he does take the water.

**Beneficence:** What is and what is not beneficent at every step of the way must be determined in the context.

**Fidelity:** Lynetta is Rodney's agent. She is also an agent of Rodney's agent—the physician. If the drink of water would increase Rodney's suffering, then Lynetta really does not face a dilemma. If it would not, then she must determine where her greater loyalty ought to lie. She must also decide what she is willing to risk. On one hand, she risks retribution from the physician. On the other hand, she risks committing a senselessly cruel act. Lynetta has a responsibility to the physician. She enjoys a position of trust in relation to the physician. It would be understandable if she did not find the position particularly enjoyable in this situation.

This would be rule bending at its highest to go against the physician's order. It would jeopardize her future plans. She can, and should, however, call the physician and talk to him about the problem.

## DILEMMA 9.1, PAGE 152

### Patient's Benefit Versus Family's Desires

**Autonomy:** If heroic measures are not taken and Martha is allowed to die, then certainly, her uniqueness will be lost along with her life. Her uniqueness will pass out of existence. This fact, however, has no ethical relevance. The ethical concept of autonomy is not the uniqueness of a person that the outside world gazes upon. It is the uniqueness of a person as the person lives it. It is the person's self-identity as he or she experiences it. Not to allow Martha to die would not preserve her autonomy. It would violate her autonomy. Not to allow Martha to die is not the same as allowing her to live. It is forcing her to continue dying.

**Freedom:** If it is Martha's desire to die and health care professionals have agreed to act as her agent, then in applying heroic measures they would violate their agreement. They would take an action for her that she would not take for herself. Any claim that they violate her right to freedom in not applying heroic measures is one of the extreme points of ethical absurdity. If another person takes over control of Martha's actions, this person certainly violates her right to freedom.

**Objectivity:** As far as making her decision is concerned, Martha has all the information she needs. Her excruciating pain and the fact that she is terminal provide this. The standard of objectivity does not enter into the picture beyond this. In her physical state, her body is reasoning for her.

**Beneficence:** In dilemmas involving passive euthanasia, people have widely differing views as to what constitutes beneficence. Ultimately, it is up to every individual to determine what constitutes "doing good or at least doing no harm." What a person believes and what a person can justify are often very different things.

Staying in the bioethical context, let us try to clarify the question of justification through a thought experiment: Try to imagine that to end Martha's life and suffering would be to harm her. Imagine that to keep her alive and suffering would be to bestow some good upon her.

Now that you have seen this in your mind's eye, let us take it one step further. Imagine a patient, Marian, who is dying a peaceful and painless death. The technology to keep Marian alive is available but is excruciatingly painful. Assume that Marian ought not to be kept alive under these circumstances, and then try to devise some justification for keeping Martha alive. Is it not absurd to keep a patient in unendurable pain alive while permitting a patient who is not in pain to die?

Suppose that ethics demands that patients such as Marian, as well as patients such as Martha, be kept alive. This supposition implies that every health care setting ought to become a combination of cemetery and torture chamber. If a person can believe this, nothing more can be said. If a person can justify it bioethically, he or she will have transformed the nature of bioethics and of modern biomedicine—not necessarily for the better.

**Fidelity:** The demands of fidelity, of course, depend on the agreement. If health care professionals agree to act as Martha's agents, and they agree to act toward her with beneficence, then they agree to act toward Martha as she would act toward herself. Martha would not act to keep herself alive. If health care professionals keep her alive in these circumstances, they break their agreement with her.

Euthanasia, even passive euthanasia as discussed in Martha's case, is a very complex and controversial subject. To illuminate the analysis we have made through the bioethical standards, we will analyze it through the elements.

**Desire:** It is inconceivable that the desire of a terminal patient in unbearable pain to continue living as long as possible could be a rational desire. The element of rational desire calls for allowing Martha to die.

**Reason:** To paraphrase the philosopher Benedict Spinoza: Reason demands nothing contrary to nature, and nature demands nothing contrary to reason. If one wages a war on one's existence (a war that one cannot win), and if one denies everything that one knows to be true, one is turning one's back on reason, on everything that person is. Reason demands that a person accept the facts of his or her existence and the reality of his world. If reason demands anything, then it demands that a person accept that which he or she knows to be true.

For people to accept that which they know to be true is for them to act in harmony with their own nature. It is for them to act in harmony with the reality of the world around them. Reason and nature demand nothing less than this.

The reality of Martha's existence calls for the exercise of reason. It calls for the biomedical professionals who are her agents to exercise reason and beneficence.

**Life:** Martha is alive only in the sense that an irrational animal is alive. Martha is not an irrational animal. The best promise life offers her is death. If Martha's life is allowed to speak for itself, then Martha ought to be allowed to die.

**Purpose:** Analyzing Martha's situation from the vantage point of purpose shows that Martha ought to be allowed to die. This is not surprising. In the context of the bioethical standard, it is an ethical purpose. It is a rational purpose. Also, not least, it is Martha's purpose for herself.

**Agency:** Every ethical agent in exercising agency should exercise it with courage and clarity of vision. If biomedical professionals are given the power to decide Martha's fate, they should decide with courage and clarity of vision, for they are her agents.

Both the bioethical standards and the elements suggest the ethical propriety of allowing Martha to die. **This is a case in which palliative sedation is in order.** Thanks to palliative and hospice care the end of one's life has been greatly enhanced.

## DILEMMA 9.2, PAGE 153

### The Demands of Justice

All four arguments given in Chapter 3 are misleading:

- The unique individual that he once was does still exist. The state of being that he once enjoyed, however, no longer exists. Even if it were true to say that "The autonomous individual no longer exists," nothing would follow from this. If one ought to do anything, this can be only because an autonomous individual does exist. If an autonomous individual does not exist, then there is nothing that one must do.
- There is no way that anyone can benefit this patient. Beneficence cannot determine what should be done. There is no way to exercise beneficence in relation to this patient.
- Life is not precious to him. Nothing is or can be of any value to him.
- The notion of autonomy involves three notions—uniqueness, rational animality, and ethical equality.

As a rational animal, the patient is specifically identical to every other human individual. Therefore, he is ethically the equal of every other human individual. Autonomy also involves ethical equality.

It is true that no one has a right to terminate the life of an autonomous individual. This is not because an autonomous individual is unique. It is not because, when one observes the individual, he or she appears different from other people. An autonomous individual acquires the right to life by virtue of being a rational animal.

Every person and the context of every person are unique. Certain general principles, such as the individual person's independence, must guide every action in any context similar to this. One must also consider the actual differences that exist in the context.

In this person's context, there are four relevant differences:

- He has requested that he be allowed to die.
- He is now permanently dependent on the efforts of others.
- None of the elements of human autonomy now characterizes him. He is conscious of no desires; he is totally out of touch with the world. He engages in no reasoning processes, nor will he ever.
- His life consists of basic physiological processes; this is not autonomous. He has no purposes. He has no power to exercise agency. Allowing his life to terminate is not the same as terminating his life.

The recognition of this patient's autonomy does not speak against allowing him to die. The bioethical standards do not demand that he be kept alive.

## DILEMMA 9.3, PAGE 157

### Physician's Orders Versus Benefit to the Patient—A Nurse's Dilemma

This case will be resolved differently than the others in the book. Its analysis will look at this case, not as what should or should not be done for Blessing, but, primarily, as one causing moral distress for the nurses. Thus, the bioethical standards will be applied to the nurses in greater detail. *What should be done for Blessing requires little analysis; she was denied all the standards. The physician did not consider the context of her life at all. The physician violated all her rights.*

**Autonomy:** The nurses' unique nature as nurses was being violated. The nurses were being treated as functionaries. *Blessing's uniqueness was never considered; an important part of the context of Blessing's life was ignored.*

**Freedom:** The physician did not consider the nurses' freedom to act for the patient at all. The physician was unconcerned about what they thought. The nurses felt helpless in the situation because legally, they were to follow the orders the physician wrote, but to do so violated the patient's right to freedom. *Blessing's right to freedom of action was denied; the physician did not even try to treat her as human.*

**Objectivity:** The nurses knew a sufficient number of the objective facts of Blessing's life, past and present, to realize that the orders they had to follow related only to the physical facts that presented and did not begin to extend to the entire context. Having to follow these orders created, for the nurses, a severe dilemma. The physician was concerned only with curing and gave no measure of caring. He was concerned only with the context of the situation and ignored the other aspects of the context, but the other aspects could have or should have guided him to a better solution. *Blessing's right to objectivity, that right to have care within the context, was denied. Granted, she was not able to deal with the objective facts then; thus, the health care professionals should have done this for her in a way that considered the entire context. She should not have been treated like a nonperson.*

**Beneficence:** The nurses strive to benefit patients, not to harm them. What they were being required to do was a form of torture. This went against every fiber of their being, and they were being forced to do it. Not being able to benefit this patient increased the moral distress the nurses felt. *Blessing was being harmed in the name of "doing what is right" to deal with her physical body. This can be right only if right is that which one can do by force.*

**Fidelity:** This standard has as its basis trust and a commitment to fulfill the agreement that one has promised and is obligated to perform. The nurses knew that the trust of all within the health care system is important for the care of patients and for the feeling that what one has done is justified within the context. The fact that the nurses could not justify what they had to do increased, even more, their feelings of moral distress. *Blessing could not possibly have any trust in the health care system, nor could she believe that anyone cared about her. She was denied the right of all the standards in regard to herself and her context.*

Each of the standards was denied to Blessing, and the possibility of acting on them ethically was denied to the nurses. There was no way to avoid severe moral distress on the part of the nurses. The only help for the nurses is to have the moral courage to do something about this and to engage with others to use strategies to decrease the moral residue that occurs. However, this is not without risks.

## DILEMMA 11.1, PAGE 185

### Playing the Odds or Betting on a Sure Thing

This is a situation that Vladimir very well might want to discuss with his nurse. If he does, it is desirable that she understand the vital and fundamental factors influencing his decision. Vital and fundamental factors, in a purposive ethic, are ethical factors.

Here the bioethical standards are irrelevant. This is not, in its most important sense, a case of a nurse dealing with a patient. Nor is this a case of a nurse helping a patient deal with another person. This is a case of a nurse acting as a sounding board to help her patient think and make a decision for himself. Vladimir needs self-awareness. His nurse can help him analyze his situation by reference to the elements of his autonomy.

**Desire:** Vladimir will have to decide whether his greater desire is to play again or to retain the gross motor movements of his hand. Then he must examine the strength of these desires against the probabilities of realizing each one.

**Reason:** Vladimir must assess the benefits and detriments of each course of action. Then he must decide on what his most reasonable course of action will be in light of his rational desires.

**Life:** Vladimir must try to ascertain what his overall lifestyle will be if either operation succeeds or fails. Then he must decide whether he is willing to take the risks of one course of action or be content with the results of the other course.

**Purpose:** In assessing all the possibilities, Vladimir will have to decide on the purposes that motivate him.

**Agency:** When Vladimir has made a decision, he ought to think about whether this decision really reflects his character and values.

There is no question of a nurse making the choice for a patient in a case like Vladimir's. Even if she is asked, it is obvious that she ought to refuse. If she is skilled, her consciousness can be a mirror in which her patient can see his ideas and values reflected.

## DILEMMA 11.2, PAGE 188

### Trauma Versus Treatment

Bioethical dilemmas are among the most complex and difficult that any human being ever faces. Wally's case is certainly among these. It will be difficult to resolve this dilemma with optimum beneficence—in such a way that Wally is done some good and no harm. If she handles it badly, a nurse can do Wally much more harm than good. A nurse who can handle this beneficently must be able to exercise a sort of ethical artistry.

**Autonomy:** Wally is in the health care system. The health care system has its own specific structures and purposes. The health care system is responsible for the health and well-being of everyone who enters it. On the other hand, Wally is young. He did not come into the health care system on his own. He was not even brought in after discussion. He is suddenly thrust into a strange environment.

Taking Wally for debriding without his consent suggests that Wally's body can be taken for treatment and his consciousness can be left behind. This interaction between Iris and Wally would be truly inhuman. Iris's momentary reflection on her own nature would show her that such inter-action is ethically undesirable. Whatever its benefits, and they are obvious, compelling Wally to go for treatment at this time would violate his autonomy.

**Freedom:** It is part of the implicit agreement that is the basis of human rights that the young shall be protected. What are the right and wrong things for Iris to do depends on the context of her relationship with Wally. It may be necessary for her to establish a rapport with Wally very quickly. There are overwhelming reasons why Wally ought to go for debriding. Nonetheless, if Iris were to take him by coercion, this would be a violation of his freedom. Badly handled, the overwhelming adversity he faces can stunt this potential. A nurse never knows how much good or harm in a person's life she can do. Her pride ought to compel her to do the best she can.

**Objectivity:** If Iris is to deal with Wally on the basis of objectivity, she will have to tell him that his mother is dead. The absence of ethical value in this is obvious. For Iris to put both burdens on Wally at one time would be fiendish. She would increase Wally's objective awareness in a context where this would decrease Wally's ability to act on objective awareness. She would abandon her own objective awareness of the nature of the health care system and the meaning of her role in it.

**Beneficence:** Beneficence calls for Iris to do as much good and as little harm as possible. Ideally, this would consist of finding a way to get Wally to treatment without inflicting force on him. It would involve telling him of his mother's death under optimum circumstances.

**Fidelity:** The nurse–patient agreement begins with an exchange of values. This may be the best way for Iris to proceed to do good and avoid harm to Wally. It may be best for her to continue this exchange. Iris needs to hang loose. She needs to bargain with Wally, to find some way to trade values with him. This will avoid the trauma to Wally that a violation of his autonomy and freedom would involve.

A skillful and effective nursing intervention here calls for Iris to treat Wally not as a "big boy" but as a human person. Although Wally is legally a minor, this is a very fine place to avoid paternalism.

Analysis under the elements of Wally's autonomy might clarify even more what is to be done.

**Desire:** Wally's desire to wait for his mother is rational. Force is irrational. Force would be a psychological assault on Wally.

Suppose Wally had been treated at the scene of the fire. He probably could have been treated without a prior discussion and without psychological harm. However, his hospital room takes him away from the noise and stress of the disaster. It suggests that now there is a chance to think and to discuss. The situation calls out for Iris to bargain with Wally. Iris should not tell Wally that his mother is alive. Besides, truth is the last thing to consider now.

**Reason:** In Wally's context, it is perfectly reasonable for him to want the comfort of his mother's presence. Effective and skillful communication and trade will have to be carried out at this level. There is probably no way Wally can reason on a more abstract level than this.

**Life:** Wally ought to be treated with the highest consideration. With the loss of his mother, he is at a point where he must begin to build his life again.

**Purpose:** For Iris to trade with Wally effectively, she must discover the nature of Wally's most rational (practical) purposes. She must discover what she can do to make Wally see his most desirable purposes under these conditions of his life.

**Agency:** The purpose of exchanging values with Wally is to enlist his desire for some purpose, to motivate his agency, and to increase his cooperation with Iris.

## DILEMMA 11.3, PAGE 191

### Rights of Children

The concept of rights is very difficult to deal with here. For purposes of bioethical analysis, rights as we have discussed is *the product of an implicit agreement among rational beings, by virtue of their rationality, not to obtain actions nor the product or condition of actions from others except through voluntary consent, objectively gained.*

- In the same way the rights agreement arises, among all people everywhere, another agreement arises. This agreement arises by virtue of the reasoning power of a parent, the undeveloped state of a child's reasoning power, the naturally dependent state of the child, and the bonds of love that exist between parent and child. It is the agreement that a parent will protect and nurture the child. It is a bond of benevolence uniting parent and child. This agreement calls for a parent to decide for a child in a situation where the child is incapable of deciding for himself. Sandy's mother does have a moral right to sign the consent form.
- Sandy's nurse has a moral right to give him the preoperative medications. She is acting as the agent of Sandy's mother. She is doing what Sandy's mother would do if she were able.
- The surgeon is also acting as her agent. He also is doing what Sandy's mother would do if she could.
- Sandy will acquire the rights that would protect him against this procedure when there is no longer a need for the parent–child agreement.
- Sandy's mother, the surgeon, and the nurse have rights that would protect them from undergoing this procedure involuntarily. With maturity, they have acquired this right.
- Sandy's mother, the surgeon, and the nurse acquired the rights that they possess when they acquired the experience and the rational capacity to decide for themselves.
- Sandy will acquire the rights that his mother, the surgeon, and the nurse possess when he acquires the experience and the rational capacity to take over his parents' role in making his vital and fundamental decisions.
- Sandy will acquire the right to decide for his children when his reason becomes more powerful than his emotions.
- Sandy's desire is not a rational desire. It is the short-term whimsical desire of a child. It is true, and Sandy knows it to be true, that his desire must give way before the parent–child agreement.

- Sandy's uniqueness cannot protect him. It will begin to protect him only when it becomes a rational autonomy. Until then, it is not sufficient for the exercise of rights. No irrational autonomy will protect Sandy's short-term urges only against his rational self-interest. He becomes ethically autonomous only when his autonomy is strong enough to protect Sandy against his whims.

## DILEMMA 11.4, PAGE 192

### Right to Be One's Own Agent

Even assuming that this is a procedure that he ought to undergo, Roger's physician and the court were not justified in the course of action they took. Roger's reasoning and decision might not have been the best, but they are not entirely irrational. Sometimes, the rights of others prevent us from doing that which we very much want to do. If this were not the case, there would be no reason for the existence of rights. Roger's rights should have prevented the physician from doing what she wanted to do.

A health care professional's role cannot give him or her extraordinary rights. These extraordinary rights would be a right to violate the rights of others. There cannot be such a thing as a right to violate the rights of others. If there were such a right, there could not be any rights at all.

The nurse's role in this situation would be to counsel Roger, to apply gentle coercion, and to offer no encouragement to Roger's physician.

Let us assume that the method by which the judge declared Roger incompetent became a method common in the legal system. It is obvious that this would make the legal system an all-powerful tyranny where no one would have any rights whatsoever. The purpose of the judicial system would no longer be to protect rights. Its purpose would be to arbitrarily establish rights for some people and to violate the rights of others. If this were permissible in this case, one would be hard-pressed to establish a point at which it is no longer permissible.

## DILEMMA 11.5, PAGE 202

### Refusing Treatments in the Context of Loss of Hope

Negative thoughts and emotions have overwhelmed Mrs. Smith's autonomy. The task is to overcome these negative emotions with positive ones. This can be done, if at all, through the elements of autonomy.

Desire can be used to inspire positive thought processes to increase her desire. It is important that the positive values that are possible to her—given a state of living that she can enjoy—overcome the influence of her immediate negative experience.

The elements of her autonomy, if she is to put her life back together, will strengthen her desire to act, her objective awareness, and her fidelity to the life that is still hers for the taking. Despair is best combated through the elements.

To inspire Jody to meet the challenges life presents and regain the possibilities her life offers would be a splendid ethical achievement. Nonetheless, there is a vast difference between achieving this entirely for Jody's sake and achieving it for the sake of others.

## DILEMMA 12.1, PAGE 211

### Is It Ever Right to Sell One's Organs?

There are a number of reasons why one might want to sell an organ. A person with masochistic tendencies might find it a gratifying means of self-mutilation. Under extraordinary circumstances, a parent might sell an organ as the only means to feed his or her starving children.

**Reason:** To give up a greater value, such as a family member's life, when it could be saved at the cost of a lesser value, such as a piece of one's liver, is irrational. To condemn one for giving or selling an organ to save a loved one's life is to make an arbitrary and indefensible judgment. To satisfy a desire for self-mutilation is disproportionate in the other direction. It would be an action that one could not justify.

**Desire:** When one possesses that which one desires, it becomes a value to him or her. One's values exist on a hierarchy. One gives up one's value in favor of another for many complex reasons. The values are one's own, and the reasons are one's own. When federal and state laws pass, the state claims ownership of the value it has taken under its control. Today the state prohibits the sale of what it owns. Tomorrow, it may find this property a valuable source of state income.

**Life:** We live only once, and life has meaning for us. Things we value give meaning to life. If we value nothing or nothing very much, then we do not value life or we do not value it very much. If we are not allowed control of the things we value, we are not allowed control of our lives. Also, along with this go our liberty and the pursuit of our happiness.

**Purpose:** Sometimes when the beams of a bridge shift and the bridge threatens to collapse, a bridge worker's foot will be caught between two girders. To save the worker's life, the foot must be amputated. Should this be illegal? Perhaps not. No one benefits but the worker. Though why this should make a difference is puzzling.

**Agency:** When we analyze a situation, when we choose an option, and when we decide on a course of action, we do all this for the purpose of protecting or maximizing our agency. What process of analysis, choice, and decision could have inspired one law covering this vast spectrum of human dilemmas?

As for Ms. Sparrow, to be so determined to sell a kidney to pay back the hospital was a very questionable motivation—a drastic step. It is certainly giving up a greater value for a lesser value. It would be unethical to become involved in this. The appropriate person, who is not the nurse, should get involved and help her solve the dilemma with a payment plan. We realize that the position we take here will not be popular. We think that selling one's organs, in most situations, should not happen, but context is all important here.

## DILEMMA 12.2, PAGE 215

### The Rights of a Confused Patient

Every health care professional is limited in the actions he or she can take. Every nurse must come to terms with this fact. Nurses today practice within a pluralistic society and in the bureaucracy of the health care system. It would be unreasonable for a nurse to expect that she can remake the system in her image. This is a dilemma where a nurse must make a judgment as to what she is willing to risk. Ethically, however, she owes her greatest fidelity to her patient.

Marilu may decide that there is nothing that she can do. Based on this decision she may do nothing. Marilu has no ethical obligation to do the impossible. She does have an obligation to know the difference between the right thing to do—the thing that her agreement calls for her to do—and the wrong thing to do. She also has an obligation to know why it is impossible to do it.

In this situation, for Marilu to continue to dispute with the physician would not make sense. It would be a formalistic action that might make Marilu look very good in her own eyes. It probably would not do much to help Lillian. The best thing for Marilu to do may be to contact Lillian's daughter and explain the situation to her. I, Gladys, did this and her daughter came and took her home.

## DILEMMA 12.3, PAGE 217

### Rights of a Patient With a Psychiatric Diagnosis

There is a strong tide of opinion that supports the idea that "Every human being of adult years and sound mind has a right to determine what shall be done with his own life" (President's Commission for the Study of Ethical Problems in Medicine and Biomedical and Behavioral Research, 1982, p. 20).

Everyone has the right to be free of outside interference. The acceptance of a person's right to determine what to do with his or her life ought to be part of the mind-set of every person involved in making ethical decisions for others.

Competency is very difficult to assess. According to the President's Commission of 1982, the assessment of competency depends on values, goals, choices, life plans, and purposes. The assessment of competency, then, is an ethical assessment. Ethics is concerned with values, goals, choices, life plans, and purposes. It is not surprising that the issue of competency makes many ethical abuses possible. The criteria for assessment that the President's Commission of 1982 has set down are ethical criteria. The criteria are ethical in the framework of a symphonological ethic. The President's Commission (1982) proposed three elements of competency. To establish competency, a person must:

1. Possess a set of values and goals that are reasonably consistent and that remain reasonably stable so that they do not radically conflict.
2. Have the ability to understand and communicate information so that it can be known that this person can appreciate the meaning of potential alternatives.
3. Have the ability to reason and deliberate about choices in light of values, so that he or she can compare the impact of alternative outcomes on personal goals and life plans (pp. 57–60).

Granted this is a very old reference, but it still holds today.

A person's decision-making capacity is impaired if it fails to, at least, minimally promote his or her desires and purposes. It is very difficult to determine incompetency. A patient who does not want to do what a nurse or physician wants him or thinks is best for him to do is not necessarily incompetent. It may be that this patient has a better outlook on the context of his life than either the nurse or the physician. With this better outlook, his judgment may be superior to that of the nurse or the physician.

On the other hand, it is not necessary to regard every statement a person makes as reflecting his desires and purposes. A child's vision is not sufficiently long range always to express his or her real desires and purposes. The same may be true of a patient in extreme pain, one in shock, or one with brain metastasis, mental retardation, or psychiatric problems. He may be able to act, at best, only on urges. The difference between desires and purposes, on one hand, and urges, on the other, is that the latter are short-term motivations whereas the former are integrated into a person's life.

The desires of the truly incompetent patient are not the result of an objective reading of the facts facing him. In this sense, they are not desires at all. The expression of his desires is the product of a type of free association.

If a person is unable to express personal desires and purposes, this, in itself, does not establish that someone else has a right to do it for him or her. The best that another person can do is to help the individual establish a longer range outlook. Ideally, a health care professional, when dealing with an incompetent patient, would be an ally to the patient—the same as if the person had a clear vision of his life purposes.

The situation of an incompetent patient is very much like the situation of a child, with one major difference: The child is in this situation a very long time; the patient, one hopes, will be in this situation a very short time.

For different reasons, neither an incompetent patient nor a child has the rational capacity to make decisions. The relationship between a health care professional and an incompetent patient is the most delicate of all bioethical relationships. It may be that this relationship calls for an agreement very similar to the parent–child agreement.

When acting for an incompetent patient, a health care professional must attempt to do for the patient what the patient would do for himself if he were able. The health care professional must try to see things from the patient's perspective. To do this, the health care professional must obtain some familiarity with a patient's situation and values. If this understanding of the patient's context cannot be obtained, then perhaps the health care professional should act toward the patient as he or she would act toward a naked, comatose stranger. This requires that he or she protect the patient against himself and other health care professionals. A health care professional can look on the treatment of a psychiatric patient either from the perspective of utilitarianism or as a triage situation.

From the utilitarian perspective, the professional's viewpoint will be on the greater number, focused on the effect of his or her action on the group—on the patient's family, the rest of the hospital staff, and so forth. The professional's goal will be the greater good for the greater number, not the welfare of the patient. This cannot fail to narcotize concern for the patient.

If the health care professional looks at the situation as though it had the same form as a triage situation, his or her viewpoint will be one of interest in the effect of his or her action on the patient. This will make the welfare of the patient the center of attention. This is where the center of attention belongs.

The legal and ethical positions of the incompetent patient are very often in conflict. Ideally, ethical decisions would be made for the incompetent patient only within the following parameters: For a health care professional to assume responsibility, make ethical decisions, and take actions for a patient, there ought to be some implicit or explicit invitation for that individual to do so. Otherwise, there is a violation of the patient's self-governance. With the violation of the patient's self-governance, there is coercion. Coercion is not ethically justifiable.

The only exception to this would be in a situation strongly analogous to that of the naked, comatose stranger. Even here, though, there is a kind of implicit invitation. There are times when the psychiatric patient is in virtually the same state as the naked, comatose stranger. Then the same conditions for treatment would hold. A radical ethical differentiation should be made between the patient who comes into the health care setting voluntarily and the patient who does not. The patient who comes in voluntarily makes an implicit agreement with the people in the health care setting. The patient who does not enter voluntarily makes no such agreement.

This is the only course of ethical action consistent with the bioethical standards. This course of ethical action is very much at odds with the laws presently governing these situations. The current laws provide the patient some protection; however, they provide much more opportunity for exploitation.

There is a very old saying, to the effect that "Where there are many laws, there is much tyranny." This is because where there are many laws people do not concern themselves with ethical thinking or ethical analysis. They come to follow the letter of the law, and, beyond this, they do whatever is convenient. It goes without saying that this holds only when the patient has not threatened or committed any criminal action. If he has, then of course the ethics of the situation are very different.

Bioethicist Morris Abram, head of the President's Commission for the Study of Ethical Problems in Medicine and Biomedical and Behavioral Research (1982), stated:

> *while recognizing the important role that the law has played in this area, the Commission does not look to the law as the primary means of bringing about needed changes in attitudes and practices. Rather, the Commission sees "informed consent" as an ethical obligation that involves a process of shared decision making based upon the mutual respect and participation of patients and health professionals. Only through improved communication can we establish a firm footing for the trust that patients place in those who provide their health care. (p. 32)*

Everyone, whatever his or her condition in life, possesses individual rights and ethical status. People possess rights by virtue of their rationality. This does not mean that someone who is irrational does not possess rights. The possession of rights is species wide. Everyone, regardless of physical or psychological conditions, possesses the right to ethical treatment. Suppose it were possible to pick and choose which members of the human species would have their rights recognized. Obviously, under these circumstances, there could be no trust among ethical agents.

Without the possibility of trust among ethical agents, no one could possibly possess rights. For this reason, every member of the species must enjoy the possession of rights. When making a decision for an incompetent patient, it is especially important to make the decision according to the values and goals of the patient. Otherwise, the bioethical standards have been violated.

Throughout history, the treatment of psychiatric patients has been harsh; fortunately, the tide is turning. Every health care professional ought to remain fully aware of the right of an individual to make decisions for his or her own life. When it becomes necessary to force a patient to do something or to restrain a patient from doing something, a health care professional should never take the situation as the status quo.

The difficulties of dilemmas involving psychiatric patients are very complex. A case study cannot capture them. In Jason's case, it certainly appears that his agency is impaired. In all likelihood, if he were in touch with his life, he would want to recover from his present condition. If it is justifiable to treat him against his expressed desires (or urges), the person who does treat him should not lose sight of the fact that the purpose of treatment is to return Jason's agency to him.

## DILEMMA 12.4, PAGE 219

### Who Gets the Donor Heart?

The ideal way to establish who is to be the recipient would be to establish that everyone concerned has an obligation to accept one person (Mr. X or Ms. Y) as the rightful recipient. Calling in Hank, a nursing assistant, to flip a coin will not establish an obligation. The judgment of an ethics committee will have some weight but not enough to establish an obligation. One of the candidates could have given a significant contribution to the hospital, but this is not sufficient to establish an obligation.

The hospital team offered both candidates an agreement—an explicit one in the case of Mr. X and an implicit one with Ms. Y. Only one accepted the offer. The hospital team offered an agreement to Mr. X in the form of a warning about his habits. He repeatedly rejected the offer, saying that it was "too hard." Had he accepted this offer, the team would have been obligated to keep the terms of the agreement and act to sustain or protect his life.

Ms. Y could be told the circumstances and wait for another heart to become available. However, she is under no obligation to do this. She was offered the same agreement as Mr. X, albeit implicitly. She accepted and kept her part of the agreement. Now the hospital team has an obligation to keep that offer.

Looking at this in another way, the heart donor has made an implicit agreement. It is unlikely that he would donate his heart, expecting it to be given to someone as indifferent to the donor's bequest as Mr. X promises to be. There seems to be a perfect meeting of the minds between the donor and Ms. Y. If Ms. Y does not feel it would be too hard to care for her new heart, she is the one morally entitled to it.

## DILEMMA 12.5, PAGE 220

### Desires of a Patient Versus Family's Request for Life-Sustaining Treatment

**Autonomy:** The Mrs. C. that the family visits can be either one of two persons. One person would not be alert and interactive but free from suffering. The other Mrs. C. would be (maybe) alert and interactive. If she were, she would undergo significant suffering. The choice is between the pleasure of small talk and the comfort of knowing that Mrs. C. is not suffering.

**Freedom:** The pleasure of planning for the future is not a real possibility. Mrs. C. has no future. There is no enjoyment that could possibly justify the suffering Mrs. C. would endure.

**Objectivity:** The family seems incapable of maintaining an objective awareness of what is transpiring. There is no reason to continue Mrs. C.'s suffering until they stumble onto the reality of the situation.

**Beneficence:** The family's desires would cause Mrs. C. positive harm and provide her no benefit. Chatting with her family, who is indifferent to what she is going through, is not a benefit. She has defined benefits in her desire to be kept pain free.

**Fidelity:** The only fidelity to the family relationship that Mrs. C. can count on is the fidelity that she exercises toward herself in refusing the desires of the family. She has to count on the health care professionals to maintain her fidelity to herself.

## REFERENCES

President's Commission for the Study of Ethical Problems and Medicine and Biomedical and Behavioral Research. (1982). *Making health care decisions: The ethical and legal implications of informed consent in the patient-practitioner relationship* (Vol. 1). Washington, DC: U.S. Government Printing Office.

Wells, H. G. (1904, April). In the country of the blind. *The Strand Magazine, 27*(160), 401–415.

# GLOSSARY

**abstract** Refers to the more general and less contextual. *John* is a concrete individual. *Boy* is an abstraction. *Male* is still more abstract. *Person* is more abstract still. "A nurse ought to be faithful to her agreement with every patient who comes under her care" is more abstract (more general and less contextual) than "This nurse ought to be faithful to her agreement with this patient."

**acceptance** Positive response to the offer of an agreement. Engagement with another agent to realize a purpose.

**action** A behavior arising in the decision of an agent to which the agent assigns a personal meaning. A behavior that an agent initiates from within and that remains under the agent's control.

**affinity** A state of approval of the character and motivations of another agent to the point of being willing to identify emotionally with the other.

**agency** The capacity of an agent to initiate and sustain action.

**agent** One who initiates action or one who is capable of taking internally generated action.

**agreement** A propensity or formal potentiality in existents to behave in specific ways when they are interacting. A shared state of awareness—a meeting of the minds—on the basis of which interaction occurs.

**analysis** The process whereby one seeks to understand a whole by examining its basic parts or a process of directed awareness aimed at understanding.

**animal** For purposes of bioethical analysis, any organism capable of moving about from place to place on its own power. This obviously includes humans.

**animality** That which an animal organism has in common with other animal organisms.

**apathy** Lack of interest in the things that a person generally considers worthy of attention.

**appropriate** Whatever gives an agent a greater power of agency is appropriate for that agent; for instance, an understanding of the nature of a dilemma is appropriate for its solution. Freedom from suffering and disability are appropriate to every human being. That which produces intelligibility in the relations between ethical causes and effects (responses). Those conditions under which an agent's virtues can flourish, that which makes an increased or more certain understanding possible, and that which supports the continuation of causal chains and enables an agent to realize his purpose is appropriate to the agent's agency.

**arbitrary** A belief, conclusion, or decision is arbitrary when it is not based on compelling evidence—when another belief, conclusion, or decision could have been chosen just as well.

**autonomy** As a bioethical standard, the independent uniqueness of every individual person. This uniqueness is the specific nature—the character structure—of that person. One's autonomy includes one's specific identity and consequent ethical equality with all other rational agents. Primarily, however, it refers to an agent's uniqueness.

**balance** The property of an interaction whereby there is a mutual exchange of values—reciprocity. Balance and proportion are maintained when there is a parity between benefit given and benefit received. Balance and proportion are lacking when there is a disparity or when a harm is returned for a benefit or vice versa. In one sense, balance and proportion are beneficence. In the same sense, they are justice.

**benefactor** An agent who acts so as to bring about a benefit to a beneficiary.

**beneficence** The act of assisting a patient's effort to attain that which is beneficial. The desire to benefit one with whom one empathizes. As a bioethical standard, the power of a patient (or professional acting as the agent of a patient) and the necessity he faces to act to acquire the benefits he desires and the needs his life requires.

**beneficiary** One who benefits from an action. The recipient of a benefit.

**benefit** Something that enhances or promotes well-being.

**benevolence** A psychological inclination to beneficence.

**bioethical standards** The character structures of a person that serve as measuring rods of the justifiability of his motives and actions.

**bioethics** A system of standards arising with the professional agreement to determine, sanction, and justify the interaction of a biomedical professional and patient.

**burnout** "A syndrome of physical and emotional exhaustion involving the development of a negative self-concept, negative job attitude, and loss of concern and feeling for patients" (Pines & Maslach, 1978, p. 234).

**caregiver strain** A deleterious effect of witnessing the suffering of patients and being unable to alleviate this suffering.

**caring** A devotion to a patient beyond that which one's professional practice demands.

**category** The aspects of professional action by which one can judge the skill or competence of that action.

**causal** Pertaining to cause and effect.

**certainty** A state, following upon analysis, where understanding has a visual quality that adds justified confidence to one's judgment. All certainty depends on what the context allows.

**character structure** Every standard taken as a virtue plays a part in structuring the individual nature of a person. Each standard, in this sense, is a character structure. The interlocked virtues that produce and explain the individual's characteristic actions are his or her character structure.

**choice** The intentional resolution of an alternative.

**codependence** This is a way of caring in which the nurse tries to find her sense of ethical worth by working to make herself and her patient mutually dependent on the other.

**coercion** The act of compelling someone, by threats or force, to act in a particular manner. The act of forcibly restraining, compelling, or controlling another person.

**cognition** The act of grasping the defining or relevant properties of an object or aspects of a situation.

**cognitive agreement** An agreement of the understanding with the object that is understood—the agreement between a knowing mind and its known object.

**coherence** A theory of truth that holds that a belief is true if it is logically coherent with the collection of one's other true beliefs.

**concept** A mental sign, held in the mind, signifying something existing in reality; the idea of that which is known. That which relates a knower to what he or she knows.

**conceptualism** The theory that concepts are formed by virtue of the similarity of similar things.

**conditions** The effect on a person of circumstances that have been brought about by oneself or another and have an effect on a person.

**conflict** The opposite of harmony.

**consequences** That which follows as the result of a cause; the moral effects of an initiated cause.

**considerations** Purposes, context, and causal progression. It includes the facts of the situation, the facts of awareness, and the facts of one's knowledge.

**context** The interweaving of the relevant facts of a situation—the facts that are necessary to act on to bring about a desired result, the knowledge one has of how to deal with these facts most effectively, and one's awareness of what is relevant.
   **(of awareness)** An agent's present awareness of the relevant aspects of the situation.
   **(interpersonal context)** A context involving more than one person.

**(of knowledge)** An agent's preexisting knowledge relevant to the situation.

**(of the situation)** The interwoven aspects of a situation that are fundamental to understanding the situation and to acting effectively in it.

**(solitary context)** A context involving only one person—the agent.

**continuity** The connectedness of events in a process. The continuing existence of a state of affairs.

**correspondence** A theory of truth that holds that a belief is true when it arises from, is formed according to, and corresponds with the state of affairs that is the object of the belief.

**courage** The habit of responding to the possible gain or loss of a value with action motivated to an appropriate degree given the worth of the value.

**cultural competence** "Cultural competence is the ongoing process in which the health care provider continuously strives to achieve the ability to effectively work within the cultural context of the client (individual, family, community)" (Montenery, Jones, Perry, Ross, & Zoucha, 2013, p. e56).

**decision** A choice made between alternative values and consequent courses of action.

**deontology** "The theory that . . . actions in conformance with . . . formal rules of conduct are obligatory regardless of their results" (Angeles, 1992a, p. 270).

**desire** One's psychological orientation toward a purpose. The capacity of an organism whereby it acts to retain its values, including its own life.

**determine** To bring something—a state of awareness or a state of being—into existence; to direct a course of action.

**determinism** The doctrine that human choices are the effects of necessitating conditions; the theory that all conscious behavior is a response to outside forces in the same way that the behavior of physical entities is a response to external forces.

**dilemma** A situation in which one faces a conflict of purposes or purposes whose value is not clear.

**doubt** The state of mind in relation to a belief when there is both reason to accept the truth of the belief and reason not to accept the truth of the belief and no objective way to decide which is valid.

**duty** An ethical sanction demanding adherence to a rule without regard to consequences.

**efficacy** The power to produce a desired result of effect.

**element** "The fundamental, essential, or irreducible constituent of an object" ("Element," 1997). Thus the roundness of a ball is an element of a ball. Its color is not.

**emotivism** The doctrine that holds feelings or emotions as forms of ethical knowledge. The doctrine that every ethical judgment is nothing more than a disguised description of a person's feelings.

**epistemology** The study of how truth is identified, how knowledge is acquired, and how knowledge is validated.

**ethical** Pertaining to ethics.

**ethical agreement** An agreement between people concerning vital and fundamental values.

**ethical noncognitivism** The theory that ethical terms cannot be defined or understood; hence ethical judgments can be neither true nor false.

**ethical nonnaturalism** Ethically good and bad properties form no part of the world in which we live. Properties in things that we consider ethical properties are not in the thing but merely in our preference or aversion.

**ethicist** One engaged in the theoretical study of ethics.

**ethics** A system of standards to motivate, determine, and justify actions directed to the pursuit of vital and fundamental goals. Ethics is not convenience, is not etiquette, is not that which brings on a state of self-satisfaction.

**evasion** The refusal or failure to give appropriate consideration to facts that ought to be factored into a decision-making process.

**evil** The evil in relation to an ethical agent is that which negates (blocks) its efficient functioning as the kind of thing it is (failure and the violation of rights, for instance, are evils); disruption of an intelligible, causal sequence in knowledge or action; inappropriate or disproportionate to the context.

**existential** Concerning human existence.

**explicit** Actually spoken or agreed to—not merely understood implicitly.

**extremes** A method of analysis through which a health care professional can clarify a bioethical context by identifying the relationships—the rights and responsibilities—of the people involved in the context.

**fidelity** Adherence to the terms of an agreement. An individual's faithfulness to his or her autonomy. For a nurse, it is a commitment to the obligation she has accepted as part of her professional role.

**flourishing** The realization of human development and its potentialities (e.g., happiness); enjoying happiness based on circumstances desirable and appropriate to one's time of life.

**foreseeable** Predictable according to that which is given in the context—probable.

**formal agreement** An agreement made between people to interact based on complementary motivations.

**formalism** The theory that ethical action is action that conforms with certain forms of behavior; an ethical formalist is one who concentrates entirely on the abstract category into which an action can be placed, without regard for the context or the effects of the action.

**freedom** As a bioethical standard, self-directedness. An agent's capacity and consequent right to take independent, long-term actions based on the agent's own evaluation of his or her circumstances.

**fundamental** Essential to making or revealing a thing as the kind of thing it is; the fundamental element of a thing is that which best explains its behavior. For instance, roundness is essential to the rolling of a ball; therefore, roundness is a fundamental property of a ball. The roundness (globularity) is also the defining property of a ball.

**fundamental element** That element in a context that determines what will occur, how it will occur, and the foreseeable outcomes.

**futile care** Treatment to be delivered that will not improve the outcome for the patient (Jonsen, Siegler, & Winslade, 2006; Kasman, 2004).

**gentle** (As in *gentle* coercion). *Simple coercion* destroys a patient's ability to act on his understanding of his situation, on his notion of self-ownership, or on his conception of benefit and harm. *Gentle coercion* involves dialogue with a view to persuading—but persuading by means of activating, or at least not destroying, a patient's understanding and self-ownership. A form of persuasion that is neither disinterested nor an attempt to take over control of a person's time and effort. Gentle coercion does not attack a person's reasoning power. It is an appeal to that person's reasoning power.

**Golden Mean** That middle state or action that is appropriate to a context and, therefore, a virtue. The extremes of excess and deficit are vices, inappropriate to the context.

**good** The good of a thing is that which assists its efficient functioning as the kind of thing it is (i.e., success, fidelity, respect for rights, and health care are all goods); appropriate or proportionate to the context.

**habit** Behavior, associations, or inclinations acquired by repetition (Angeles, 1992b).

**hedonism** The ethical theory that only those actions that produce pleasure in the agent are appropriate ethical actions, pleasure being the only value worthy of pursuit.

**implicit** Understood but not as a focus of intention. Understood without being openly expressed; that of which one is not consciously aware but which can be brought to conscious awareness.

**indeterminate** That which is not subject to precise analysis and identification.

**indirection** That which characterizes bargaining with a patient in a way that avoids predictable conflict.

**in-general** Describes an action one takes in a way that is appropriate to a situation of a type in which it is taken rather than a way that is specifically appropriate to the concrete situation.

**integrity** A virtue that characterizes an ethical agent in one's fidelity to one's own objective values and agreements—fidelity to oneself; the causal connection between experience, belief, description, and action.

**intelligibility** That aspect of an object or state of affairs whereby it is recognizable as the kind of thing it is. (If the fundamental nature of a state of affairs is easily recognizable, then the state of affairs is intelligible; if any aspect of a state of affairs makes the state of affairs recognizable, then that is its fundamental aspect.)

**intelligible** Structured in such a way as to be understandable.

**intention** The state of affairs that an agent acts to bring about; a mental act of attention to an object.

**interaction** A chain of actions arising from agreement and interwoven in a cause-and-effect sequence.

**interpersonal ethics** Ethics as it pertains to interaction between two or more people. A system of standards arising with an agreement to motivate, determine, and justify the implicit presuppositions of interaction.

**interwoven** Systematic; composed of interacting, interrelated, or interdependent facts that form a complex whole (e.g., sweaters are made up of interwoven strands of yarn; ethical contexts of the interweaving of circumstances and awareness).

**introspection** The act of directing one's attention back into one's own subjectivity; the act of reflecting back onto one's own psychological processes.

**intuitionism** Any theory that attributes ethical insight to a spontaneous event vis-à-vis a process, for example, the theory that ethical agents possess an ethical sense analogous to the five senses.

**justice** The concept of justice can, perhaps, be best understood by an analogy to a much more basic concept—the concept of physical causality. Physical objects act and interact based on what their nature permits them to do—and they cannot act contrary to this. Justice, then, is to ethical agents as causality is to physical objects. Physical objects cannot interact acausally or unjustly. Ethical agents, however, have the power to choose, and they can choose either appropriately (so that intelligible cause-and-effect relationships are maintained—which is justice—or in such a way that the intelligible cause-and-effect relationships between actions and reactions are lost—this is injustice).

**justifiable** That in a choice or decision that makes it subject to approval upon being explained.

**justification** A description in terms of how something meets a purpose—the purpose as formulated in a decision or agreement; demonstration that something corresponds with the terms of an agreement.

**justify** To describe or explain in terms of or as related to an agreed-upon purpose.

**lenses** The bioethical standards serve as a sort of lens insofar as analysis conducted on their basis serves to reveal the justifiability of motivations, decision, choices, and so forth.

**life** The process wherein an organism generates and sustains actions directed toward the attainment of its needs and purposes according to its potential; a process whose natural product is flourishing.

**logical** According to the demands of understanding; intelligible.

**logical positivism** The theory that statements have cognitive value if, and only if, they are, at least in principle, verifiable by sense experience.

**meaning** In ethics, relation to a purpose. The meaning of X to an agent is the way X assists or hinders an agent's purpose or an agent's flourishing.

**metaphysics** In the tradition—"The study of being qua being" (Aristotle, as quoted in McKeon, 1941); the study of what is real in reality. For instance, that everything is what it is, that nothing is what it is not; a demonstration of why something is what it is. Or that something has a foundation in reality. For instance, symphonology has a foundation in reality because, throughout reality, agreement produces harmony. The lack of agreement either produces nothing or produces discord.

**moral courage** The ability to do what is right or moral despite elements that would influence a person to act in another way (Lachman, 2011).

**moral distress** The physical or emotional suffering one experiences when constraints (internal or external) prevent one from following the course of action that one believes is right (Pendry, 2007, p. 217).

**more or less** Out of context; inexact; without a purpose.

**mores** Rules or standards of behavior as related to a certain society; the ethical conventions of a society.

**motivation** The reason that an agent takes an action. For instance, the desire not to get wet is the motivation for opening one's umbrella; fear is one's motivation for taking flight; and the desire to gain benefits only possible or more easily acquired through cooperation is one's motivation for entering into an agreement.

**natural agreement** An agreement among things that they will interact according to the nature of each. For instance, the wind will carry a leaf. Natural agreements arise through the nature of each existent.

**necessary** It is probably not necessary to define *necessary*, but if a certain state of affairs, A, can be an actual state of affairs only if another state of affairs, B, is actual, then B is necessary to A. This is the thrust of *necessary* throughout the book.

**normative** "Having to do with an established standard of behavior" (Runes, 1983); having to do with ethics.

**nurse** (or any health care professional) The agent of a patient, doing for the patient (given education and experience) what he would do for himself if he were able.

**nurturing** Affording professional treatment to bring a patient to a better state of life, health, and well-being.

**objective** Existing apart from a perceiving subject; having actual existence or reality, as in objective awareness.

**objective awareness** Awareness directed outward to the characteristics necessary to establish cognition of an object.

**objectivity** As a bioethical standard, a desire to know something as it is in itself and apart from distorting conditions or misleading prejudgments; a patient's need to achieve and sustain the exercise of his objective awareness.

**obligation** A condition that (ethically) necessitates the obliged to perform some action.

**offer** The state of mind of another ethical agent that seems to promise to serve a purpose if one engages with it.

**paradox** A description of a state of affairs that apparently cannot exist, but which, in fact, can exist.

**passion** A behavior that an agent undergoes through a force external to oneself and not as the outcome of his or her act of self-determination.

**paternalism** The practice of assuming an authority that one does not possess. The acting toward one as if you were a parent and he or she were your child.

**patient** One who has lost or suffered a decrease in agency. One who is unable to take the actions his survival or flourishing requires. An agent but in relation to a biomedical professional. One whose actions are affected by the actions of an agent.

**perfect agreement** An objective agreement is an agreement to interact made between two agents when their interaction is based on an objective awareness of the circumstances influencing their interacting and its foreseeable result. A perfect ethical agreement is an objective agreement where each agent is objectively certain that the other is the right person with whom he or she should be interacting.

**perfection** Intrinsic desirability, appropriateness to survival and flourishing.

**person** A rational animal, independent, able to act based on decisions and agreements and able to discover meaning in things.

**power** A capacity to bring about a state of affairs.

**practical reason** Intelligent in matters of ethics; when the aim of ethics is action.

**precondition** A condition that must exist before something else can occur. That which relates to something else in such a way that it is necessary to the existence of that second thing. Parents are the precondition of a child, language is a precondition of literature, and objectivity is a precondition of an agreement.

**presupposition** Very much like precondition but having more to do with the context of one's knowledge. That which must be assumed if that of which it is a presupposition is assumed. For example, knowledge of the fact that Paul is or was a child presupposes knowledge of the fact that Paul had parents. Knowledge of the fact that a culture has produced literature presupposes knowledge of the fact that the culture possesses a language. Knowledge of the fact that one has formed an agreement presupposes knowledge of the fact that one is free to form an agreement.

**pride** The objective conviction that one is worthwhile. The pleasure that one takes in one's virtues.

**principle** The motivating ground of an action. A basic fact, truth, or law from which other facts, truths, or laws proceed. A basic cause from which other causes arise.

**probability** When the evidence for an alternative significantly outweighs the evidence against it, the first alternative is more probable than the second—foreseeability.

**professional** One who has, by virtue of education, training, and experience, the ability to enter a profession and to act effectively in it.

**proper** Appropriate to a context; meeting a requisite standard.

**proportion** A measure of benefit or value between one action or the product of the action in comparison with another action, or the product of another action according to reciprocity. In one sense, balance and proportion are beneficence. In the same sense, they are justice.

**purpose** That state of affairs that is the object of an action that desire motivates; the psychological condition that accompanies an orientation toward bringing about this state of affairs.

**rational** Tending to appropriate proportions; well reasoned; appropriate to the context.

**rational self-interest** An agent's rational self-interest is defined in terms of one's understanding of one's individual nature against the background of what is needed for personal development. It also requires a complete acceptance of the nature, motivations, and self-interest of one's "trading partners."

**realism–moderate** The theory that concepts are formed through the abstract sameness of things.

**reason** The faculty of thinking, thinking being a process of awareness directed toward (a) what is relevant, (b) what is appropriate, (c) what is balanced, and (d) what is proportional in the demands of a context and the agent's responses to these demands.

**reciprocity** An appropriate balance between value given and value received. A balanced interchange of benefits or values.

**relevant** Necessary to the understanding of a context. Serving to bring about balance and ethical proportion. (Something is relevant to a context if one cannot fully understand the context without it.)

**responsibility** The ethical link connecting an agent to the consequences of the changes he or she has caused to come about.

**rights** The product of an implicit agreement among rational beings made and held by virtue of their rationality not to obtain actions nor the products or conditions of actions from one another except through voluntary consent objectively gained. *Rights* means, in one sense, the product (freedom from aggression) of an agreement (not to aggress). In another sense, rights is the agreement itself. In either sense, the generic term (freedom from aggression; agreement) is singular. Therefore, the term *rights* is a singular term. It is a grave ethical mistake to regard the term *rights* as a political rather than a more fundamental ethical term and to regard it as plural—an ever-changing product of legislation.

**ritualistic ethic**  An ethical system that holds that ethical principles are right or wrong without regard for the desires, choices, and purposes of the people involved or the consequences of ethical action.

**sameness**  Although individual things are not the same as individuals, they are the same as members of the same genus. John and Mary are merely similar to each other as individuals; as members of the genus *PERSON*, they are the same.

**sanction**  In ethics, agreement or cooperation in a broad metaphorical sense. For instance, criminals do not have the sanction of reason. Nature sanctions actions taken with foresight. Reality does not sanction irresponsible actions.

**sequentiality**  Pertaining to a series of future events, intelligibly and causally linked to a series of past events.

**sincerity**  The quality of one's motivation in forming an agreement when one is fully committed to the agreement.

**social relativism**  The theory that the customs, beliefs, and practices of a society determine what is ethical and what is unethical.

**solitary ethics**  A system of standards to motivate, determine, and justify decisions and actions taken in the pursuit of an agent's own vital and fundamental goals.

**standard**  That by which the ethical appropriateness of an action can be measured. Various standards that have been proposed are Socrates, knowledge of that which is beneficial; Plato, the Form of the Good; Aristotle, the actions that noble and virtuous people would take; Aquinas, happiness; Spinoza, the preservation and enhancement of the agent's life; Kant, duty; Bentham, the greatest good for the greatest number; Ayn Rand, the preconditions of "man's life qua man."

**sufficient**  One thing, A, is sufficient to another thing, B, if the existence of A, in and of itself, makes necessary the existence of B. For instance, the existence of lightning is sufficient to the existence of thunder. Thunder cannot exist without lightning. Lightning cannot exist without producing thunder. Desire is not sufficient to action—one may feel desire without acting. But action is sufficient to justify a belief in the existence of desire. Action is a behavior motivated by desire; action implies desire.

**symphonology**  A system of ethics based on the terms and presuppositions of agreement. In any specific case, this will be the agreement that establishes the nature of the relationship between the parties involved in interaction.

**system** The interrelationships of the elements that make up a whole.

**tacit** That which is hidden from direct view; relying on focal and subsidiary awareness and unspoken but ever-present knowledge guides us to comprehension of something real; based on experience. "We know more than we can say" (Polanyi, p. 4).

**telishment** The practice of reducing crime by subjecting criminals to death by slow torture and revealing to potential criminals what their fates will be by gently torturing an innocent person to death.

**term** A condition or stipulation that defines the nature and limits of an agreement.

**triage** A triage situation is a situation calling for choices to be made when the benefits that one can bring about in the situation are limited. The choices may be choices among benefits, beneficiaries, or both.

**truth** The relationship of correspondence between an idea and the object of the idea.

**uncertainty** The mental context of a dilemma. The right or best course of action may be action A or action B, but the superiority of one over the other is not clearly evident to the person who has to make the choice.

**uniqueness** Difference from others of the same kind.

**utilitarianism** "The theory that one should act as to promote the greatest happiness (pleasure) of the greatest number of people" (Angeles, 1992c).

**utility** Greatest good for the greatest number.

**value** The object of an action that an autonomous desire motivates; that which is instrumental in the realization of a purpose.

**vice** The opposite of virtue. A habit produced by an inferior or corrupt character. A habit established on irrational desire.

**vicious** Tending to vice; unable to live rightly and well.

**violate** To violate a standard is to ignore or act against the character structure that the standard signifies. More generally, whenever one ignores or acts against that which is appropriate to an agreement, one violates the agreement.

**virtue** A human excellence. According to a purposive ethic, *virtue* refers to a person's ability to act to fulfill his or her rational desires.

**virtuous** Tending to virtue; habituated to living rightly and well.

**vital** Essentially related to the preservation or enhancement of life, as, for instance, a vital need or a vital desire.

**vital agreement** An agreement between the life of a living thing and the organic conditions necessary to its life or survival. It is life's agreement with itself.

**volition** The power to take uncompelled and purposeful actions.

**vulnerable** Unprotected, capable of being harmed.

**whim** A decision made on the analysis of subjective factors. A decision motivated by one's feelings or attitudes apart from the context.

**wisdom** Prudent judgment as to how to use knowledge in the everyday affairs of life (Angeles, 1992d).

**Note:** The various philosophic systems that we have described above are not complete descriptions. In some cases, we would not claim ballistic accuracy. Our purpose is not to provide the reader a complete understanding of contemporary philosophy but to include everything that separates symphonology from it. However, the descriptions of the ethical systems are reliable.

## REFERENCES

Angeles, P. A. (1992a). Deontology. In *Dictionary of philosophy* (2nd ed.). New York, NY: HarperCollins.

Angeles, P. A. (1992b). Habit. In *Dictionary of philosophy* (2nd ed.). New York, NY: HarperCollins.

Angeles, P. A. (1992c). Utilitarianism. In *Dictionary of philosophy* (2nd ed.). New York, NY: HarperCollins.

Angeles, P. A. (1992d). Wisdom. In *Dictionary of philosophy* (2nd ed.). New York, NY: HarperCollins.

Efficacy. (n.d.). In *Merriam-Webster's online dictionary*. Retrieved June 10, 2014, from http://www.merriam-webster.com/dictionary/efficacy

Element. (1997). *American heritage dictionary* (3rd ed.). Boston, MA: Houghton Mifflin.

Jonsen, A. R., Siegler, M., & Winslade, W. J. (2006). *Clinical ethics: A practical approach to ethical decisions in clinical medicine* (6th ed.). New York, NY: McGraw-Hill.

Kasman, D. L. (2004, October). When is medical treatment futile? A guide for students, residents, and physicians. *Journal of General Internal Medicine, 19*(10), 1053–1056. doi: 10.1111/j.1525-1497.2004.40134.x

Lachman, V. D. (2010, September 30). Strategies necessary for moral courage. *OJIN, 15*(3). doi:10.3912/OJIN.Vol15No03Man03

McKeon, R. (Ed.). (1941). *The basic works of Aristotle.* New York, NY: Random House.

Pendry, S. P. (2007). Moral distress: Recognizing it to retain nurses. *Nursing Economics, 25,* 217–221.

Pines, A., & Maslach, C. (1978). Characteristics of staff burnout in mental health settings. *Hospital Community Psychiatry, 29,* 233–237.

Polanyi, M. (1966). The tacit dimension. Garden City, NJ: Doubleday.

Precondition. (1997). *American Heritage Dictionary* (3rd ed.). Boston, MA: Houghton Mifflin.

Runes, D. D. (Ed.). (1983). Normative. In *Dictionary of Philosophy.* New York, NY: Philosophical Library.

Segen, J. C. (2012). Cultural competence. In *The Dictionary of Modern Medicine.* Park Ridge, NJ: Partheon Publishing Group.

Spinoza, B. (1949). *Ethics.* J. Gutmann (Ed.). New York, NY: Hafner. (Original work published 1675).

# APPENDIX

## THE ICN CODE OF ETHICS FOR NURSES

*An international code of ethics for nurses was first adopted by the International Council of Nurses (ICN) in 1953. It has been revised and reaffirmed at various times since, most recently with this review and revision completed in 2005.*

## PREAMBLE

Nurses have four fundamental responsibilities: to promote health, to prevent illness, to restore health and to alleviate suffering. The need for nursing is universal.

Inherent in nursing is respect for human rights, including cultural rights, the right to life and choice, to dignity and to be treated with respect. Nursing care is respectful of and unrestricted by considerations of age, colour, creed, culture, disability or illness, gender, sexual orientation, nationality, politics, race or social status.

Nurses render health services to the individual, the family and the community and co-ordinate their services with those of related groups.[1]

## THE ICN CODE

The *ICN Code of Ethics for Nurses* has four principal elements that outline the standards of ethical conduct.

## ELEMENTS OF THE CODE

### 1. NURSES AND PEOPLE

The nurse's primary professional responsibility is to people requiring nursing care.

---

In providing care, the nurse promotes an environment in which the human rights, values, customs and spiritual beliefs of the individual, family and community are respected.

The nurse ensures that the individual receives sufficient information on which to base consent for care and related treatment.

The nurse holds in confidence personal information and uses judgement in sharing this information.

The nurse shares with society the responsibility for initiating and supporting action to meet the health and social needs of the public, in particular those of vulnerable populations.

The nurse also shares responsibility to sustain and protect the natural environment from depletion, pollution, degradation and destruction.

## 2. NURSES AND PRACTICE

The nurse carries personal responsibility and accountability for nursing practice, and for maintaining competence by continual learning.

The nurse maintains a standard of personal health such that the ability to provide care is not compromised.

The nurse uses judgement regarding individual competence when accepting and delegating responsibility.

The nurse at all times maintains standards of personal conduct which reflect well on the profession and enhance public confidence.

The nurse, in providing care, ensures that use of technology and scientific advances are compatible with the safety, dignity and rights of people.

## 3. NURSES AND THE PROFESSION

The nurse assumes the major role in determining and implementing acceptable standards of clinical nursing practice, management, research and education.

The nurse is active in developing a core of research-based professional knowledge.

The nurse, acting through the professional organisation, participates in creating and maintaining safe, equitable social and economic working conditions in nursing.

## 4. NURSES AND CO-WORKERS

The nurse sustains a co-operative relationship with co-workers in nursing and other fields.

The nurse takes appropriate action to safeguard individuals, families and communities when their health is endangered by a coworker or any other person.

## SUGGESTIONS FOR USE OF THE ICN CODE OF ETHICS FOR NURSES

The *ICN Code of Ethics for Nurses* is a guide for action based on social values and needs. It will have meaning only as a living document if applied to the realities of nursing and health care in a changing society.

To achieve its purpose the *Code* must be understood, internalized and used by nurses in all aspects of their work. It must be available to students and nurses throughout their study and work lives.

## APPLYING THE ELEMENTS OF THE ICN CODE OF ETHICS FOR NURSES

The four elements of the *ICN Code of Ethics for Nurses*: nurses and people, nurses and practice, nurses and the profession, and nurses and co-workers, give a framework for the standards of conduct. The following chart will assist nurses to translate the standards into action. Nurses and nursing students can therefore:

- Study the standards under each element of the *Code*.
- Reflect on what each standard means to you. Think about how you can apply ethics in your nursing domain: practice, education, research or management.
- Discuss the *Code* with co-workers and others.
- Use a specific example from experience to identify ethical dilemmas and standards of conduct as outlined in the *Code*. Identify how you would resolve the dilemmas.
- Work in groups to clarify ethical decision making and reach a consensus on standards of ethical conduct.
- Collaborate with your national nurses' association, co-workers, and others in the continuous application of ethical standards in nursing practice, education, management and research.

**Element of the Code # 1:** NURSES AND PEOPLE

| Practitioners and Managers | Educators and Researchers | National Nurses' Associations |
|---|---|---|
| Provide care that respects human rights and is sensitive to the values, customs and beliefs of all people. | In curriculum include references to human rights, equity, justice, solidarity as the basis for access to care. | Develop position statements and guidelines that support human rights and ethical standards. |
| Provide continuing education in ethical issues. | Provide teaching and learning opportunities for ethical issues and decision making. | Lobby for involvement of nurses in ethics review committees. |
| Provide sufficient information to permit informed consent and the right to choose or refuse treatment. | Provide teaching/learning opportunities related to informed consent. | Provide guidelines, position statements and continuing education related to informed consent. |
| Use recording and information management systems that ensure confidentiality. | Introduce into curriculum concepts of privacy and confidentiality. | Incorporate issues of confidentiality and privacy into a national code of ethics for nurses. |
| Develop and monitor environmental safety in the workplace. | Sensitise students to the importance of social action in current concerns. | Advocate for safe and healthy environment. |

**Element of the Code # 2:** NURSES AND PRACTICE

| Practitioners and Managers | Educators and Researchers | National Nurses' Associations |
|---|---|---|
| Establish standards of care and a work setting that promotes safety and quality care. | Provide teaching/learning opportunities that foster life long learning and competence for practice. | Provide access to continuing education, through journals, conferences, distance education, etc. |
| Establish systems for professional appraisal, continuing education and systematic renewal of licensure to practice. | Conduct and disseminate research that shows links between continual learning and competence to practice. | Lobby to ensure continuing education opportunities and quality care standards. |
| Monitor and promote the personal health of nursing staff in relation to their competence for practice. | Promote the importance of personal health and illustrate its relation to other values. | Promote healthy lifestyles for nursing professionals. Lobby for healthy work places and services for nurses. |

**Element of the Code # 3:** NURSES AND THE PROFESSION

| Practitioners and Managers | Educators and Researchers | National Nurses' Associations |
|---|---|---|
| Set standards for nursing practice, research, education and management. | Provide teaching/ learning opportunities in setting standards for nursing practice, research, education and management. | Collaborate with others to set standards for nursing education, practice, research and management. |
| Foster workplace support of the conduct, dissemination and utilisation of research related to nursing and health. | Conduct, disseminate and utilise research to advance the nursing profession. | Develop position statements, guidelines and standards related to nursing research. |
| Promote participation in national nurses' associations so as to create favourable socio-economic conditions for nurses. | Sensitise learners to the importance of professional nursing associations. | Lobby for fair social and economic working conditions in nursing. Develop position statements and guidelines in workplace issues. |

**Element of the Code # 4:** NURSES AND CO-WORKERS

| Practitioners and Managers | Educators and Researchers | National Nurses' Associations |
|---|---|---|
| Create awareness of specific and overlapping functions and the potential for interdisciplinary tensions. | Develop understanding of the roles of other workers. | Stimulate co-operation with other related disciplines. |
| Develop workplace systems that support common professional ethical values and behaviour. | Communicate nursing ethics to other professions. | Develop awareness of ethical issues of other professions. |
| Develop mechanisms to safeguard the individual, family or community when their care is endangered by health care personnel. | Instil in learners the need to safeguard the individual, family or community when care is endangered by health care personnel. | Provide guidelines, position statements and discussion fora related to safeguarding people when their care is endangered by health care personnel. |

## DISSEMINATION OF THE *ICN CODE OF ETHICS FOR NURSES*

To be effective the *ICN Code of Ethics for Nurses* must be familiar to nurses. We encourage you to help with its dissemination to schools of nursing, practising nurses, the nursing press and other mass media. The Code should also be disseminated to other health professions, the general public, consumer and policy-making groups, human rights organisations and employers of nurses.

## GLOSSARY OF TERMS USED IN THE *ICN CODE OF ETHICS FOR NURSES*

**Co-worker**
Other nurses and other health and non-health related workers and professionals.

**Co-operative relationship**
A professional relationship based on collegial and reciprocal actions, and behaviour that aim to achieve certain goals.

**Family**
A social unit composed of members connected through blood, kinship, emotional or legal relationships.

**Nurse shares with society**
A nurse, as a health professional and a citizen, initiates and supports appropriate action to meet the health and social needs of the public.

**Personal health**
Mental, physical, social and spiritual wellbeing of the nurse.

**Personal information**
Information obtained during professional contact that is private to an individual or family, and which, when disclosed, may violate the right to privacy, cause inconvenience, embarrassment, or harm to the individual or family.

**Related groups**
Other nurses, health care workers or other professionals providing service to an individual, family or community and working toward desired goals.

# INDEX